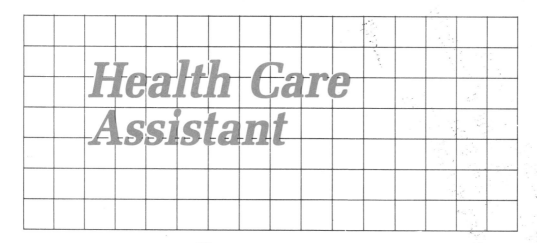

Health Care Assistant

Myrna Iwiles:

Congratulations for being selected an an outstanding student of the Nurses' Aide Program. We, the faculty and staff of the Educational Opportunity Center of Westchester applaud you and wish continued success.

Leonard Harper

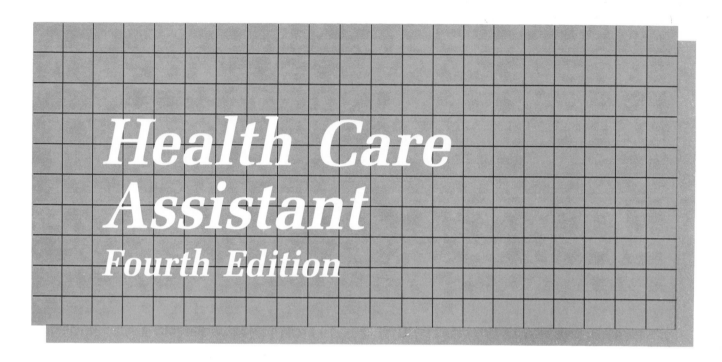

Health Care Assistant
Fourth Edition

Esther Caldwell, MA, PhD

Consultant in Vocational Education (CA)

Barbara R. Hegner, MSN, RN

Professor
Nursing and Life Science Department
Long Beach City College (CA)

❖ *Delmar Publishers Inc.* ®

NOTICE TO THE READER

Cover design: Hardy House

Delmar Staff:
  Administrative Editor: Adele M. O'Connell
  Production Editor: Carol A. Micheli

For information address Delmar Publishers Inc.
  2 Computer Drive West, Box 15–015
  Albany, New York 12212

Printed in the United States of America
Published simultaneously in Canada
by Nelson Canada,
A division of International Thomson Limited

Library of Congress Cataloging in Publication Data

Caldwell, Esther.
  Health care assistant.

  Rev. ed. of: Health assistant. c1981.
  Includes index.
  1. Nurses' aides. 2. Care of the sick. I. Hegner, Barbara R. II. Caldwell, Esther. Health Assistant. III. Title. [DNLM: 1. Nurses' Aides. 2. Nursing Care. WY 193 C147h]
  RT84.C3   1985   610.73'0698   84-26021
  ISBN 0-8273-2453-7
  ISBN 0-8273-2454-5 (Instructor's guide)

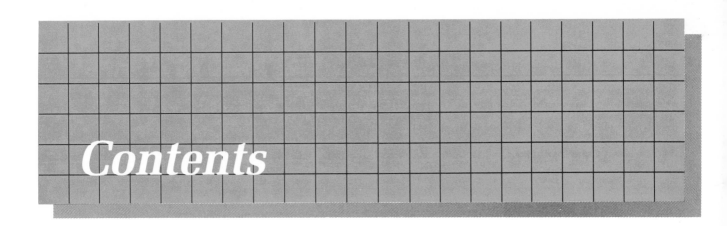

Contents

Section Eight   *Measuring and Recording Vital Signs*   204

Section Nine   *Principles of Nutrition and Fluid Balance*   226

Section Twelve　The Expanded Role of the Health Care Assistant　418

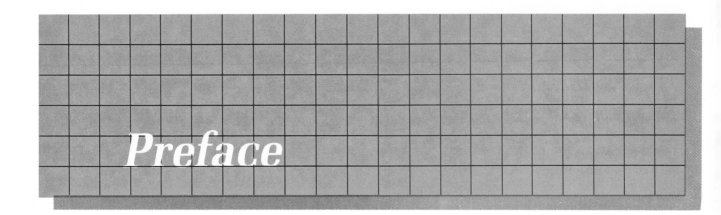

Preface

Presently, over one-half of all health service jobs are held by professional nurses, paraprofessional nurses, and an increasingly large percentage of nursing care assistants. The preparation of this last group of people to function as well-trained and competent health care assistants is becoming especially important today as the professional members of the nursing staff assume greater responsibility for the more technical and complex aspects of patient care and less of the day-to-day responsibility.

In many health care facilities, the greatest portion of basic, routine care is given by ancillary staff members who are carefully selected and trained specifically for their role within the health care team. Although these ancillary workers provide patient care, they are not prepared or trained to practice nursing. The name given to these health care workers varies with the institution, but they are usually designated as health care assistants, nursing assistants, nurses aides, ward aides, or orderlies.

Health Care Assistant, Fourth Edition, is designed to provide beginning students with the initial skills and background knowledge necessary to allow them to function effectively as both an integral part and a necessary member of the health care team. Health care assistants who are already employed in the field will also find this text a useful, up-to-date reference that will refresh their knowledge and enhance their understanding of specific patient needs and care practices.

This new edition of *Health Care Assistant* has been totally reorganized in order to present the necessary information in a logical, step-wise manner, progressing from simple concepts to more complex ones, and from general information to specific applications. Related information has been grouped together in order to enhance the student's comprehension of the material. Because basic anatomical principles and medical terminology are so necessary to the job, they are now presented early in the text so that students can use the knowledge as a guide in their study of subsequent units. New units on care of the elderly and chronically ill and on maternal-infant care reflect not only current changes in the population being cared for, but also the expanded role of the health care assistant. Throughout the text the content has been thoroughly updated and expanded, with new illustrations, patient care procedures, and more indepth explanations of patient needs and current care practices.

Even the physical format of the text has been changed in order to facilitate learning. Larger illustrations promote understanding of important principles and procedures, and the expanded format permits you, the student, to make notes in the margins and to complete the review sections in the text itself, in order to test your mastery of the information that was presented in the unit. Additional pedagogical features that appear in the Fourth Edition include:

- Patient care procedures, which are now identified in the Table of Contents and highlighted in color within the units

- Topical outlines that introduce the material to be presented within each unit
- Glossary of terms
- Comprehensive performance evaluation chart
- Final, comprehensive examination

In addition, some of the most important features—learning objectives, unit summaries, suggested learning activities, review questions, and lists of key terms introduced within each unit—have been retained from the previous edition and expanded upon. The questions within each unit and the self-evaluation questions that appear at the end of each section of the text offer a variety of review methods that encourage students to test their mastery of the information, as well as their verbal and written skills.

This new edition of *Heath Care Assistant* also presents information introducing some advanced techniques which may be performed by health care assistants in some facilities. It should be emphasized that both instructors and students should familiarize themselves with the policies and regulations established by their state and the health care agency in which they practice before undertaking these technical procedures. In many cases, specialized training will be necessary in order to safely and effectively perform these procedures. The related information presented in this text is intended to serve as an adjunct to such specialized training, as well as a reference for review.

A concerted attempt has been made to ensure that the information within *Health Care Assistant* is accurate and that it reflects up-to-date practices and procedures. However, because of the dynamic nature of the health care field, the reader is encouraged to keep abreast of changes mandated by the state, initiated by the health care agency, or recommended by medical researchers.

Unit 1 Community Health Care Facilities

OBJECTIVES

As a result of this unit, you will be able to:

- Explain the health responsibilities of the community agencies.
- Discuss the interrelationships between agencies from the local level to the international level.
- Name the types of facilities available for patient care.

Health care assistants or nursing assistants play an important role in the care of people who are ill or who cannot fully take care of themselves. The care you will give to these persons will be under the direction and supervision of licensed, professionally-trained health care workers, such as doctors and nurses. As a health care assistant, you will carry out this care in a variety of community settings.

NEEDS OF THE COMMUNITY

Citizens who live in a common area and share common health needs form a *community*. Provisions for disposal of wastes, assurance of safe drinking water, healthful foods, protection from disease and health care are important to every person within a community. Safe drinking water, disposal of wastes, and food control are mandated by public health laws and enforced by government agencies.

Health care is provided by specially-trained workers in clinics, doctor's offices, homes for the aged, and hospitals. Nursing assistants help provide this care mainly in hospitals and homes for the aged: sometimes called *convalescent homes or long-term care facilities*.

When illness or accidents strike, when a baby is born, or when people get older and unable to care for their own everyday personal needs, workers in some type of community agency provide care for them. This care may be short-term or long-term, and can range from:

- emergency care which may save a life,
- to a routine checkup to identify minor problems before they become life-threatening,
- or surgery to repair an injured body or remove a diseased organ.

COMMUNITY AGENCIES

Since you will be part of the health care team, you should have an understanding of the different types of health care agencies.

There are two broad categories of community agencies: governmental, or tax supported, and nonofficial, or nonprofit, which receive their support through voluntary contributions. These two types of community agencies provide the numerous services both required and desired by the citizens.

Nonprofit Agencies

The American Heart Association, the American Respiratory Disease Association and the Diabetic Association are examples of nonprofit agencies. Many of the agencies have *logos* or symbols which help to identify them. They use their resources to conduct research into the causes and care of specific conditions.

Through the work and efforts of some of these agencies, many of the causes of disease have been identified and cures or preventive techniques have been developed. For example, the National Foundation of the March of Dimes was once dedicated primarily to the control and elimination of poliomyelitis, a severe, crippling, viral disease. Now that this has been successfully brought under control by immunization, this agency has now turned its attention to understanding, preventing, and correcting birth defects.

Governmental Agencies

Governmental agencies set standards, collect statistics, and are organized on the local, state, national, and international levels. The national health-related agency in the United States is called the United States Public Health Service. Its international counterpart is called the World Health Organization.

Records and statistics are gathered by agencies on the local level. They are compiled and compared at the state and national levels. From this information, patterns of disease and other health problems are charted. These statistics provide vital information which help health care providers at all levels address the specific health needs of either a community, a nation, or the world.

Information and regulations for control of these health problems then move from the national level back down to the local level, where they are

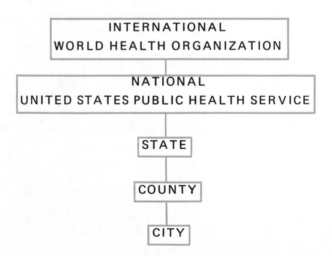

FIGURE 1-1.   Organization of health agencies

put into action. The county health department is an example of a governmental agency that is responsible for the supervision of local health needs. The types of programs conducted depend on the needs of the community, but immunization, sanitation inspections, maternal and child health investigations and conferences, free chest X-rays, and statistical services are only a few of the many services that the health department can offer to the citizens.

The World Health Organization is an international organization that is concerned with world health problems. It was founded in 1948 and meets annually in Geneva, Switzerland, its home office. Its concerns are worldwide and include compiling statistics, publishing health information, investigating serious health problems, and providing medical consultants whenever the need arises. Through the work of the WHO, smallpox, once a dreaded, world-wide disease, is believed to have been completely eliminated throughout the world.

HEALTH CARE FACILITIES

Patient care facilities are also called health care agencies. These facilities include both hospitals, Figure 1-2, and long-term care facilities: convalescent homes and homes for the aged. The health care field calls persons receiving health care *patients*.

Hospitals

Some hospitals are small, serving the needs of an individual community and others are extremely large, operating as part of a complex medical center. In some large facilities, highly-sophisticated machinery and treatments are available, while other hospitals focus largely on research or teaching.

Some hospitals only take care of patients with special conditions or care for special age groups. Two examples of these are *orthopedic* and children's hospitals, Figure 1-3.

Rehabilitative hospitals offer service to patients after an acute period of illness or trauma. The rehabilitative hospital helps the patient return to self-care to the maximum extent possible.

Government hospitals provide care for service personnel and their

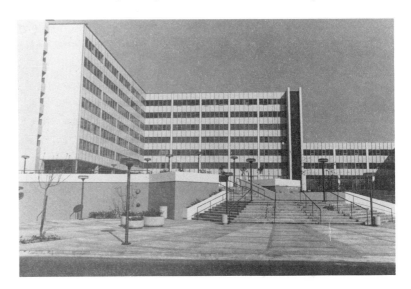

FIGURE 1-2. A large medical center in a metropolitan area handles a variety of different cases.

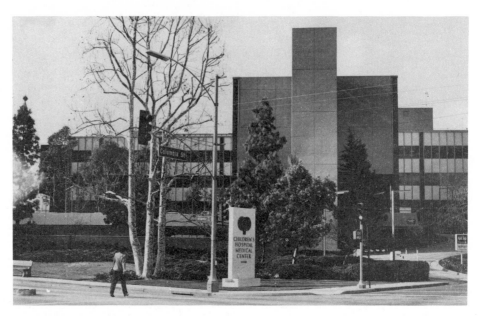

FIGURE 1-3.   A special facility within a medical center cares for sick children.

dependents, and are governmentally owned.

The entire care of a patient may be provided within one facility. Conversely, patients requiring specialized care may need to be transferred by ambulance or helicopter from one facility to another, Figure 1-4.

Most hospitals, however, whether they are privately or governmentally owned, small or large, are general in scope and provide care for patients of all ages with varied health problems. The common denominator is that *all* hospitals need trained health workers at *all* levels.

HOSPITAL DEPARTMENTS. Hospitals are organized into different departments that function in much the same way that individual family members function to benefit the family.

Very large medical centers have many diverse departments, including nuclear medicine, research, orthopedic rehabilitation, Figure 1-5, respiratory care, and social services. Smaller hospitals have fewer departments, but common departments are likely to include emergency (ER), surgery (OR), obstetrical (OB), intensive care (ICU), laboratory (lab), radiology (x-ray), and central supply (CS).

Patient service areas may also be further segregated. For example,

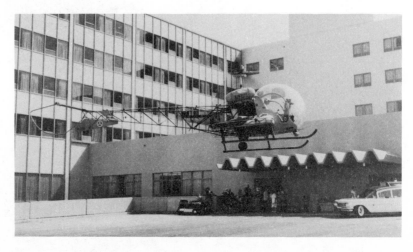

FIGURE 1-4.   Helicopters may be used to transport patients from one facility to another or from the scene of an accident to a hospital.

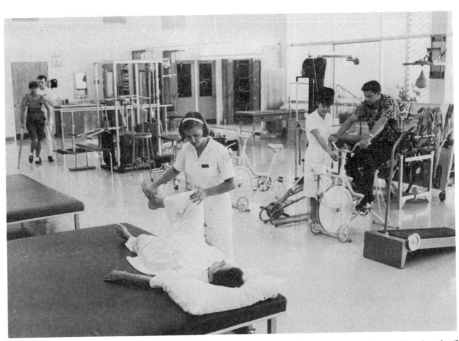

FIGURE 1-5. The rehabilitation department helps patients return to maximum levels of self-care.

patients with female problems that require surgery may be on a gynecological unit (Gyn or Ob-Gyn) while patients undergoing regular surgery may be cared for on the surgical unit. Before and after surgery both types of patient remain on their respective wards, but are moved to the operating room for the surgical procedure. From the operating room, the patient is usually kept in the recovery room (RR) until they have regained consciousness.

Many *ancillary*, or supportive, *departments* are needed to support the work going on in the patient care units. These include the dietary depart-

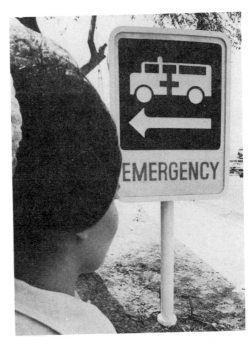

FIGURE 1-6. The emergency room (ER) is ready at all times to meet emergency needs for health care.

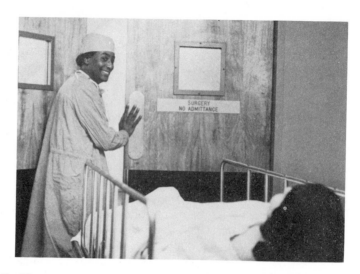

FIGURE 1-7.   The operating room (OR) or surgery is a special department within a hospital.

ment which provides meals for both patients and staff, the housekeeping department that cares for the overall cleaning of the hospital, and the maintenance department which sees to the care and repair of equipment.

The volunteer department is an *auxiliary department* within the structure of many hospitals. Its people contribute greatly to overall patient care, Figure 1-8. They deliver mail and flowers, escort patients to therapy areas or other departments, write letters for patients, cheer up and support patients and their families, provide reading materials and puzzles, and run gift shops and bazaars with the proceeds going toward the health care facility.

You will become familiar with the location and function of all the different departments within your health care agency as you proceed with your education.

Long-term Health Care Facilities

In the United States, the growing size of the aging population has resulted in an increase in the number of extended-care facilities, and health

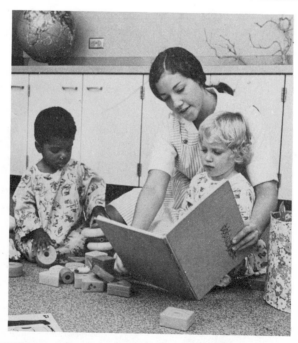

FIGURE 1-8.   Volunteers contribute important support activities.

care assistants provide a major portion of this care. In the next twenty years, this need will become even more evident. As the general population increases, the demand for health care also increases. New facilities are opening every day.

Extended-care facilities may be custodial care units providing for the basic physical and life needs of the patients in their care or may encompass a much more elaborate complex. All have nursing and dietary departments. In some, rehabilitation departments and recreational services are available. Although equipment for respiratory therapy and other medical treatments are available, much equipment is in the form of disposables so that central service departments are not needed. Most offer some degree of in-service education and training to their personnel.

An ombudsman who is a nurse, social worker, or trained volunteer functions as patient advocate and takes care of the social service needs of the patient.

The best extended-care facilities make an effort to create an atmosphere which is not hospital-like since, for many patients, the facility becomes the patient's home.

JOB PLACEMENT

Health care assistants carry out important functions in various health agencies. You will become a skilled and valuable worker in your community as you practice the activities taught in your health care assistant class and perfect the procedures. As a trained health care assistant, you will be employed in one of the community health facilities this unit has described.

Summary

Official and unofficial agencies work together to provide for the health needs of the citizens of the community. Information gathered at the local level is compiled by state and federal agencies. Plans formulated at the national level are transmitted to the local agencies for action. Health agencies employ health care assistants in large numbers to provide patient care.

SUGGESTED ACTIVITIES

1. Visit your local health department. Discuss range of health-oriented activities that are conducted by the department.

2. Discuss examples of the facilities available for patient care in your community. How many of them employ health care or nursing assistants? What are their job responsibilities?

3. Discuss the community's responsibility for the health of its citizens.

4. Discuss how information gathered in the community about health problems can be of value to people throughout the world.

5. Look at magazines, newspapers, and outdoor advertising to try to discover the logos of different health associations or health care agencies.

VOCABULARY

Learn the meaning and correct spelling of the following words and abbreviations.

agency	convalescent home	OB
ancillary	facility	OR
auxiliary department	ICU	orthopedic hospital
CS	logo	rehabilitative
community	long-term care facility	

UNIT REVIEW   **A. Brief Answer.**

1. An example of a local tax-supported health agency is:

2. Name three agencies in the community that are supported by voluntary contributions.
   a.
   b.
   c.

3. The three types of patient care facilities named in this unit are:
   a.
   b.
   c.

4. Five functions of the local health department are:
   a.
   b.
   c.
   d.
   e.

5. Who directly supervises the health care assistant's work?

6. Describe the difference between a nonofficial and an official health care agency.

7. Why are statistics that detail the number of people affected by a particular disease important?

8. What hospital departments are designated by the following abbreviations?
   ER _____
   OR _____
   CS _____
   ICU _____

B. Completion. Fill in the names of the missing levels of health agencies.

International
City

Unit 2 Role of the Health Care Assistant

OBJECTIVES

As a result of this unit, you will be able to:

- Identify the members of the nursing team.
- Dress properly for the job.
- Name the job responsibilities of an assistant.
- Make a chart showing the lines of authority an assistant follows.

Throughout recorded history, ill people have been helped to regain health through nursing care. In ancient Egypt the lady of the house directed this care, assisted by helpers. These helpers were the first health assistants.

Today, professional nurses plan the nursing care of patients based on the doctor's orders. To provide nursing care, the professional registered nurse has the assistance of the registered technical nurse, the licensed vocational or licensed practical nurse, and the trained health care assistant. This group is called the nursing team.

THE NURSING TEAM

The Registered Nurse

The *registered nurse* has passed a state-required examination to become registered and has either (1) a 4-year college education with a baccalaureate degree, (2) an associate of arts degree from a junior college, or (3) a diploma from a hospital nursing school. All have been trained, in varying degrees, to coordinate the many aspects of patient care. Because they are registered, all of these nurses use the initials RN after their names.

The Licensed Practical/Vocational Nurse

The *licensed vocational* or *licensed practical nurse* has generally completed a 1-year training program and has passed a licensure examination administered by the state. She is identified by the initials LVN or LPN.

Health Care Assistant

The health care assistant—you in this case—are being trained to assist with the care of patients under either an RN's or LPN's supervision. Because the assistant's responsibilities are not as great, the basic training period is usually about 6 weeks, but growth and learning will continue throughout your lifetime as a caregiver. In the hospital, the assistant is called by one of the following names: nurse's aide, nursing assistant, health care assistant, ward attendant, or orderly.

ROLE OF THE HEALTH CARE ASSISTANT

The assistant works directly with the patient, giving physical care and emotional support. That makes the health care assistant an important

9

person who can contribute much to the comfort of the patient. Important observations made during the delivery of care are reported to the nurse and are recorded on the patient's chart. Remember that although this care is always given under the direction of a registered nurse or licensed vocational/practical nurse, not all health care facilities assign the same tasks to the assistant, Figure 2-1.

State Regulations

Health care assistants must be sure to understand the scope of the specific tasks they will be expected to carry out, as well as the state regulations that govern their clinical practice. Some states are moving toward greater control over the work performed by the health care assistant. These states are passing laws which spell out the duties and responsibilities of the assistant, as well as the basic education and level of *competency* required for practice. Be sure you are familiar with any specific state regulations or legislation that relate to your role as an assistant.

Lines of Authority

Health care assistants receive their assignments from the team leader or head nurse. Upon completion of their assignment, they report to this same person. This represents the assistant's immediate line of authority and communication, Figure 2-2.

If the hospital is a large one, the assistant may function on a team whose leader is a licensed practical nurse or a registered nurse. In this case, the assistant's immediate superior is the team leader. The team leaders receive their instructions from the head nurse. The head nurse is responsible for the total care of a certain number of patients. Sometimes this includes all the patients on a wing, a unit, or a floor of the hospital. Supervisors are responsible for several head nurse units. They receive their authority and direction from the director of nursing. Hospitals vary in the complexity of their staffing.

Assistants should learn the lines of authority in their health care facility, as shown in Figure 2-3. As a student, your immediate authority is a supervisor or your teacher, or someone designated as your supervisor.

Authority for nursing care is passed from the doctor to the supervisor, the head nurse, or the team leader, and then to the assistant. When the responsibility for an assignment is accepted, the assignment must be fully understood and the assistant must be capable of handling it. *If there is any doubt, it should be discussed with the team leader.*

Admit, transfer and discharge patients	Care for patients with IVs
Answer lights	Measure intake and output
Ambulate and transport patients	Care for isolation unit
Bathe patients	Assist with special procedures
Make beds	Carry messages accurately
Assist patients with bedpans, urninals, and commodes	Pass nourishments
Apply binders	Give oral hygiene
Chart	Care for patients with oxygen therapy
Clean patient unit and utility room	Assist with physical examinations
Apply hot and cold compresses	Position patients
Change and pass drinking water	Provide postmortem care
Give enemas	Give preoperative and postoperative care
Care for equipment	Shave male patients
Care for equipment	Collect speciments
Feed patients and pass trays	Test urine and feces
	Determine vital signs

FIGURE 2-1. Common duties of health care assistants

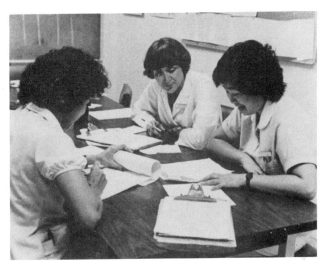

FIGURE 2-2. The nursing leader gives report to the members of her team.

Guidelines for the Health Care Assistant

Never attempt to perform a task for which you have not been properly trained. If you feel unsure of carrying out a procedure that was part of your training program, inform the nurse. Do not feel embarrassed. It is

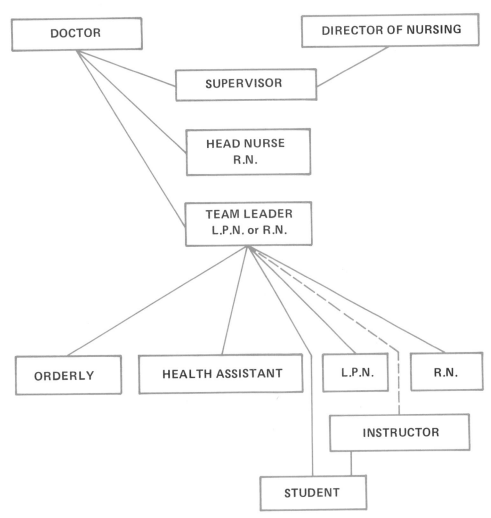

FIGURE 2-3. Lines of authority for nursing care

better to ask for clarification and supervision than to make an error and injure a patient, Figure 2-4.

If another health care worker asks you to perform a task that is clearly out of your scope of training such as starting an intravenous infusion, be prepared to refuse, explaining in a courteous manner that this is a task for which you have not been technically or legally prepared. Report the incident to your nurse so that your scope of duties can be clearly understood by all staff members.

On the other hand, be willing to learn new skills under the close supervision of your nurse. This will increase your ability to provide good, safe nursing care. If, for example, your nurse suggests a new way to lift a patient that is different from that which you have learned in your program, listen and watch carefully as the instruction is given. Seek supervision as you practice the new technique until both you and your supervisor feel you can do it safely on your own.

Not everyone can be a health care assistant. Assistants are special people: they are interested in others, they take pride in themselves, and they are willing to learn the skills necessary to care for those who are ill.

This interest in and care for people can be a valuable asset to the entire nursing team—far indeed from the stereotyped "bedpan passer." You are, after all, the person whom the patient sees most often; and in that capacity you have the chance to observe and hear many things which the other team members will not. By transmitting these observations to your supervisor, you are likely to give the other team members a valuable insight to the patient's illness and attitude toward that illness. For example, haven't you already observed that the patient's attitude toward the attending doctor or nurse is much less relaxed than it is with you, the health care assistant? For that same reason, the patient is far more likely to tell you of "minor complaints" that may possibly not be minor at all.

PERSONAL HEALTH AND HYGIENE

Good personal grooming is essential since the assistant is in close contact with patients, Figure 2-5. Because the work of the assistant, although rewarding, is not physically easy, it is particularly important that all body odors be controlled. A daily bath and the use of an antiperspirant/ deodorant are essential. The health care assistant should also recognize that strong perfumes, aftershave lotions, and cigarette odors are often offensive to patients.

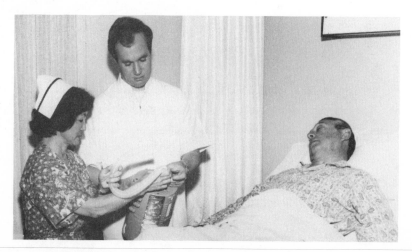

FIGURE 2-4. Always ask for clarification if you are unsure how to proceed with patient care.

Hair and fingernails should be kept short and clean. If nail polish is used by female assistants, it should be clear, not colored.

Stockings and socks should be freshly laundered. Shoes and shoelaces should be cleaned daily. Fatigue will be lessened if shoes give proper support to the feet and are well-fitted.

Jewelry is not part of the health care assistant's uniform, as it is a ready medium for bacteria to grow. There is also the possibility of jewelry causing injury to the patient or to the assistant, especially if the patient is confused or is a young child. Most health care agencies do permit the members of the nursing staff to wear a wedding ring and a watch with a second hand. The watch is used in monitoring the condition of patients.

Uniforms

Some hospitals today allow health care workers great leeway in selecting the type and style of their uniforms. Traditionally, patients were able to identify the various types of health care workers by their uniforms, including caps. Today, it is often very difficult to distinguish between a physiotherapist, registered nurse, physician, or social worker. It is no wonder that newly-admitted patients are often confused as to whom they should approach for information or help. To help avoid this confusion, some states and many health care facilities require personnel to wear a name badge or photo identification tag at all times while on the job.

If your health care facility requires that you wear a uniform, it should only be worn while on duty. If your health care agency does not provide facilities for changing your uniform before and after going on duty, be sure to wear a cover-up as you travel to and from work. Upon arriving home, remove your uniform, fold it inside out, and put it into the laundry. Wearing a fresh uniform every day should become a habit.

Your Attitude

Being a health care assistant requires enthusiasm and great energy. A well-nourished person who receives the proper rest is better able to per-

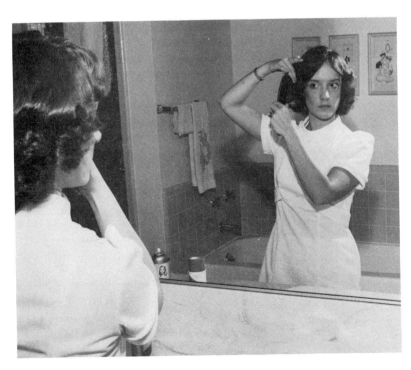

FIGURE 2-5. Good grooming begins with a clean body and hair.

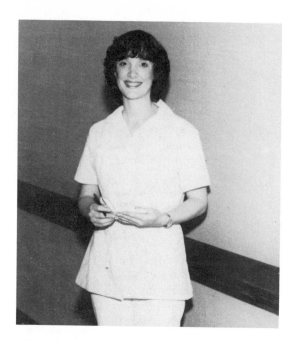

FIGURE 2-6.   The health care assistant who is well-groomed reflects pride in herself and in her work.

form efficiently. Make sure that you get adequate rest, as well as recreation, so that you can perform your duties well.

Above all, remember that your patients' safety and comfort is your main concern. Try to keep in mind their needs and feelings. After all, would you feel confident if you were ill and the assistant caring for you had long fingernails that could scratch you, or that could collect dirt and possibly infect your surgical incision? Or, how would you feel if the assistant who was preparing you for surgery kept having to push the hair out of his eyes; or if the assistant assigned to give you a backrub wore clanking bracelets on her wrists?

Remember, too, that how you look reflects the pride that you have in yourself and in your work. Well-groomed nursing assistants who pay attention to the details of their person and appearance show others, especially their patients and co-workers, that they are likely to have the same pride and caring attitude in their work, Figure 2-6. If you observe good grooming and personal habits, patients will feel more secure and confident, and other staff members will regard you as mature and reliable.

Summary

The health care assistant has specific responsibilities, but they may vary depending upon the employing agency. The lines of communication and authority within the health care agency must be clearly understood. Procedures and policies established by the health care agency should be followed carefully. Proper appearance and personal hygiene are essential qualities of health care assistants since they work in such close contact with patients and co-workers. In all situations, the health care assistant is ultimately responsible for his or her own actions and appearance.

SUGGESTED ACTIVITIES

1. Discuss the responsibilities of the health care assistant listed on page 10. List those you might be asked to perform in the health care facility to which you are assigned.

2. Discuss the importance of good grooming. How does it affect the patient's opinion of the health care facility? How does it affect your co-workers' opinion of you? What does your personal appearance say about you?

3. Investigate the laws and regulations which control the education and practice of health care assistants in your state.

VOCABULARY   Learn the meaning and correct spelling of the following words and abbreviations.

competency   LVN/LPN   RN
health care assistant nursing team   scope of practice

UNIT REVIEW   **A. Clinical Situations.** Briefly describe how a health care assistant should react to the following situations.

1. You are asked by a co-worker to start an IV.

2. A superior offers to demonstrate a different way to safely perform a skill that you have already learned.

3. You observe that some of your co-workers have unkempt hair and long fingernails.

B. Completion.

1. In the health care facility, the person who assists the LPN and the RN in giving patient care is called a _____ or _____.
2. When in doubt about the proper action to take, the assistant should check _____.

3. In the space provided, list the missing members of the nursing team:

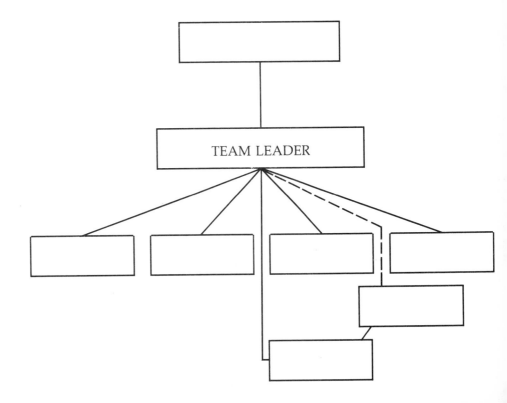

TEAM LEADER

4. Check the positive and negative grooming traits of a health assistant.

Trait	Yes	No
a. long hair		
b. clean shoelaces		
c. cigarette odor		
d. bright nail polish		
e. unpolished shoes		
f. dangling earrings		
g. light lipstick		
h. long fingernails		
i. use of antiperspirant/deodorant		

Unit 3 Ethical and Legal Issues Affecting the Health Care Assistant

OBJECTIVES

As a result of this unit, you will be able to:

- Discuss the ethics involved in the preservation of life.
- Identify the kind of information that is considered to be confidential.
- Demonstrate tactful refusal of a tip offered by a patient.
- Describe the legal responsibilities of a health care assistant.
- Recognize ethical and legal situations and take the proper course of action.

The ethical code of medicine is a set of rules which guides the conduct of all those who care for the sick. This is a moral rather than a legal code, established for the protection of the patient. It is just this code which is addressed in the Patient's Bill of Rights, which is spelled out in Unit 8. When you assume responsibility for nursing care, you, too, voluntarily agree to live up to the ethical code.

ETHICAL ISSUES

Preservation of Life

One of the most basic rules of *ethics* is that life is precious. Everyone involved in the care of patients puts the saving of life and the promotion of health above all else. It is not always easy to keep this rule in mind when you are caring for a patient who is dying, especially if you know your patient is in pain or when your patient seems to have limited potential for a prolonged, productive life. You must do everything you possibly can to make the patient comfortable and give emotional support to the family.

Probably at no other time in history have the questions of medical ethics been under such scrutiny. When is life gone from a person on a life support system? How much heroic effort should be given in situations of terminal illness? How valid are "Living Wills" written by terminally ill patients who wish no extraordinary means to be employed in the event their heart stops or their breathing ceases? These and many other medical-legal questions swirl all around us today and will eventually be decided under the law.

Still, one fact is very clear—the major role of medicine and all members of the health care team is to preserve life when possible and make comfortable those whose lives may not last much longer.

Confidential Information

One of the most basic rules of ethics concerns what you see and hear as you work in a health care facility. Much of this information is of personal concern to the patient and must be kept in strictest confidence, Figure 3-1.

When you are upset or under pressure, you sometimes find yourself telling a friend something that in a calmer moment you would never have

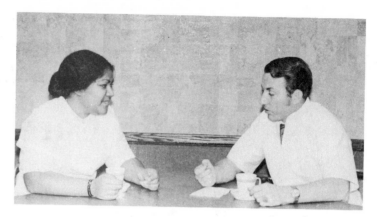

FIGURE 3-1. Information about patients is confidential and must not be discussed casually with others.

said. The sick person is under great stress and may confide in you, for the same reasons. The ethical code forbids you from repeating this information or using it for your own personal gain. If you believe that the information is important to the *welfare* of the patient, you should promptly report the matter to your immediate supervisor. Only that information that has a direct bearing on the patient's care and well-being may be repeated.

For instance, the patient who is worried about the care of her children at home might be greatly helped if the supervisor contacted a social worker. The repetition of facts, however, must be made only to your supervisor and not within the hearing of visitors or other patients. Remember, your intent is not to gossip but to share information that will benefit the patient.

There may be the temptation to "talk shop" with your co-workers at lunch or breaktime. Discussing patients in this way is considered gossiping, and is ethically wrong.

Patient Information

Patients, and sometimes their visitors, will question you about their condition or treatment. You will learn to evade these inquiries tactfully by stating that you do not know all the details of the treatment or patient's condition. Inquiries should be redirected to a doctor or nurse who can prop-

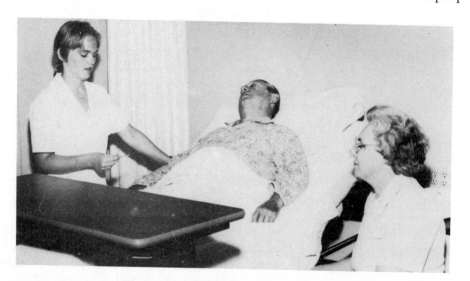

FIGURE 3-2. Information about the patient should not be given to family members.

erly answer these questions. It is the privilege of each doctor to decide how much information should be given to an individual patient.

Never give information concerning the death of a patient to the patient's family. *Always* let the nurse or physician relate this information. Refer any such questions to your supervisor. Treated with tact, a refusal of this kind is rarely resented by the patient, or family.

It is also not wise to discuss a patient's condition while in the patient's room, even if the patient is unresponsive. The patient may be able to hear everything that is said.

Tipping

Patients are charged for the services they receive while in the hospital. The salary you are paid is included in that charge. It is a fact that inpatient care is costly and that everything possible must be done to promote cost containment. Since the service you give depends on need and does not depend upon the patient's race, creed, color, or ability to pay, there is no place for tipping within this system. Sometimes patients offer a "little something" to you. A firm but courteous refusal of the money is usually all that is necessary to assure the patient of your meaning, Figure 3-3. Small gifts may, however, be accepted.

Respecting Religious Beliefs

Patients of all faiths and with varying beliefs are admitted to the hospital. These individual religious differences must be respected. A visit from a patient's minister, priest, rabbi, or spiritual advisor can be very helpful because many ill patients desire the support of their clergy, Figure 3-4.

Report all requests for clergy visits to the nurse, who can make the necessary contacts and arrangements. You should know the type of chaplain services available in your facility, whether a chapel for ambulatory patients is open, and whether religious broadcasts are available. You should never encourage patients to move in any religious direction, but you should always make sure they know the options available to them within the facility.

It may be necessary for you to assist a member of the clergy when he or she visits the patient. Regardless of your own personal beliefs, you must be respectful, courteous, and helpful, assuring privacy.

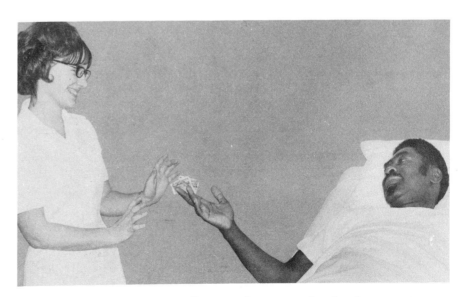

FIGURE 3-3. Tips must be courteously refused.

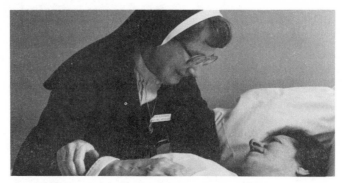

FIGURE 3-4.   A visit from clergy or other members of the religious community can be very reassuring and helpful to the patient.

LEGAL ISSUES

Negligence

Assistants are trained workers and can normally be expected to perform in certain ways. When an assistant fails to give care that is expected or required by the job, that assistant is guilty of *negligence*. For example, if a hospital has a policy that bedrails be up at night and an assistant, preparing a patient for bed, forgets—or is in too much of a hurry—to put up the bedrails and the patient falls, the assistant is negligent.

Malpractice

Malpractice occurs when an assistant improperly gives care or gives care in which there has been no formal instruction. The assistant would also be guilty of malpractice if an enema solution of a higher temperature than required was prepared and it burned the patient. Starting an intravenous infusion is a procedure for which assistants are not prepared, so an assistant who starts an infusion is also guilty of malpractice.

Reporting Illegal and Dishonest Acts

Because of the nature of their work, people employed in hospitals must have the highest degree of honesty and dependability. Despite careful screening, sometimes dishonest people are hired and things begin to disappear. These range from washcloths to money or drugs. If such an act is observed, whether major or minor, it should be reported immediately to the supervisor. Not reporting such an act is considered *aiding and abetting* the crime.

As a health care assistant, the opportunities for poor practice, illegal activities, and neglect are ever-present. Resist the temptation to lower your standards. Honesty and integrity are the hallmarks of the successful health care worker.

Writing or Witnessing a Patient's Will

Sometimes patients ask members of the staff to write a will for them. All matters of this nature should be promptly reported to the supervisor. Writing a will is a legal matter for which none of you are prepared or trained. Signing a will as a witness can lead to difficult legal complications and should likewise be avoided. There are legal aspects to everyday living as well as to every job. As a citizen you do not have problems if the law is obeyed. As a health assistant you will not have problems if you follow the hospital policies as outlined in the hospital's procedure book. Perform only those services that you have been taught and know the proper lines of authority.

RESTRAINTS

It is sometimes necessary to restrain the movement of patients. Whenever employed, restraints must always be applied in accordance with a specific physician's order which indicates the extent of restraint and the rationale.

Restraints are only applied for the purpose of protecting the patient or to protect others from the patient. Application of restraints without proper authorization or justification constitutes false imprisonment.

The health care assistant must be very careful never to apply restraints on his or her own initiative and to carefully observe and care for any patient who is restrained.

Summary

All persons giving care to the ill must voluntarily agree to live up to an ethical code. The ethical code protects the patient by prohibiting the discussion of personal matters, and by assuring the preservation of life and the promotion of health.

Patients receive service based on their need, not their ability to pay. Therefore, the acceptance of tips is not permitted.

The religious needs of all patients must be considered and respected.

Health care assistants have legal responsibilities, also. There should be no toleration of negligence, malpractice, or dishonest acts. There need not be concern about legal complications as long as prudent judgment is exercised and policies are followed.

SUGGESTED ACTIVITIES

1. Discuss why the basic rule of medical ethics is concerned with the preservation of life.

2. Discuss types of information that must be kept in confidence and those which should be reported to your supervisor.

3. If there are members of your class of different faiths, discuss the special need each would have if hospitalized.

VOCABULARY

Learn the meaning and correct spelling of the following words and phrases.

aiding and abetting	gossip	malpractice
confidential	living will	negligence
ethics		

UNIT REVIEW

A. Clinical Situations. Briefly describe how a health care assistant should react to the following situations.

1. A patient offers a tip to you for some special service you performed.

2. The patient asks you what his last laboratory blood work showed.

3. The visitor wants to know if her father *really* has cancer.

B. Completion.

1. An assistant should not accept a tip because _____.
2. An ethical code differs from a legal code in that _____.
3. The _____ is the person who is responsible for deciding what information is to be given to a patient.
4. Information about a patient must be kept _____.
5. Restraints must never be applied without _____.

Section One
Self-evaluation

A. Choose the phrase which best completes each of the following sentences by encircling the proper letter.
1. An example of a tax-supported community agency is the
   - a. Heart Association.
   - b. Association for the Blind.
   - c. health department.
   - d. Tuberculosis Association.
2. The official international health agency is called the
   - a. International Health Association.
   - b. World Health Organization.
   - c. World Health Service.
   - d. International Health Service.
3. Your daily assignment is usually given to you by the
   - a. assistant.
   - b. director of nursing.
   - c. team leader.
   - d. doctor.
4. If a patient asks you to write his will you had *best*
   - a. refuse bluntly.
   - b. avoid answering immediately.
   - c. refer the matter to the doctor.
   - d. suggest the patient talk with the team leader or supervisor.
5. One of the following is *not* part of your job.
   - a. Starting IVs
   - b. Collecting specimens
   - c. Assisting patients to ambulate
   - d. Giving enemas
6. Personal information about patients
   - a. may be discussed during coffee break.
   - b. must never be discussed outside the hospital.
   - c. may be discussed with other patients.
   - d. may be used for your own advantage.
7. When a patient offers you a tip for your services, you should
   - a. refuse in a firm, courteous manner.
   - b. accept the tip and share it with the other team members.
   - c. refuse and act shocked that the offer was ever made.
   - d. accept and then return the tip to a member of the patient's family.
8. A case of negligence would arise if a patient
   - a. who has bathroom privileges falls when you are out of the room.
   - b. falls because you forgot to wipe up water you had spilled on the floor.
   - c. develops an infection when you perform a procedure you have not been taught.
   - d. develops an important symptom which he does not report to the nursing team.
9. A case of malpractice would arise if a patient is injured because you
   - a. forgot to follow the hospital policy to put up siderails at night.
   - b. carried out a special procedure in which you had not been instructed.
   - c. failed to wipe up some water on the floor.
   - d. failed to report a defective electrical wire.
10. When you care for a patient of a different faith than your own, you are obliged to
    - a. help the patient understand your faith.
    - b. show the patient how wrong his faith is.
    - c. respect his religious beliefs.
    - d. arrange to have your clergyman make a visit.
11. Important characteristics for the health assistant include
    - a. interest in others.
    - b. willingness to learn.
    - c. good personal grooming.
    - d. All of the above.

12. Part of good grooming includes
    a. clean shoes every week.
    b. fingernails long and polished.
    c. daily bath.
    d. wearing expensive jewelry.
13. Lines of authority are important. Your immediate line of authority is
    a. a peer.
    b. a staff LVN.
    c. your team leader.
    d. the doctor.
14. The patient has written a "living will." You know this means
    a. you will inherit money.
    b. a member of the clergy must be called at the time of death.
    c. the desire is for no extraordinary means be employed in the event of death.
    d. the desire is for every means possible to be used to sustain life.
15. You learn something personal about a patient from his chart. You should
    a. keep quiet about the information.
    b. share it with other patients.
    c. share it with co-workers during coffee break.
    d. let the patient know what you have learned.
16. You observe a co-worker stealing supplies and fail to report it. You are guilty of
    a. malpractice.
    b. aiding and abetting.
    c. gossip.
    d. loyalty.
17. A patient tells you he is worried about being a "husband" after his prostatectomy. You should
    a. talk to his wife about the problem.
    b. report to your team leader.
    c. share the information with a co-worker.
    d. call the doctor.
18. When the patient's clergyperson comes for a visit, you should
    a. move other patients out of the room.
    b. draw the curtains for privacy.
    c. ask his visitor to remain.
    d. report to your team leader.
19. Health assistants function as health care workers in
    a. acute hospitals.
    b. long term care facilities.
    c. homes.
    d. All of the above.
20. The service which you give to a patient is determined by the patient's
    a. race.
    b. need.
    c. color.
    d. creed.

B. Match Column I with II.

Column I	Column II
21. Maternity department	a. OR
22. Surgery department	b. OB
23. Emergency care department	c. ICU
24. Central service department	d. CS
25. Intensive care department	e. ER

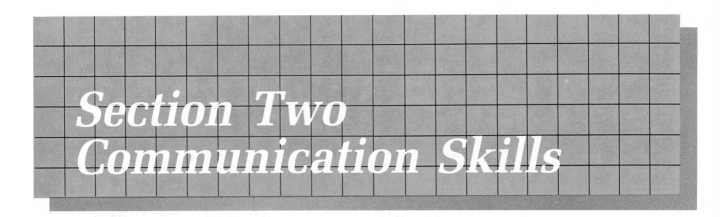

Section Two
Communication Skills

Unit 4 Principles of Communication

OBJECTIVES

As a result of this unit, you will be able to:

- Answer the telephone according to the procedure described.
- Give an oral report about a patient to the team leader.
- Chart information about the patient if hospital policy permits.
- Block print the alphabet and numbers.

Communication is a two-way process by which information—whether it be facts or feelings—is shared. In order for communication to occur, both a "sender" and a "receiver" of the information is required. There are several levels on which communication can take place. Information can be transmitted orally, in a written form, or through body language.

Health care assistants communicate with their patients, with their co-workers, and with their supervisors within the health care setting. As a health care assistant, you will need to receive and transmit information regarding your observations and care of patients, your interactions with patients, and your feelings.

As a health care assistant who is also a member of a nursing team, it is imperative that you express your observations, thoughts, and feelings to your co-workers and supervisors in a proper, clear manner if good interpersonal working relationships are to be maintained. Remember that it's very hard, and possibly dangerous, to work with someone that does not, or can not communicate well and effectively.

OBSERVATION

Observing patients is an important part of your responsibility as a health care assistant. Observing means more than just looking at a person. To properly carry out observation techniques, you must use all your senses, noting anything unusual or out of the ordinary and then reporting these findings to the nurse or team leader, Figure 4-1.

Your eyes are your major asset when making patient observations. The more carefully and consistently you make visual observations, the more skill you will develop in quickly identifying unusual situations and responses. Do not, however, neglect the valuable information that reaches you through your other senses. For instance: you might note a change in skin color, a more rapid respiration, or the slowing of a pulse. You might

25

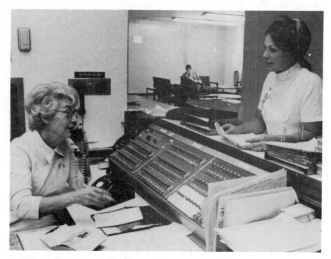

FIGURE 4-1.   Important observations should be reported at once.

smell a strange odor, hear a moan, or feel an unusual lump in the skin.

Observations of the patient are of paramount importance, but you must also make observations of the environment and equipment which pertain to patient care and treatment. For example, you must check infusion bottles and lines (tubes), such as IVs, to be sure your patient is receiving the ordered treatment. Inaccurate flow rates, blood in the tube, or a filled drip chamber are reportable observations. Drainage tubes have to be checked for flow, and the drainage must be assessed for character, amount, and any change. Equipment must also be checked to be sure it is functioning properly and that power sources are intact.

Certain patient conditions make some observations of particular significance. For example, the skin color and respirations of the patient with pneumonia would be important clues to the patient's status and to the progression of the disease.

Experience and practice will enhance your skill in quickly recognizing unusual situations and changes in your patient's condition. As you become more experienced, you will make many observations automatically upon entering any patient unit. You will quickly note equipment failure, drainage and infusions, body positions, and the general appearance of both the patient and the unit. You may be able to sense a problem or change even before you actually discover its nature. To be of use, though, your observations must be communicated *effectively* and *accurately*.

ORAL COMMUNICATION

Answering the Phone

At some time while you are on duty it may be necessary for you to answer the unit phone. Your answer should be made in the following manner:

Identify the unit
Identify yourself and your position

For example, if you are in the west wing on the fifth floor of the hospital and your name is Mrs. Brown, you might answer in this way, "5-west, Mrs. Brown, health care assistant, speaking." Answering the telephone in this way lets callers know immediately if this is the unit they want and if you are an appropriate person to take their call. This is especially important in health care settings, since misspent minutes can mean endan-

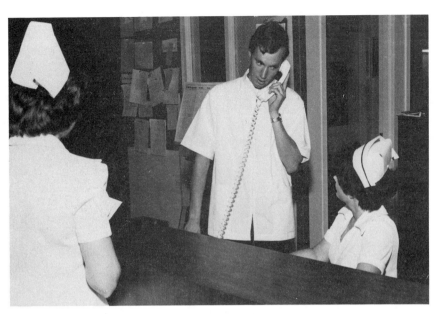

FIGURE 4-2. Oral communication includes use of the telephone to report and request important information.

gering a life. For the same reason, a health care assistant should never use the facility's phone to make personal calls.

Report

The *oral report* is often used to make sure that all members of the health care team fully understand the nursing care that has been planned for each patient. The health care team on the oncoming shift takes report from those who have cared for the patients during the previous shift.

From the report, you should learn the following information regarding each of your patients:

- name and location
- *diagnosis* (name of the patient's condition) and doctor
- special instructions for patient care

If there is any doubt in regard to your assignment, clarify it with your charge nurse or team leader before you start to work.

Usually, you will make a report about your patient to the charge nurse or the team leader just before the end of your shift. Be sure to include the identification and location of each individual patient as you give your report so there is no chance of misunderstanding. Discuss the care you gave and any special observations you have made. Your observations about the patient must be presented in a brief, but complete and accurate manner. You should report only what you observe, do for the patient, or are told by the patient. Information should be reported on only one patient at a time.

If, for some reason, you are unable to complete your assignment, make sure that your team leader knows exactly what remains to be done. You should never leave your assigned location without giving a report to your team leader.

WRITTEN COMMUNICATIONS

Nursing Care Plan

Many people are involved with the total care for each individual patient. To ensure common goals and expectations, to provide continuity of

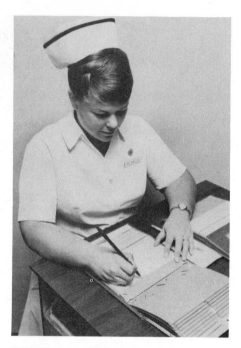

FIGURE 4-3. Working from the nursing care plan and kardex, the charge nurse plans for the patient's care.

care, and to enable assessment and planning, the patient's needs are documented in the *nursing care plan.* Nursing care plans are evaluated and revised periodically to reflect the patient's condition and progress.

Nursing care plans are now a required part of patient's records. Working from these plans, the charge nurse or team leader makes individual assignments for patient care.

Nursing care plans are frequently kept in a special carrier called the *kardex,* Figure 4-3. Using the kardex as a guide, oral reports and assignments are passed on to other team members, Figure 4-4.

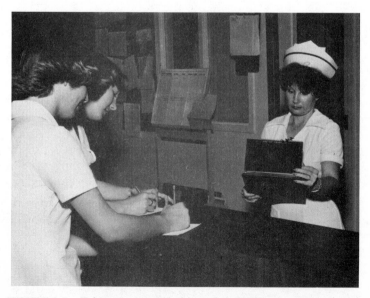

FIGURE 4-4. Taking report includes oral and written communication.

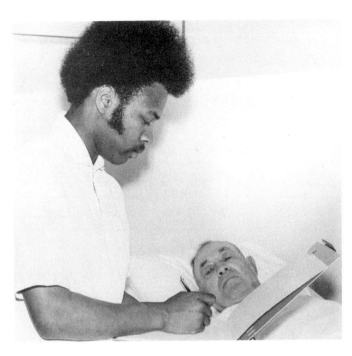

FIGURE 4-5. Charting important observations

The Patient's Chart

Charting is the process by which information regarding each patient is recorded in writing. Many members of the health care team, including health care assistants, may be responsible for charting, Figure 4-5. The chart is a legal document. It may be called to court and read as evidence in cases of lawsuits.

COMPONENTS OF THE CHART. Every patient has a chart. The chart usually consists of individual blanks which are filled with information concerning the patient. The following forms are usually included in the basic chart:

- A front sheet with information regarding sex, marital status, admission diagnosis, and employment
- A physical examination and a history record (maintained by the physician)
- A daily progress report (maintained by the physician)
- A graphic chart for recording TPR
- Nurses' notes on which pertinent information regarding the patient is made by the nursing staff

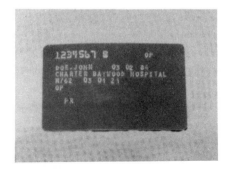

FIGURE 4-6. The addressograph resembles a charge card. It is imprinted on every sheet of the patient's record.

Other record forms are added according to the patient's condition. All records are dated and identified with the patient's name, location, physician, and hospital number. Many hospitals now use addressograph cards

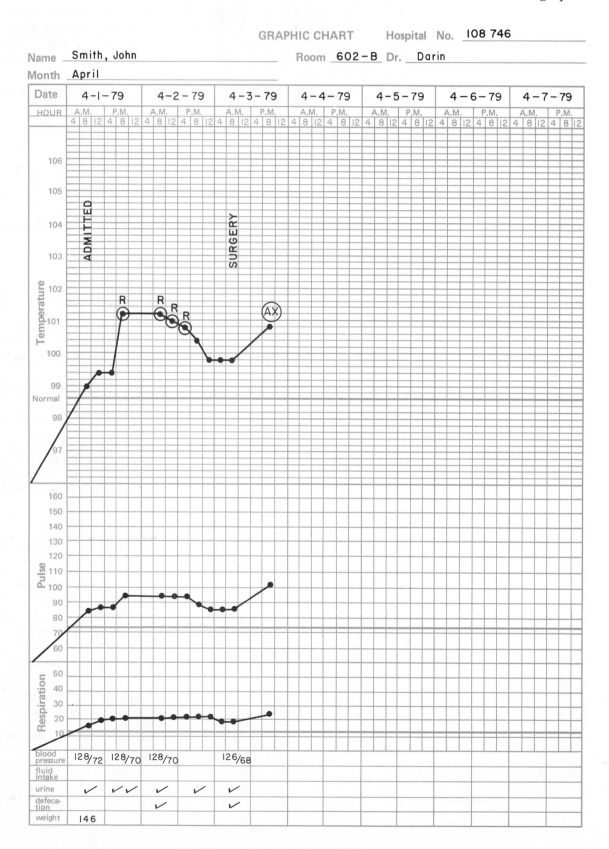

FIGURE 4-7.   Sample of a graphic chart

which provide this information. If this is the policy at your facility, be sure every sheet is individually stamped, Figure 4-6. The two records that will be of most concern to you are the graphic chart and the nurses' notes.

THE GRAPHIC CHART. The graphic chart varies in form, but it always has two basic markings: the time in blocks across the top and numbers relating to temperature, pulse, and respiratory rates along one side. Sometimes, blood pressure, voiding, and defecation are also charted on this sheet. Temperature, pulse, and respiration rates (TPRs) are plotted by placing solid dots on the lines which correspond to the readings and the time the read-

Hospital <u>City General</u>   Case Number <u>108746</u>
                                              Doctor <u>W. Darin M.D.</u>
Name <u>Smith, Robert J.</u>   Room or Ward <u>602 - B</u>

NURSES' NOTES

Date	Time	Temp.	Pulse	Resp.	Urine	Stool	Treatment or Medication	Nourishment	Remarks
4-1-69	7 30 A.M.	99	84	20					65 yr. old male adm. to rm.
									602-B via wheelchair
							B/p 128/72		c/o "Cramp like abd. pains"
							wt. 146 lbs.		abd. distended
	8				150 ml				to lab.
	8 15						C B C }		ordered
							Hinten }		Dr. Darin notified
									J. Mathews, Ass't
	9 30						Darvon Comp. 65 mg.		P.O.
	11 30						*Error J. Mathews Ass't*	tea and dry toast	appetite good
	11 30							tea and dry toast	refused
	12	99.4	88	18					c/o increased pain and
									abd. disten.
	1						Harris Flush		given c̄ tap H₂O - 105°
									lg. amt. flatus expelled
									J. Mathews, Ass't
	4	99.4	88	22	150 ml		B/p 128/70		Coughing-had some diffi-
									culty holding thermometer
									in mouth
									R. Jones, Ass't

FIGURE 4-8. An example of nurses' notes

ings were taken. The illustration of the Graphic Chart shows 8 AM, T. 99,
P. 84, R. 18, 12 noon, T. 99.4, P. 88, R. 20.

Some hospitals chart rectal temperatures in red, while others reserve
red ink for all night charting (7 PM–7 AM). An (R) should be placed above
a rectal temperature reading and an (AX) above an axillary temperature
reading. A sample graphic chart can be found in Figure 4-7.

NURSING NOTES. How much routine care to be charted depends on individual hospital policy. However, anything out of the ordinary should always be charted. Charting errors should never be erased. A single red line
should be drawn through the error or a circle drawn around it with the

---

PROGRESS SHEET

DATE ___Dec. 31___	NOTES
3 P.M.	PROBLEM: PAIN IN CHEST
	S: "I HAVE A TERRIBLE PAIN IN MY CHEST. I'M GOING TO DIE."
	O: GRASPS CHEST
	A: IN PAIN, EXPRESSING FEAR OF DEATH
	P: CHARGE NURSE NOTIFIED IMMEDIATELY B. LESLIE, H.A.
3:05 P.M.	S: "HURRY UP, I'M GOING TO DIE"
	O: LABORED BREATHING
	A: MEDICATION NEEDED TO RELIEVE PAIN
	P: NITROGLYCERINE 0.4 MG. SUB LIQ. GIVEN
	E: MEDICATION RELIEVED CHEST PAIN AND BREATHING IS LESS LABORED. P. RYDER, R.N.
Atlantic Hospital	Bruce, James 123456 146-B S. White, M.D. Patient Record

FIGURE 4-9.   A sample charting using the SOAPE approach

word "error" carefully printed and initialed. In other units of this text, specific patient procedures are introduced. These procedures and their effects need to be charted by making a notation of their completion on the patient's chart. An example of nurses notes can be seen in Figure 4-8.

Some health care facilities are taking a new approach to charting. All health team members use the same record to record observations and pertinent information about the patient. This record form is called a Problem-oriented Record (POR). Each recording is organized around a strength or problem of the patient. It includes a *subjective statement* (a feeling expressed by the patient—"I feel so hot."), an *objective observation* (an observation made by a team member—"My patient looks flushed and is sweating a great deal."), an *assessment* (judgment about what was observed—"She may have a fever."), a *plan* for meeting the patient's needs, and an *evaluation* as to the success or failure of the plan. The first letter of each concept spells SOAPE. The health assistant is usually only involved in recording subjective and objective observations and reporting to the team leader. Figure 4-9 shows a sample charting using the SOAPE approach. Notice the date, the time, and the signature of the person recording is also included for each recording. Since each hospital tends to modify these basic techniques of charting, be sure you know which form or modification is used at your facility.

GENERAL GUIDELINES FOR CHARTING. Charting must be both accurate and legible. Unless writing in script is permitted by your facility, written notations should be printed in block letters and properly spaced. Basically, block printing involves making letters with straight strokes and circles, Figure 4-10.

Notes may be charted in different colored ink, according to shift. If this method is used in your facility, be sure to use the proper color for the time you are on duty.

Since all of the information you will be charting refers to a particular patient, you need not use the term "patient" in your report. Notations should be short phrases, not complete sentences. Each entry you make in the patient's chart should be followed by your signature and title, including your first initial and full last name, Figure 4-8.

Increasing numbers of hospitals are using computers to make recordkeeping easier. Charting in international time is becoming increasingly common for use with these machines. Using this system, time is not indicated as AM or PM. Twelve midnight (12 AM) is recorded as 2400. The new day begins at 2400 hours or 12:00 AM. For this reason, only the minutes are recorded for the first hour of the new day, e.g., 12:10 AM is recorded as 0010; 12:10 PM is recorded as 1210, as seen in Figure 4-11.

NONVERBAL COMMUNICATION

Nonverbal communication is the process by which information is communicated through the use of one's body, rather than through speech or writing. This kind of communication, called *body language*, can tell you a great deal about your patient. A patient who is in pain may be somewhat protective of the affected area. Tears or an unwillingness to make eye contact with you may be indicative of depression. Some of the other ways your patients may "talk" to you through their body language may be through their:

- Posture
- Hand/body movements
- Activity level
- Facial expressions

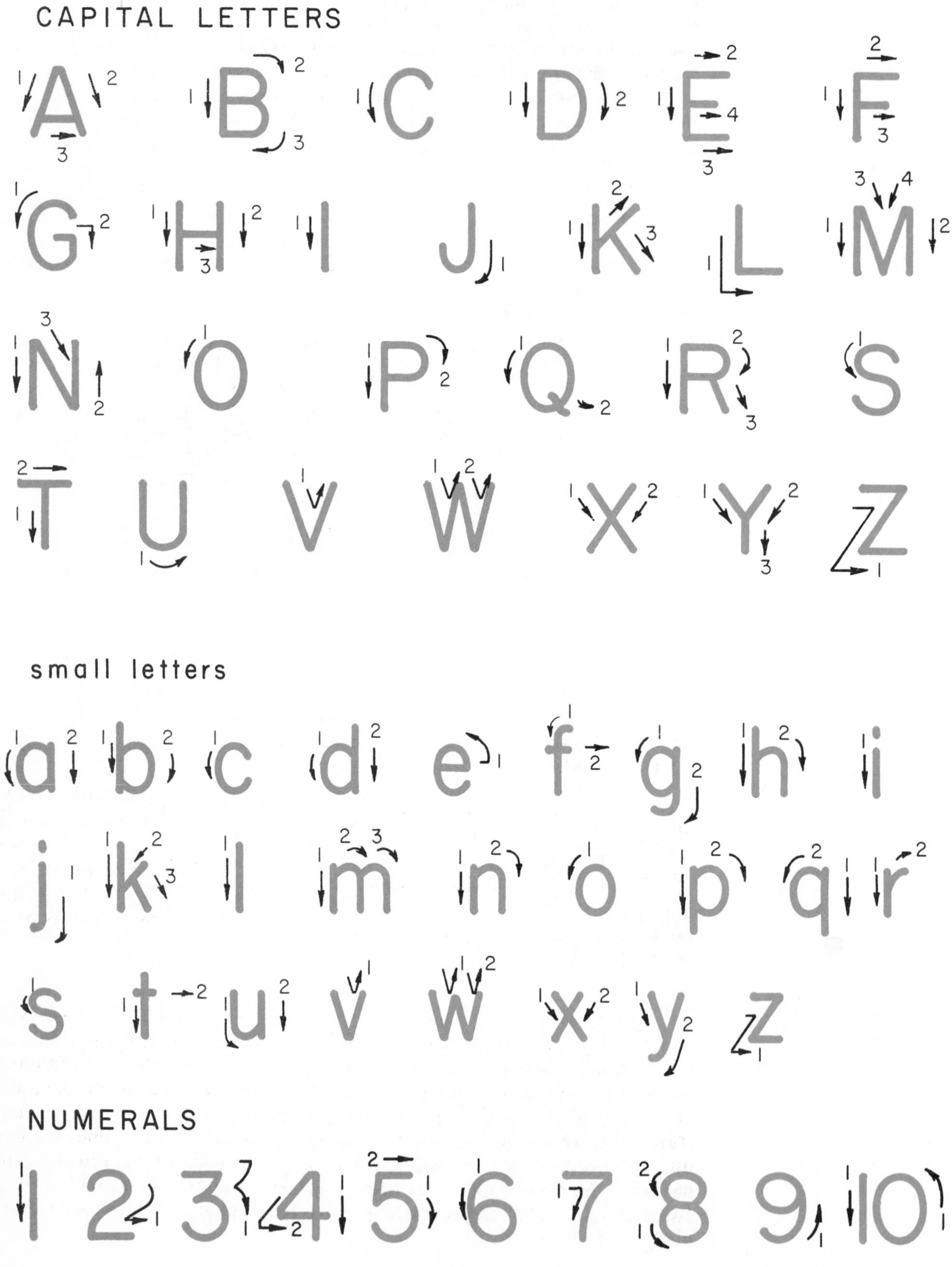

CAPITAL LETTERS

small letters

NUMERALS

FIGURE 4-10.   Block printing *(Reproduced courtesy of the University of Texas, Industrial Education Department).*

Unit 4 Principles of Communication | 35

AM	INTERNATIONAL TIME	PM	INTERNATIONAL TIME
12 midnight	2400	12 noon	1200
1	0100	1	1300
2	0200	2	1400
3	0300	3	1500
4	0400	4	1600
5	0500	5	1700
6	0600	6	1800
7	0700	7	1900
8	0800	8	2000
9	0900	9	2100
10	1000	10	2200
11	1100	11	2300

FIGURE 4-11. Time conversion chart

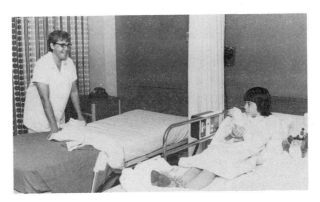

FIGURE 4-12. The body language of this assistant demonstrates her real interest in and positive feelings toward the patient.

- Overall appearance
- Body position

You should remember, too, that your body language also has meaning for your patient, Figure 4-12. When you are in a hurry and your patient wants to talk with you, do you glance at your watch frequently? When your patient seems to take a long time to change his hospital gown, do you roll your eyes or tap your foot impatiently? Do you avoid eye contact with the patient who is dying? All of these nonverbal signals tell your patients how you feel about caring for them.

Summary

Communication—whether oral, written, or nonverbal—is a two-way process of sharing information. One of the most important responsibilities of health care assistants is to observe and communicate with their patients. Their observations and interactions may then be recorded in the patient's chart or reported to their supervisor. The patient's chart is a legal document. Notations should be accurate, clear, concise, and legible. Both graphic and nursing notes may be recorded in the patient's chart by the health care assistant. Assistants should remember that their patients are also observing them and that their body language provides patients with valuable clues about their attitudes.

SUGGESTED ACTIVITIES

1. Investigate the procedure for giving and receiving oral reports in your hospital.

2. Role play answering the phone properly.

3. Examine a sample chart that is used in your hospital.

4. Practice printing the abbreviations and combining forms from the preceding unit in a legible form.

5. Discuss with your classmates how you would interpret the body language of the two patients pictured below.

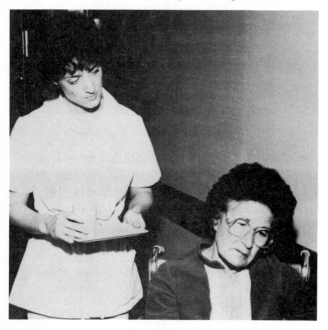

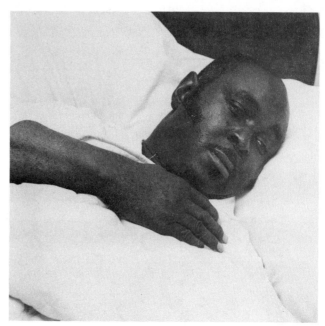

(Photo used with permission of Eli Lilly Co.)

VOCABULARY   Learn the meaning and correct spelling of the following words and phrases.

assessment	diagnosis	objective observation
body language	graphic chart	oral report
communication	kardex	SOAPE
charting	nursing care plan	subjective statement

UNIT REVIEW   A. **Brief Answer.** Answer the following questions.

1. What is a patient's chart?

2. What parts of the charting may be the health care assistant's responsibility?

3. How are notes recorded on the chart?

4. How should your signature appear on the chart?

B. **Clinical Situations.** Briefly describe how a health care assistant should react to the following situations.

1. You find it necessary to leave your unit for two hours.

2. You discover that you made an error in charting the day before.

C. **Completion.** Record the following information on the practice graphic chart provided.

	DAY 1	DAY 2	DAY 3
8 AM	99.6—88—20	98.6—72—18 (axillary)	97.2—68—16
12 noon	99.4—84—18	98.4—72—16	97.6—64—16
4 PM	99.4—80—18	101.4—82—20	99 —72—18
8 PM	101 —92—20 (rectal)	101.6—88—22	99.8—74—18
12 midnight	102.2—96—22 (rectal)	103 —92—20	100 —80—18

GRAPHIC CHART   Hospital No. _____

Name _____ Room _____ Dr. _____

Month _____

Date																					
HOUR	A.M.		P.M.		A.M.		P.M.		A.M.		P.M.		A.M.		P.M.		A.M.		P.M.		A.M.		P.M.

Temperature: 106, 105, 104, 103, 102, 101, 100, 99, Normal, 98, 97

Pulse: 160, 150, 140, 130, 120, 110, 100, 90, 80, 70, 60

Respiration: 50, 40, 30, 20, 10

blood pressure
fluid intake
urine
defecation
weight

Unit 5 Basic Anatomy and Medical Terminology

OBJECTIVES

As a result of this unit, you will be able to:

- Name the parts of the body, the body systems, and the organs.
- Use the correct terms to describe the relationship of body areas.
- Write the abbreviations commonly used in hospitals.
- Write the meanings of the various abbreviations used in hospitals.
- Recognize and use the most common prefixes, suffixes, and combining forms used in medical terminology.

All nursing care is directed toward helping patients reach optimum health and independence. Health is a state of well-being where all parts of the body and mind are functioning properly. Disease is any change from the healthy state and takes many different forms. Medical science is the study of disease and its effects on the human body. You can understand these effects better when you have a clear picture in your mind of a normal and properly-functioning body.

BASIC ANATOMY AND RELATED TERMINOLOGY

The *anatomy* (structure) and *physiology* (function) of the human body, Figure 5-1, is most easily understood if it is studied in a systematic, orderly manner. Special terms are used to describe the relationship of one part of the body to another. Imaginary lines or *planes* help us to better see these relationships. Whenever we describe the relationship of body parts, keep in mind the body as it looks in the anatomical position, Figure 5-2A.

Planes

- Transverse—lines drawn from side to side
  Superior—body parts above the line
  Inferior—body parts below the line
- Midline—line drawn through the center of the body from head to floor, Figure 5-2B. It divides the body into two equal sides.
  Medial—body parts close to the midline
  Lateral—body parts away from the midline
- Frontal—line drawn to divide the body into back and front
  Anterior (ventral) body parts in front of the line
  Posterior (dorsal) body parts behind the line, Figure 5-2C
- *Proximal* and *distal*—terms used to show the relationship of the part to its point of attachment to the body. The arm and hand are attached to the body at the shoulder. Because the hand is further away from the shoulder than the wrist, the hand is described as distal to the wrist; the wrist is proximal to the hand. The fingers are away from the point of body attachment at the shoulder. They are distal to the elbow which is closer to the point of attachment (shoulder).

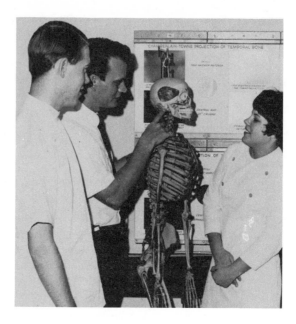

FIGURE 5-1. An understanding of normal anatomy and physiology helps us better understand the illness which affects our patients.

Cavities

Within the solid-looking body are spaces called *cavities*, which contain vital organs like the heart, stomach, and brain, Figure 5-3.

The thoracic and abdominal cavities are separated by a large, dome-shaped muscle that is called the *diaphragm*, Figure 5-4. The cavities are lined with tissue sheets called *membranes*. The membranes divide the cavities into sections by forming inner walls. The membranes help to separate the organs and prevent undue friction (rubbing). Within the *thoracic cavity* the membranes which surround the lungs are called *pleura*. Those which surround the heart are called *pericardium*.

The *meninges* are continuous membranes which line both the *cranial* and *spinal cavities*. Notice that the abdominal cavity is divided by the *peritoneal membrane* into the peritoneal cavity (surrounded by the peritoneum), the *pelvic cavity*, and the *retroperitoneal space* (behind the peritoneum). The abdominal cavity is also divided into four regions, or *quadrants*, as illustrated in Figure 5-5.

Cells

Cells are the microscopic basic units of life. On a tiny scale the living cell carries out the same functions as the body. These functions include:

- Respiration
- Nutrition
- Elimination
- Energy production
- Reproduction

The structure of cells varies but always includes three main parts:

1. *Nucleus*—directs the activities of the cell and plays an important role in reproduction.
2. *Cytoplasm*—a jelly-like substance which carries out the activities of the cell.
3. *Cell Membrane*—controls passage of materials that enter and leave the cell.

FIGURE 5-2.

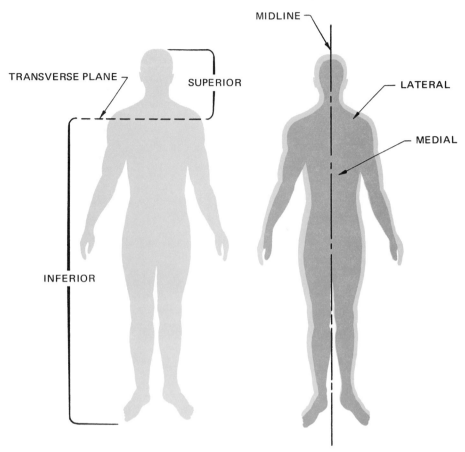

TRANSVERSE PLANE

SUPERIOR

INFERIOR

A. Body in anatomical position

MIDLINE

LATERAL

MEDIAL

B. Showing midline

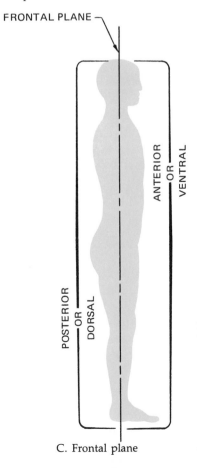

FRONTAL PLANE

ANTERIOR OR VENTRAL

POSTERIOR OR DORSAL

C. Frontal plane

CAVITY	ORGANS	
Cranial	Brain, pineal body, pituitary gland	
Spinal	Nerves, spinal cord	
Thoracic	Lungs, heart, great blood vessels, thymus gland	
Abdominal		
Peritoneal	Stomach, small intestine, most of large intestine, liver, gallbladder, pancreas, spleen	
Pelvic	Male Seminal vesicles, prostate gland, ejaculatory ducts, urinary bladder, urethra, rectum	Female Uterus, oviducts, ovaries, urinary bladder, urethra, rectum
Retroperitoneal Space	Kidneys, adrenal glands, ureters	

FIGURE 5-3. Body cavities

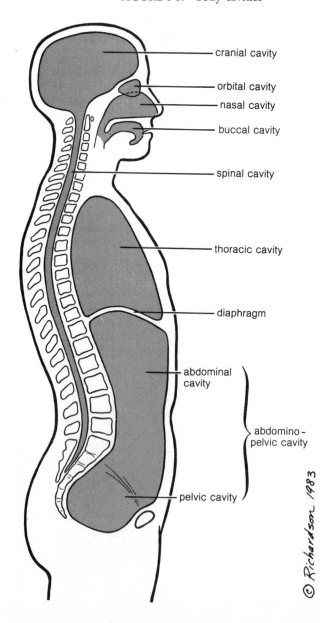

FIGURE 5-4. Side view of body cavities

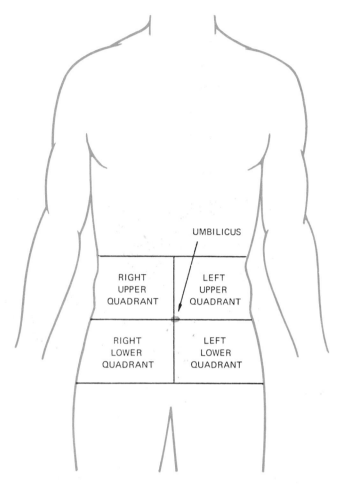

FIGURE 5-5.   The abdominal quadrants

Tissues

Tissues are special groups of cells which carry on particular activities. There are four basic tissue types:

1. *Epithelial tissue* covers the body as skin and lines the body cavities as membranes. The cells are close together and are specialized for absorption, secretion, and protection.
2. *Connective tissue* is found throughout the body. It holds other tissues together. The many forms of connective tissue include blood, bone, fibrous, and elastic types.

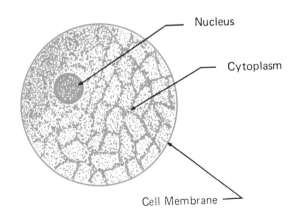

FIGURE 5-6.   Animal cell structure

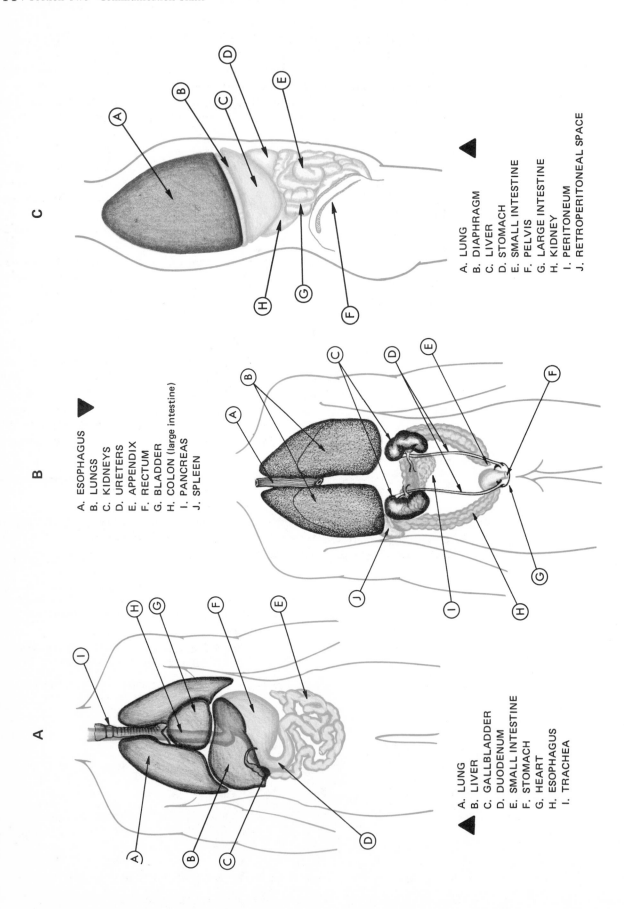

C

A. LUNG
B. DIAPHRAGM
C. LIVER
D. STOMACH
E. SMALL INTESTINE
F. PELVIS
G. LARGE INTESTINE
H. KIDNEY
I. PERITONEUM
J. RETROPERITONEAL SPACE

B

A. ESOPHAGUS
B. LUNGS
C. KIDNEYS
D. URETERS
E. APPENDIX
F. RECTUM
G. BLADDER
H. COLON (large intestine)
I. PANCREAS
J. SPLEEN

A

A. LUNG
B. LIVER
C. GALLBLADDER
D. DUODENUM
E. SMALL INTESTINE
F. STOMACH
G. HEART
H. ESOPHAGUS
I. TRACHEA

FIGURE 5-7.   The major organs of the body: (A) anterior view, (B) posterior view, (C) lateral view

3. *Muscular tissue* has cells which have the special ability to shorten (contract) and to lengthen (relax). When muscles are attached to bones, they enable the body to move. Some muscles help to form the walls of organs. Heart muscle is a highly specialized tissue.

4. *Nervous tissue* extends from the brain and spinal cord throughout the body. This tissue carries messages and regulates body functions.

Organs

Groups of different tissues acting together to carry out a specific function are called organs, Figure 5-7. For example, the stomach is an organ which aids in digestion. It is made up of nervous, connective, muscular, and epithelial tissues.

Most organs are found in pairs, and is peculiar to this group that if one of the organs is surgically removed, the other will operate alone to perform the necessary functions. Even when the organ is singular, like the stomach, from one-third to one-half can be excised without interfering with its routine function.

Systems

When several organs combine to perform a special function, they are called a system. The digestive system, for instance, includes that: tongue, pharynx, esophagus, salivary glands, intestines, liver, gallbladder, stomach, and pancreas. Figure 5-8 provides a list of the names of the body systems, together with the organs included in each. Notice that some organs function in more than one system. For a more detailed discussion of the various body systems and the disorders that affect each of them, see Section Eleven of this text.

MEDICAL TERMINOLOGY

Medicine has its own special language, called *terminology*, in which the words are formed by building on common *roots*. The root is often derived from Greek or Latin. For example, the stem or root word "oma" is

SYSTEMS	ORGANS	
Circulatory	Heart, arteries, veins, capillaries, spleen, lymph nodes, lymphatic vessels	
Endocrine	Parathyroid, pituitary gland, thyroid gland, pineal body, ovaries, adrenal gland, thymus, testes, islands of Langerhans	
Gastrointestinal	Mouth, esophagus, intestines, gallbladder, pharynx, stomach, appendix, liver, pancreas, teeth, tongue, salivary glands	
Integumentary	Skin, hair, nails, sweat and oil glands	
Musculoskeletal	Bones, joints, muscles, tendons, ligaments	
Nervous	Brain, spinal cord, nerves, ganglia	
Reproductive	Male Testes, epididymis, urethra, seminal vesicles and ducts, ejaculatory ducts, prostate gland, bulbourethral glands, penis, spermatic cord	Female Breasts, ovaries, oviducts, uterus, vagina, Bartholin glands, vulva
Respiratory	Nose, pharynx, larynx, trachea, bronchi, lungs, sinuses	
Urinary	Kidneys, ureters, urinary bladder, urethra	

FIGURE 5-8. The systems of the body

derived from the Greek word for tumor. It may be used to form a variety of words. For example, an adenoma is a glandular tumor, a lipoma is a fatty tumor, and a chondroma is a tumor composed of cartilage cells. Many of the words have common endings (suffixes) or common beginnings (prefixes). By learning some of the more common suffixes and prefixes, it is possible to put together many new words.

Give special attention to the exercises and activities in this unit. You will find that by learning the new words and parts of words in this unit, it will be easier for you to recognize the meanings of the medical terms you will meet in the rest of this text and those in common use in your hospital.

Shortened forms of words (often just letters) are called abbreviations. You are already familiar with abbreviations such as RN—registered nurse and LPN—licensed practical nurse. You will soon become familiar with additional abbreviations that are common to the world of medicine.

Each hospital also has *special* abbreviations that it uses, so learn these abbreviations too. Be sure to check with the procedure policy of your facility to determine which abbreviations have been approved for use. A good medical dictionary is a very helpful tool also.

Medical Combining Forms

A medical combining form is part of a word which has a specific meaning. For example, the combining form *cyte* means cell. *Cytology* is the study of cells. A leuko*cyte* is a white blood cell. Poly*cyt*osis is an illness in which there are too many red and white blood cells. No matter where the form *cyte* occurs in a medical word, it refers to cells; it may be a prefix, a suffix, or a root word. Remember:

- A prefix is a term added to the *beginning* of a word to change or add to the meaning of the word.
- A suffix is added to the *end* of a word to change or add to its meaning.
- In medicine, the root of a word generally indicates the condition which is being treated, studied, or is otherwise directly named by the term.

COMMON ABBREVIATIONS

Lists of abbreviations and their meanings follow. They have been grouped in related units of ten for easier learning. Other abbreviations will be presented in the following units where they find their greatest application.

Time Abbreviations

a.c.	—before meals
p.c.	—after meals
AM	—morning
PM	—evening or afternoon
h.s.	—hour of sleep (bedtime)
hr.	—hour
b.i.d.	—twice a day
t.i.d.	—three times a day
q.i.d.	—four times a day
q.2h.	—every 2 hours

Places or Departments

OR	—operating room
Lab	—laboratory
ICU	—intensive care unit
OPD	—outpatient department

OB   —obstetrics
EENT   —eye, ear, nose, and throat
GU   —genitourinary
GI   —gastrointestinal
ER   —accident or emergency room
CS   —central supply
Gyn   —gynecology
Ped   —pediatrics

Patient Orders

A.D.L.   —activities of daily living
p.r.n.   —whenever necessary
stat.   —at once
ad. lib.   —as desired
dc   —discontinue
spec.   —specimen
Noct.   —at night
O₂   —oxygen
tinct.   —tincture
q.s.   —sufficient quantity
ung.   —ointment (oint.)
$\overline{ss}$.   —one-half
$\overline{c}$ —with
$\overline{s}$ —without
gtt.   —drops
lb.   —pound
wt.   —weight
ht.   —height
N.P.O.   —nothing by mouth
p.o.   —by mouth
per   —by
liq.   —liquid
B.M.   —bowel movement
P.O.   —postoperative
preop.   —preoperative
pt.   —pint (500 ml)
L   —liter (1,000 ml, quart)
amt   —amount
Rx   —treatment (take)
Dr.   —doctor
Dx   —diagnosis

Physical and History

CHF   —congestive heart failure
RHD   —rheumatic heart disease
ASHD   —arteriosclerotic heart disease
CO   —coronary occlusion
MI   —myocardial infarction—refers to death of tissues due to loss
           of blood supply
CVA   —cerebral vascular accident—also known as a stroke
URI   —upper respiratory disease
PID   —pelvic inflammatory disease
MS   —multiple sclerosis
STD   —sexually transmitted disease

Roman Numerals		
	I	—1
	II	—2
	III	—3
	IV	—4
	V	—5
	VI	—6
	VII	—7
	VIII	—8
	IX	—9
	X	—10

Measurements and Volume		
	oz	—ounce ℥
	dr	—dram ʒ
	c	—centimeter
	cc	—cubic centimeter
	ml	—milliliter
	L	—Liter

Weight/Height		
	lbs	—pounds
	in	—inches
	kg	—kilogram

Temperature		
	F	—Fahrenheit
	C	—celsius or centigrade
	°	—degree

PREFIXES

a—from, without. **Example:** asepsis—without infection

ante—before. **Example:** antemortem—before death

anti—against, counteracting. **Example:** antidote—a substance which counteracts the effects of a poison

contra—against, opposed. **Example:** contraindicate—against the usual treatment

dys—pain or difficulty. **Example:** dysuria—painful urination

erythro—red. **Example:** erythrocyte—red blood cell

hyper—above; excess of. **Example:** hypertension—high blood pressure

hypo—under; deficiency of. **Example:** hypotension—low blood pressure

poly—many. **Example:** polyglandular—affecting many glands

pseudo—false. **Example:** pseudoparalysis—apparent loss of muscular power without true paralysis

SUFFIXES

algia—pain. **Example:** neuralgia—pain in nerve

asis or *osis*—state, condition, process. **Example:** leukocytosis—excess number of leukocytes (white blood cells)

cele—turmor or swelling. **Example:** cystocele—protrusion of urinary bladder into vagina

cyte—cell. **Example:** erythrocyte—red blood cell

ectomy—excision, surgical removal. **Example:** appendectomy—removal of the appendix

emia—blood. **Example:** glycemia—sugar in the blood

itis—inflammation. **Example:** appendicitis—inflammation of the appendix

oma—tumor. **Example:** lipoma—fatty tumor

ostomy—creation of an opening. **Example:** colostomy—surgical opening into the large bowel (colon)

otomy—cutting into. **Example:** laparotomy—surgical incision into the abdomen

OTHER MEDICAL COMBINING FORMS

aden—pertaining to a gland. **Example:** adenitis—inflammation of a gland

bio—pertaining to life. **Example:** biopsy—inspection of living organism (tissue)

cardi—pertaining to the heart. **Example:** cardialgia—pain in the heart

chole—gall. **Example:** cholelithiasis—gall stones

crani—pertaining to the skull. **Example:** craniotomy—surgical opening of the skull

cyt—pertaining to a cell. **Example:** cytometer—a device for counting and measuring cells

hyster—pertaining to the uterus. **Example:** hysterectomy—excision of the uterus

neo—new. **Example:** neoplasm—any new growth or formation

path—disease. **Example:** pathology—science of disease

pneum—lung. **Example:** pneumococcus—organism causing pneumonia

tox or *toxic*—poison. **Example:** hemotoxic—causing blood poisoning

Summary

The human body has a definite form and structure. Groups of different tissues acting together to carry out a specific function are called organs. The organs are grouped into systems which carry on the body functions. A careful study of the healthy body provides a foundation for learning about the changes which take place in disease.

Medical terminology refers to special words, abbreviations, and word combinations which are used to convey meanings to members of the hospital staff. Some words and abbreviations are fairly standard. The more common ones have been presented in this unit. Hospitals and other health agencies may have individual ways of abbreviating. Familiarity will be gained through repeated usage.

You will have many opportunities to increase your familiarity with medical terminology as you practice how to report and chart.

SUGGESTED ACTIVITIES

1. Study a model of the human body if one is available.

2. Practice locating body areas in relation to the planes described in the unit.

3. Discuss the reasons why a general knowledge of body structure and function is valuable to those who give basic bedside care to patients in the hospital. Why should the assistant learn correct medical terminology?

4. Practice writing the abbreviations in this unit, together with their meanings.

5. Investigate special abbreviations that are used in your health care facility.

6. Pronounce each form after your instructor to be sure you are saying it correctly.

VOCABULARY Write the meaning and correct spelling of the following words in your notebook, using the prefixes, suffixes, and combining forms you have learned. Then check your work by looking up the words in a medical dictionary.

adenoma	dorsal	pericardium
anatomy	epithelial tissue	physiology
anterior	erythema	planes
antitoxin	hyperadenosis	pleura
body cavity	hypofunction	pneumonectomy
cardiac	hysteralgia	posterior
cardiocele	lateral	proximal
cardiopneumatic	membranes	pseudoanemia
cell	muscular tissue	pseudoappendicitis
connective tissue	nervous tissue	system
contrastimulant	neuropathy	terminology
cranial	nucleus	tissue
cytoplasm	organ	ventral
distal		

UNIT REVIEW **A. Brief Answers.** Answer the following questions.

1. What is the medical term for each of the following phrases?
   a. above another part
   b. below another part
   c. near to the midline
   d. away from midline
   e. in front of the frontal plane

2. What are the names of four body cavities?

3. What are the names of the four membranes that line body cavities?

4. a. What is a cell?

   b. What is tissue?

5. Nine systems are given in this unit. List them and given an example of one organ in each system.

B. Clinical Situations. Briefly describe how a health care assistant should react to the following situations.

1. The nurse tells you to allow the patient to "ambulate ad. lib."

2. The nurse hands you a patient's urine sample and says, "Get this to the lab stat."

C. **Matching.** Match the abbreviations in Column 1 with their meanings in Column II.

Column I

_____ 1. a.c.
_____ 2. b.i.d.
_____ 3. OR
_____ 4. p.r.n.
_____ 5. p.o.
_____ 6. stat.
_____ 7. Noct.
_____ 8. c̄
_____ 9. ung.
_____10. s̄

Column II

a. three times a day
b. whenever necessary
c. night
d. before meals
e. operating room
f. by mouth
g. after meals
h. without
i. twice a day
j. at once
k. ointment
l. with

D. **Define the following combining forms.** Then circle the prefix or suffix which you have learned.
   1. erythrocyte _____
   2. dysuria _____
   3. pneumonitis _____
   4. adenopathy _____
   5. craniotomy _____

E. **Sentence Rewrite.** Rewrite the following sentences, using the proper abbreviations.
   1. Mr. Jones was sent to the operating room for emergency surgery after examination in outpatient department—ear, nose, and throat clinic.

   2. Patient had a bowel movement at eight o'clock this morning. A specimen was sent to the laboratory by order of Doctor Adams.

   3. Mrs. Merriweather was sent from the emergency room to obstetrics at ten-thirty this evening.

   4. Discontinue hot soaks. Apply hot water bottle as necessary. Bathroom privileges.

   5. Record intake and output. Scheduled for Operating Room 4 at nine o'clock Wednesday morning. Nothing by mouth after midnight tomorrow. Give pre-operative care for prostatectomy.

Unit 6 Classification of Disease

OBJECTIVES

As a result of this unit, you will be able to:

- Define disease and list some possible causes.
- Identify disease-related terms.
- Distinguish between signs and symptoms.
- List ways in which a diagnosis is made.
- List four modes of therapy.
- List six major health problems.

DEFINITION

Disease is any change from a healthy state. The disease (pathology) may be a change in structure or function, or it may be the failure of a part of the body to develop properly, Figure 6-1. Each disease has a cause *(etiology)*, probable outcome *(prognosis)*, and a usual set of signs and symptoms.

Causes of Disease

Many factors may contribute to the development of disease in the body. The immediate or direct cause is known as the *exciting* etiology (cause). For example, an injury from a fall may cause a bone to break; the blow of the fall is the exciting cause of the broken bone.

There are many different kinds of exciting etiologies, some originating outside the person's body: *exogenous*, while others originate from factors within: *endogenous*.

Traumas are mechanical injuries that damage the tissues of the body. These traumas may be so extensive that the cells forming the tissues die. Physical agents of many kinds can traumatize and seriously injure the body tissues. These include extremes of temperature, radiation, unusual pressure, electric shock, foreign bodies, chemical agents, and harmful microorganisms or their products. Since each of these causes of disease originate outside the body, they are referred to as exogenous etiologies.

The Disease Process

The body is like a complex chemical factory that depends upon delivery of adequate oxygen and nutrients to the active cells. Moreover, chemicals produced by some cells make the functioning and chemistry of other cells possible. Lack of adequate blood supply *(ischemia)* to a body tissue prohibits the delivery of these essential elements. As a result, the normal chemistry of the cells cannot be carried out.

Ischemias usually originate from factors within the body. For example, a blood clot *(thrombus)* which has formed within the blood vessel wall can block a blood vessel. The ischemia would be an endogenous cause of disease since without blood, and the vital oxygen it carries, cells cannot function, become diseased and die.

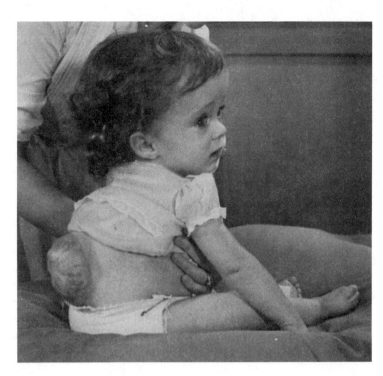

FIGURE 6-1.   This child has spina bifida and meningocele (a protrusion of the spinal cord and its covering) due to a defect (congenital) in the formation of the spinal column. *(Photo reproduced courtesy of the March of Dimes Birth Defects Foundation)*

People are sometimes born without the necessary chemicals to carry out important body functions. This might occur when someone is born with tissues that cannot produce enough insulin (a hormone) and therefore cannot utilize sugar properly. This disease, diabetes mellitus, also has an endogenous etiology.

Predisposing factors set the stage for an exciting etiology to cause a disease state, Figure 6-2. Malnutrition, age, fatigue, heredity, and certain occupations make it easier for disease to develop. A young child that is malnourished and underweight is much more apt to develop an infection than one who is well nourished. The germs causing the infection are the

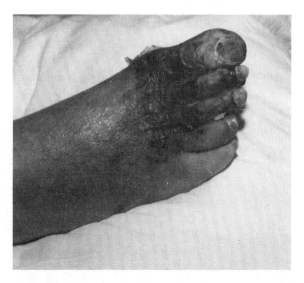

FIGURE 6-2.   Diabetes is a predisposing cause in the development of gangrene of the toes.

Signs	Symptoms
Skin color	Nausea
Rapid pulse (Tachycardia)	Dizziness
High blood pressure (Hypertension)	Pain
Vomiting	Anxiety

FIGURE 6-3.

exciting cause but the age and nutritional state of the child contributed to the development of the infectious process.

Signs and Symptoms

Signs and symptoms are evidence of disease processes going on within the body, Figure 6-3.

Signs of a disease are objective: they can be seen by others. The color or condition of the skin is an example of a sign of disease, Figure 6-4. *Symptoms* are subjective: they are felt by the patient, who tells us about them. Pain is a symptom common to many pathological conditions.

Complaints of pain provide good clues to the type of pathology going on in the body. It is not enough for the health care assistant to simply note that the patient has pain. It is important to learn from the patient the kind (character) of the pain, its exact location, intensity and duration, and to report this information promptly to the nurse or team leader. All observations of signs and symptoms must be noted and reported because they help to determine proper treatment.

The development and course of different diseases vary greatly. The signs and symptoms of an infected finger may develop rapidly, last a relatively short period and then, as the body controls the process, recovery is seen. This type of disease process is classified as an *acute* disease. Another example of acute disease is shown in Figure 6-5. Other organisms, such as those causing tuberculosis, may cause an infection in the lungs which remains with the patient for years. A prolonged disease is known as a *chronic* disease. Chronic disease states often have periods when the patient experiences the signs and symptoms and periods when evidences of the disease are less pronounced or disappear altogether. Rheumatoid arthritis is such a disease, since at times the affected joints are red, hot to touch, swollen and painful; at other times the signs and symptoms seem to go away.

COMPLICATIONS. Diseases such as measles or mumps—which are usually acute and follow a rather predictable cause—are sometimes made more serious by the development of pneumonia. The pneumonia makes the original process more harmful and is regarded as a *complication*. As you learn

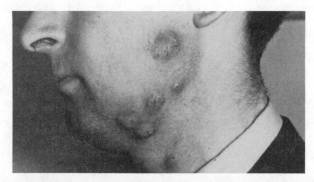

FIGURE 6-4. This patient shows the signs of ringworm on his face. *(Photo reproduced courtesy of the Center for Disease Control, Atlanta, GA)*

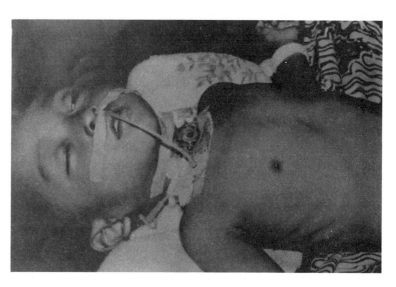

FIGURE 6-5. This child in Indonesia is suffering from an acute infectious disease called diphtheria, which is caused by a microorganism. *(Photo reproduced courtesy of the World Health Organization)*

more about patients and their illnesses, you will begin to associate specific signs and symptoms with a particular disease state.

DIAGNOSIS AND THERAPY

Before the physician can prescribe the proper treatment for the patient, he or she must determine what disease process is going on. Naming the disease process is known as establishing a *diagnosis*. In order to do this, the patient is examined, a history of previous illness is taken and reviewed, and various laboratory tests are performed.

The doctor then compiles all the information, matches it to possible diseases and then names the process. Once the diagnosis is confirmed, it is often possible to predict the course of the disease and probable prognosis and to determine the most appropriate *therapy* (treatment).

There are four basic approaches to therapy: surgery, chemotherapy, radiation, and supportive care.

Surgery

Surgery is used to remove unhealthy tissue, Figure 6-6, repair damaged tissue, and substitute functional tissue or artificial materials for that tissue which is beyond repair. For example, a *herniorrhaphy* is a surgical procedure to repair a weakened area of the abdominal wall and *coronary bypass* procedures replace unhealthy blood vessels with healthy ones from the patient's own body.

Chemotherapy

Chemicals or drugs of many kinds are given to patients to interfere with harmful processes or to promote and improve body function. *Antibiotics* are given to control infections and digitalis is given to improve heart function. Special drugs may be given that interfere with the growth of cancer cells and aspirin may be given to reduce pain and lower temperature.

Radiation

Radiation is a technique used for both diagnosis and treatment. X-rays are often taken to examine the patient for possible broken bones. Controlled exposure to active rays brings about disorganization and destruction

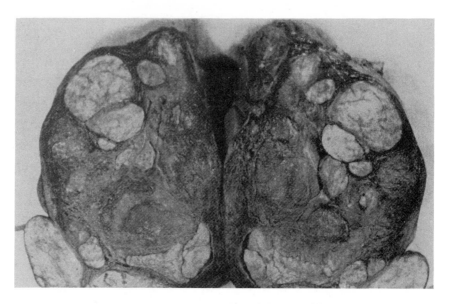

FIGURE 6-6.   A dissected uterus showing pathological changes. *(Photo courtesy of W. B. Saunders Company)*

of abnormal tissues such as tumors that could be life threatening, Figure 6-7.

Supportive Care

Supportive care seeks to aid the body in its attempts to overcome the disease process. It includes therapies to reduce signs and symptoms and the discomforts the patient feels. Rest and proper nutrition, proper positioning to aid circulation and breathing, all contribute to the body's own attempt to control the effects of the disease.

Body Defenses

The body has a natural line of defense against disease. Unbroken skin serves as a mechanical barrier. The acidity of certain body secretions such as perspiration, saliva, and stomach juices slows the growth of microorganisms. White blood cells surround and destroy anything foreign which

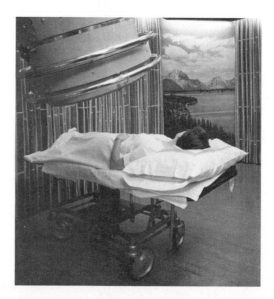

FIGURE 6-7.   Neoplasia are treated by radiation, surgery, and drug therapy.

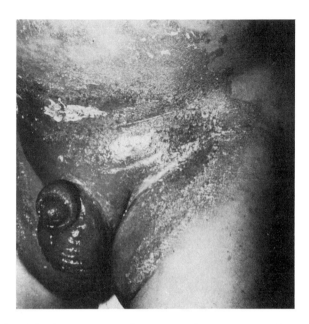

FIGURE 6-8.   This baby has a severe inflammation due to a yeast infection. *(Photo courtesy of the Center for Disease Control, Atlanta, Ga, by L. Matlovski.)*

does gain entrance into the body. Special body cells produce chemicals called *antibodies* which protect the body against specific infections.

INFLAMMATION. The process of inflammation, which we often associate with infections such as boils and abscesses, is really an important part of the body's natural defenses, Figure 6-8. When anything foreign enters the body, small blood vessels (capillaries) in the area get bigger (dilate), bringing more blood to the infected part. In the blood are white blood cells and other protective substances. Fluid (serum) and white blood cells pass through the capillary into the area and a wall is gradually built up around the foreign object. As the white blood cells try to destroy the invader, pressure builds up to force the material to the surface of the body. The inflammatory process takes place to some extent in the body whenever injury occurs. The signs and symptoms of acute infection are:

- Redness
- Swelling
- Heat
- Loss of function

MAJOR DISEASE STATES

There are many diseases that threaten the human body. Examples of some major disease groups are listed below. They include:

- **Congenital Disorders**: Those conditions are present at birth and are due either to genetically-inherited conditions or abnormalities that developed as the baby was formed. For example, *sickle cell anemia* is passed from parents to child through inheritance and results in improperly formed red blood cells. *Clubfeet* are sometimes the result of poor position during the growth of the baby in the mother's uterus.
- **Trauma**: These are injuries to tissues such as those due to exposure to unusual pressure or extremes of temperature. A fractured bone can be due to trauma when someone is thrown from a motorcycle and strikes his leg against a curbstone.

- **Chemical imbalances**: These include abnormal states of either too much or too little fluid in the body. For example, a patient might retain fluid in the body when the heart does not pump strongly enough. Important chemicals and fluids are sometimes lost from the body through perspiration, vomiting, or excess urination. These conditions make the normal functioning of the body difficult. Nutritional imbalances such as overweight or underweight are included in this group of diseases.
- **Infections**: These include the effects of the invasion of microorganisms in the body. The microorganisms which cause disease are called *pathogens* and include bacteria and viruses as well as other forms.
- **Ischemias**: This condition can affect any body part since all tissues need a blood supply to survive. Inadequate blood supply (ischemia) leads to diminished levels of oxygen and if unrelieved leads to a state of no oxygen (anoxia) and death of the tissue. A blood vessel of the heart, blocked by a blood clot would not be able to deliver the normal blood supply resulting in loss of heart function (heart attack).
- **Neoplasia**: The word neoplasm means "new growth;" it is another term for tumor. Neoplasms are becoming an increasingly important kind of disease. There are two types of these new growths. One type of tumor is called *benign* or nonmalignant. The benign tumor usually grows slowly and does not spread. It doesn't usually cause death unless it is located in a vital area such as the brain. The other type of tumor is called a *malignant neoplasm* or cancer. Cancers grow rapidly and spread to other parts of the body *(metastasize)*. They often cause death. You will care for many patients who are suffering from either metastic neoplasms or benign tumors.

Early detection of cancer can often result in total cure. The earlier the cancer is found, the higher the rate of cure. Pain is not usually an early symptom. Early signs and symptoms of malignancies include:

- Change in bowel or bladder habits
- **A** sore that does not heal
- Unusual bleeding or discharge
- Thickening or lump in breast or elsewhere
- Indigestion or difficulty in swallowing
- Obvious change in wart or mole
- Nagging cough or hoarsness

Note that the first letter of these early signs and symptoms spell out **CAUTION.**

Although neoplasms may be treated through surgery, radiation, chemotherapy, or a combination of all three, remember: the best and most successful treatment is early detection.

Summary

Disease has many forms and causes. Signs and symptoms are important indications of the presence of disease and must be carefully observed, reported, and recorded. Major disease states include congenital disorders, traumas, chemical imbalances, infections, isch-emias, and neoplasia. Once the diagnosis has been made, the therapy is prescribed and may include surgery, chemotherapy, radiation, or supportive care.

SUGGESTED ACTIVITIES

1. Discuss the signs and symptoms you have observed of a disease in your own body.

2. Discuss common disease states and describe their treatment.

3. Practice specific information about a patient complaint of pain.

VOCABULARY Learn the meaning and correct spelling of the following words.

benign
capillary
dilate
direct cause (of disease)
etiology
inflammation
malignant
malnutrition
metastasize
neoplasm

objective signs
pathology
predisposing cause (of disease)
prognosis
sign
subjective symptoms
symptom
therapy
trauma

UNIT REVIEW

A. **Brief Answer.** Answer the following questions.
  1. What are the early signs and symptoms of cancer?

  2. Why is early treatment important for patients with cancer?

  3. Name three natural defenses of the body.

  4. What are the signs and symptoms of inflammation?

  5. What is the difference between predisposing and direct cause of disease?

  6. Name four modes of therapy.

  7. Describe four major disease states.

B. **Clinical Situations.** Briefly describe how a health care assistant should react to the following situations.
  1. Your patient says her head aches.

  2. Your patient has a bluish discoloration of his skin.

Section Two
Self-evaluation

A. Define the following words.
1. a cell
2. an organ
3. a system
4. neoplasm
5. etiology

B. Match Column I with Column II on planes and relationships.

Column I	Column II
6. above	a. midline
7. back	b. transverse
8. structure	c. frontal
9. divides the body into right and left sides	d. posterior
10. away from the midline	e. anterior
11. front	f. inferior
12. divides the body into upper and lower parts	g. superior
13. divides the body into back and front	h. anatomy
14. posterior	i. physiology
15. below	j. lateral
	k. medial
	l. dorsal

C. Choose the phrase which best completes each of the following sentences by encircling the proper letter.
16. The tissue specialized to carrry messages is called
    a. epithelial.
    b. connective.
    c. muscular.
    d. nervous.
17. The tissue specialized to protect, secrete, and absorb is
    a. epithelial.
    b. connective.
    c. muscular.
    d. nervous.
18. Included in the gastrointestinal system is/are
    a. stomach.
    b. ovaries.
    c. testes.
    d. adrenals.
19. Included in the respiratory system is/are
    a. lungs.
    b. stomach.
    c. ovaries.
    d. liver.
20. Included in the urinary system is/are
    a. gallbladder.
    b. kidneys.
    c. spinal cord.
    d. uterus.
21. Included in the nervous system is/are
    a. oil glands.
    b. larynx.
    c. joints.
    d. brain.
22. The small intestine is found in the
    a. peritoneal cavity.
    b. pelvic cavity.
    c. spinal cavity.
    d. thoracic cavity.
23. One part of the patient's record that is of concern to the health assistant is the
    a. graphic chart.
    b. progress report.
    c. physical report.
    d. history report.

24. Each entry made on the nurse's note should include
    a. date.
    b. time.
    c. signature.
    d. All of the above.
25. If your hospital uses international time and your watch reads 12:30 PM, you should properly write
    a. 0030.
    b. 1230.
    c. 2430.
    d. No answer is correct.

Unit 7 Meeting Basic Human Needs

OBJECTIVES

As a result of this unit, you will be able to:

- List some emotional and physical needs of patients.
- Define self-esteem.
- List the main reasons patients have difficulty sleeping.
- Describe the stages of human development.

Each of us has things that are necessary for us to live successfully. These are called "needs" simply because we cannot get along without them. When a patient is admitted to the hospital, those needs come too. The difference now is in the way these needs are expressed and fulfilled. Expression and fulfillment have to be different because of the hospital environment and the illness. Remember that the basic needs remain the same, regardless of how they are expressed or how they have to be met because of an individual's level of development or state of health.

HUMAN GROWTH AND DEVELOPMENT

Human beings grow (change physically) and develop (change socially and psychologically) on a *continuum* that begins at birth and ends at death. Not all persons progress at the same rate in both areas but there are several fairly well-defined periods of development, Figure 7-1.

As individuals move through each successive level of development, they change in both their physical appearance and in their developmental skills. Each level presents tasks that must be mastered before moving on to the next level. Sometimes, growth spurts occur and developmental skills must catch up.

Neonatal and Infant Period

This period is characterized by rapid physical growth. A newborn infant with an average length of 20 inches and an average weight of 7 pounds at birth gradually develops into an infant who has learned to crawl, sit, stand, and take first steps. Emotional attachments move from self-awareness and parental attachment to ties with other family members. Systems

```
Neonate  . . . . . . . . . . . . . . . . .  Birth to 1 month
Infancy  . . . . . . . . . . . . . . . . 1 month to 2 years
Toddler  . . . . . . . . . . . . . . . . 2 years to 3 years
Preschool  . . . . . . . . . . . . . . 3 years to 5 years
School Age  . . . . . . . . . . . 5 years to 12 years
Preadolescent  . . . . . . . . . . 12 years to 14 years
Adolescence  . . . . . . . . . . . 14 years to 20 years
Adulthood  . . . . . . . . . . . . . . 20 years to 50 years
Middle Age  . . . . . . . . . . . . 50 years to 65 years
Later Maturity  . . . . . . . . . 65 years to 75 years
Old Age  . . . . . . . . . . . . . . 75 years and beyond
```

FIGURE 7-1. Stages of growth and development

that are relatively immature at birth become more stabilized, and alertness and activity increase. Teeth form, and verbal skills begin to develop. The mother of the infant is the central figure of emotional attachment.

Toddler Period

The toddler period is a busy, active phase. It is a period in which exploration and investigation are paramount. It is also a period in which motor abilities develop and vocabularies and comprehension increase. Control is gained over elimination, and social awareness of rights and wrongs are introduced.

Attempts at socialization and discipline are often fraught with frustration and negative responses on the part of the toddler as awareness of self as a separate person grows.

Brief periods of separation from mother are tolerated, but she still remains the source of security and comfort.

Play may be in the company of other children but with no interaction. This age group is very possessive and "no" and "mine" are a major part of their vocabularies.

Reaching the end of this period, the toddler is able to walk, run and display motor skills that include feeding himself and riding toys. Vocabularies, though still limited, have increased so that words are put together and articulation is clearer.

Preschool Years

The 3- to 5-year-old builds on the motor and verbal skills developed in the toddler. Growing less reliant on mother, this age group begins to recognize their position as a member of the family unit and their uniqueness from other members. Sibling rivalries develop and attachment to the father is now seen.

Cooperative play is gradually increased and, as language skills improve, many questions are asked. Imagination begins to develop, and sexual curiosity is awakened.

By the end of this period socialization has progressed to the point that children not only are more cooperative but almost eager to follow established rules within limits and to interact with family members and peers.

School-age Children

The school-age child is able to communicate, and development of small motor skills enable tasks, such as writing, to be mastered. The child's sense of self increases, and peer relationships develop. The proper social behavior is reinforced through games, simple tasks, and play.

Sex-differentiated friends are chosen, and groups like scouts are joined, serving to further identify the individual as a person of a particular sex.

Preadolescent Period

Preadolescence is a transitional stage and a period of great uncertainty. Hormonal changes stimulate the secondary sex characteristics. Not yet in a period of sexual functioning, the individual feels on the threshold of tremendous change. Mood swings, feelings of insecurity, and a growing awareness of the opposite sex are predominant. Arms and legs seem out of proportion to the rest of the body.

Adolescence

Adolescence is marked by the gradual development of sexual maturity and a greater appreciation of the individual's own identity as a male or a female person. Conflicting desires for the freedom of independence and the security of dependence make this an often-troublesome period.

Gradually, as the developmental tasks are successfully mastered, the adolescent is able to make comparisons between the values he or she has been taught and reality. Adolescents establish their own system of coping and are able to make independent judgments and decisions.

Early Adulthood

Early adulthood is marked by independence and usually the choice of a mate, and the establishment of a career and family life. Health is usually optimal during this period. Friends are chosen to form a support group.

Middle Age

Middle age is frequently associated with final career advancement, terminating in retirement. Children, reared during the period of adulthood, begin to leave home to enter their own adult period. Health is usually still at good levels but some slowing may be seen. Futures are somewhat more in question, but more time can usually be devoted to leisure activities.

Pressures at this period are often financial, as the middle-aged person may still have responsibilities for their own aging parents as well as for their children. The financial needs often complicate the planning of the individual's own retirement.

Later Maturity

Later maturity is marked by a gradual loss of vitality and stamina. Physical changes signal the aging process as sight and hearing diminish and hair often turns grey. Chronic conditions develop and persist. This is a period of gradual losses: loss of mate, loss of friends, loss of self-esteem. Depression and introspection are often experienced. The longer independence can be maintained, the more positive the changes during this period.

Support groups, established in the adult and middle years, can provide valuable assistance and social contacts. Persons in later maturity can function as important role models for younger age groups.

Old Age

Old age is frequently characterized by failing physical status and growing dependency. The person in old age must deal with illness, loneliness, loss of friends and loved ones and the realization of their own mortality. Success in this final period depends upon the mechanisms of coping which the elderly have developed over the years and the degree to which an emotional and physical support system is available.

BASIC HUMAN NEEDS

Developmental skills and physical growth may vary during the life span, but the basic human needs experienced by every individual remain

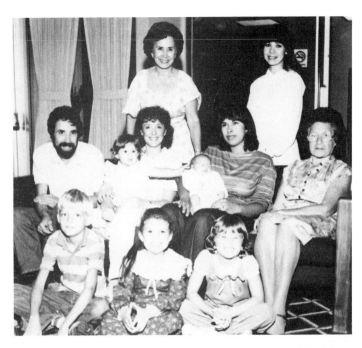

FIGURE 7-2. The characteristics of different age groups are reflected in this group picture.

remarkably constant, Figure 7-2. These needs include the need to communicate, to have one's emotional and spiritual well-being assured, and to have certain fundamental physical needs fulfilled. At times, one need may become more pressing than others, but as human beings, *all* of the basic needs must be met for successful survival. It is imperative, therefore, for health care assistants to keep their patients' basic needs in mind at all times.

Communication

One of the most basic needs of all people is the need to understand others and to be understood themselves. This is called communication when it is successful. We usually try to communicate verbally. Sometimes we do this also by the *way* we say the words, by the *tone* of our voice, by the *expression* on our face, and sometimes by *touch*, Figure 7-3. Even the way we stand or reach out says a lot. We know it is not always easy to find the right words to express our thoughts and feelings. Consequently we, the nursing staff, must be constantly aware of the patient's need to communicate effectively too.

If all members of the nursing staff are interested and unhurried in talking with their patients, they make it easier for patients to express their needs. This approach also makes it easier for the staff to find proper ways to fulfill those needs.

Emotional Needs

Even more basic than the need to communicate is the need to protect our self-esteem. All individuals—you, your co-workers, and your patients—have in their own minds an idea of how they appear and wish to appear to others. This idea is referred to as *self-esteem*. A person's self-esteem must be protected at all costs.

For instance, a person might visualize and project to others the image of a very self-reliant person, capable of making important decisions, and able to care for self and family. Suddenly that same person is scantily dressed in a hospital bed, having a stranger taking care of the most intimate physical functions, and even deciding the time to eat and bathe. This set of

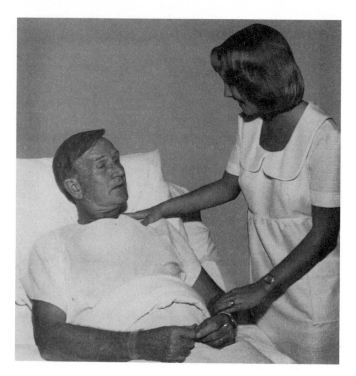

FIGURE 7-3.   Successful communication is a two-way exchange.

circumstances threatens even the most secure person's self-esteem, Figure 7-4.

How the patients respond to this threat to their self-esteem depends on two things. First, it depends on how often each patient has had these feelings of helplessness before, and how well they have dealt with them. Second, it depends on you and your ability to appreciate those feelings.

One patient may feel frustrated and angry and may not even know that it's fear. The patient may act out these feelings by complaining about the hospital, the staff, roommates, you or the food. In fact, every aspect of the care may be cause for complaint. Be open and receptive to these actions, recognizing the underlying feelings.

Still another patient may react quite differently to the same emotional stress. That difference produces a person who may be quiet and withdrawn, completely cooperative and non-complaining, Figure 7-5. The whole

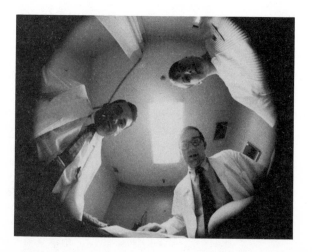

FIGURE 7-4.   Have you ever wondered how we look from the patient's point of view?

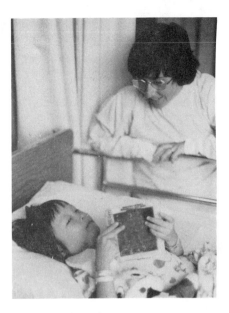

FIGURE 7-5.   It sometimes takes a great deal of patience to break through a wall of fear and frustrations.

behavior displayed presents a false front to hide the feelings of inadequacy to the situation. Be just as aware of these patients' needs for caring support.

DEALING WITH THE FEARFUL PATIENT. The experienced assistant does not take remarks personally. The assistant realizes that the patient's complaints and refusal to cooperate may be a way of saying, "I need to be reassured and protected." By giving the patient an opportunity to talk, and by listening carefully to everything that is said, it is possible to convince the fearful patient to *decide* to assume some personal care whenever possible. If help in feeding, shaving, or other such personal matters is needed, the assistant acts in a very gentle, efficient manner and assures the patient's privacy at all times.

To handle these situations successfully, it is necessary to recognize that this patient is a person with individual likes and dislikes. Give the quality of care that takes these likes and dislikes into consideration. Whenever possible, an attempt should be made to help the patient find ways to occupy all the empty time while in the hospital, Figure 7-6. Boredom alone

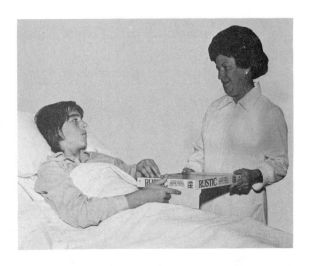

FIGURE 7-6.   Activities help to pass the time during convalescence.

can lead to irritability. Some hospitals have volunteers who bring books and other activities directly to the bedside.

Patients in the hospital relinquish a good bit of control over their lives. They literally put their lives and well-being into the hands of care givers. In exchange, the patient assumes that certain of their rights will be assured. These rights include the right of privacy.

Privacy may be provided by means of curtains or screens which are placed around the bed. Remember to knock and say the patient's name before entering a room. Speak, also, to the patient before entering a screened area. Privacy must be provided for the patient who is bathing, uses the bedpan, has treatments, or is visited by clergy. Be prompt at other times to recognize a patient's need for privacy and to provide it.

Patients must feel assured that their privacy will be protected to the extent that even though you perform the most intimate procedures for them, you will do so in a way that neither exposes them unnecessarily nor embarrasses them. They must also be secure in knowing that personal information coming to your knowledge will not be revealed to others, and that you will always treat them with the courtesy you would extend to a guest in your home.

Understanding what patients are really trying to tell us is one of the most difficult parts of giving nursing care. When we are successful, it is probabbly the most rewarding. With this in mind, always remember to treat the patient as a unique individual.

Spiritual Needs

The spiritual needs of the patient are often greater when he is fearful and ill, Figure 7-7. The assistant should be prepared to act on requests for clergy visits and spiritual support without imposing personal beliefs on the patient. The patient may want to visit with a familiar clergy member, or may ask about the chaplain or clergy service available at the health care facility. During these visits, the health care assistant should provide privacy by drawing the curtains or closing the door if this is possible and desirable.

Some hospitals ask clergy from the community to make visits to patients who desire a visit, but who do not know a particular minister, priest or rabbi. Larger hospitals have chaplain residencies for people preparing for a clergical career. The residencies provide an opportunity to serve pa-

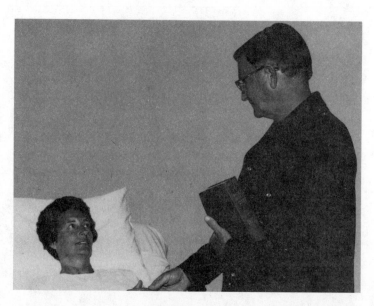

FIGURE 7-7. A minister's visit is very comforting to the patient.

tients' spiritual needs while offering training for the chaplains.

Chapels are open in some hospitals and both visitors and ambulatory patients often find comfort in visiting them. Religious services are sometimes broadcast to patients' rooms from these chapels.

Familiarize yourself with the services available to your patients. When asked, share this information but do not urge any particular service. Patients should feel free to make their own choices.

Physical Needs

You will also be concerned with the physical needs of your patients. They are the need to to be sheltered, to breathe, to eat, to sleep, and to eliminate waste products.

SHELTER. In the health care facility, the need to be sheltered is considered when the proper environment is maintained. Some examples include making sure the bed is secure and the siderails are up, that beds are left in the lowest, horizontal position, and that provisions are made to keep the patient safe and warm. These seem like simple requirements, but it is often the extra bit of attention to safety details that provides the patient with a real sense of security. Protection is the basis of this first physical need. Every patient has the right to feel cared for and safe.

OXYGEN. Most of us take breathing for granted. We hardly give it more that a passing thought until it becomes difficult. While there are many reasons which cause people to have difficulty in breathing, when they do have difficulty, the need is always the same. The body cannot live without *oxygen* found in the air. It may be necessary, therefore, to supply the patient with an increased amount of oxygen and moisture. Oxygen by cannula or mask may be used for this purpose, Figure 7-8. Sometimes this need can be met by adjusting the overbed table in such a way that the patient, supported by pillows, is able to lean on it. This position is called the *orthopneic* position.

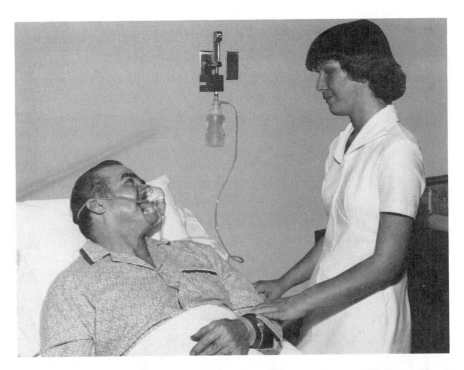

FIGURE 7-8. Oxygen may be delivered by a mask that is specially designed

FOOD. Appetites are known to lag in the hospital. Inactivity, hospital odors, pain and the illness itself all contribute to a decreased appetite and intake of fluids.

Some patients have to be fed because of their condition. Some may be given only special foods. Some are unable to take food in the usual way. Some patients are given liquid nourishment through a tube which has been passed through the nose and into the stomach. Feeding through a tube is called *gavage*. Nourishment may also be given through a sterile tube into the veins, a process known as *intravenous infusion* (IV).

Since patients receive nourishment in such a variety of ways, you need to see to the special needs of each individual person. There are, however, some general points to keep in mind.

Appetites are improved when food is served at the proper temperature in pleasant surroundings. Close bathroom doors and use room deodorants. Make sure that unneeded equipment is removed from sight. Prepare patients by allowing them to wash hands and face and assisting them to sit up in bed or get out of bed if permitted. Offer the tray in a calm, pleasant manner, even if the nourishment is not what *you* prefer. Even a bland diet offered in this way is more acceptable. Be available to assist if needed but allow the patient to do just as much as he/she is able for themselves.

SLEEP. Noise and pain are the chief reasons patients have difficulty sleeping. Control noise whenever possible. Handle equipment carefully, reduce volume on televisions, limit conversation with co-workers, and use a lowered voice.

A few extra moments of your time to give a soothing back rub, a change of position, and a neat bed are often good ways to induce sleep. Sometimes medication is needed to help the patient sleep. The assistant should have the patient completely prepared for sleep before the professional nurse administers medication so the patient will not have to be disturbed after being medicated.

Worry also plays a role in a patient's sleeplessness. Patients worry about many things: what the future will bring, how much the hospitalization will cost, who is taking care of their home and work responsibilities. You will not have the answers to all these pressing concerns. You can listen, however. Share these concerns with the nurse. This is not gossiping and the nurse may be able to enlist the aid of other members of the staff in solving the problems. With worries reduced, patients will rest easier.

ELIMINATION. To remain healthy, the body must be able to eliminate perspiration, *urine*, and *feces* properly. Baths help get rid of perspiration and keep the skin healthy. The release of urine from the bladder is known as *voiding*. Expelling the feces (stool) from the bowel is called *defecating*.

Encourage the patient to drink fluids and, if possible, eat foods high in bulk. When additional help is needed, the insertion of a sterile tube (known as a catheter) into the urinary bladder, helps to promote urine elimination. The sterile catheter may be left in the bladder to provide constant drainage. The tube is then attached to a bag which collects the urine. *Enemas*, laxatives, and *suppositories* help the bowels get rid of solid wastes in the form of feces.

Patients who are unable to use the usual toilet facilities need help in using bedpans, *urinals*, and bedside *commodes*. Always remember that the patient's right to privacy should be respected. Keep exposure to a minimum, screen the unit and leave until the patient is finished. Leave a signal bell close at hand.

A male attendant usually cares for the personal needs of the male patient. If a male attendant is not available for this procedure, however, the female assistant should perform this service for the patient with efficiency and tact. A bedpan or urinal should always be given to the patient as soon as it is requested. Because bedpans are uncomfortable, be sure to check and remove it promptly when the patient is finished.

PHYSICAL ACTIVITY. People, by nature, are active beings. When illness occurs it frequently limits activity and the health facility must devise ways to promote activity for these individuals. The capability of the patient and the goals of treatment must be kept in mind when the activity level of any patient is established.

Activity promotes generally-improved functioning of all systems. Circulation and respiration are increased, muscles, bones, and joints function more adequately, and the body as a whole responds in a positive way.

When patients are unable to carry out activity independently, such as ambulating, getting in and out of bed and using the bedpan or commode, the health care assistant may have to assist them. Be sure you are aware of the patient's limitations, as well as the degree and type of activity allowed. Do not allow patients to become either overstressed or fatigued.

Summary

Individuals develop at varying rates, yet there are some well-defined developmental stages through which each person passes. Certain developmental skills are characteristically acquired at certain stages of life—from birth to death—and a person's success in mastering these skills affects the progress of their development. Regardless of their developmental level, people have common basic emotional and physical needs. The way these needs are expressed vary, especially when a person is ill. The nursing staff must be sensitive to these individual needs and devise ways of successfully providing for them.

SUGGESTED ACTIVITIES

1. Discuss the possible reactions of individuals at varying developmental levels to hospitalization.

2. Role play situations in which patients show fear, anger, and frustration. Show how the assistant should respond to these situations.

3. Discuss ways the assistant can help patients protect their self-esteem.

4. Discuss ways of meeting basic needs in the hospital.

VOCABULARY

Learn the meaning and the correct spelling of the following words and phrases.

commodes	intravenous infusion	self-esteem
continuum	orthopneic	suppositories
enemas	parallel play	urinals
feces	preadolescence	urine
gavage		

UNIT REVIEW

A. Brief Answer.

1. List five developmental stages and the characteristics of each.

2. List and describe five basic emotional or physical needs.

B. Clinical Situations. Briefly describe how a health care assistant should react to the following situations.

1. Your patient indicates a need for spiritual support.

2. Your patient is complaining of an inability to sleep at bedtime.

3. Your patient complained loudly about his care, the food, and the other patients in the room.

C. Completion. Complete the following sentences.

1. Self-esteem means _____.
2. The chief reasons patients have difficulty sleeping are _____, _____ and _____.
3. Waste products that need to be eliminated from the body are _____, _____, and _____.
4. Gavage is a technique used to _____.
5. An experienced health care assistant never takes a patient's remarks _____.

D. Matching. Match the person with the appropriate chronologic age by matching Columns I and Column II

Column I	Column II
1. Old age	a. 70 years old
2. Adolescence	b. 16 years old
3. Later maturity	c. 7 years old
4. Schoolage	d. 35 years old
5. Adulthood	e. 80 years old

Unit 8 Interpersonal Relationships

OBJECTIVES

As a result of this unit, you will be able to:
- Adjust and react appropriately to various situations.
- Demonstrate dependability.
- Discuss understanding of human relationships.

Interpersonal relationships simply mean any and all interactions between people. You develop interpersonal relationships with everyone you know. Some are deep and lasting, and some are only casual. But to some degree, you react to others and they react to you. Friendship is a good example of an interpersonal relationship that is satisfactory to two people.

Much of the satisfaction that an assistant derives from work is due to the quality of relationship that is developed with other staff members and patients. Some people call this the ability to "get along" with others.

Similarly, good relationships with others begin with your *own* personality and attitudes. If you are a warm and accepting person with positive attitudes, others will respond in the same way. If you walk down the street and someone smiles at you, without thinking, your reaction is to smile back. Most human relationships are like this.

PERSONAL AND VOCATIONAL ADJUSTMENTS

There is a certain amount of personal adjustment that you will have to make to your new work situation. Hospital rules and orders from supervisors must be obeyed promptly *even if you do not agree with them*, simply because they are written for the protection and welfare of the patient. For the same reason, the ability to accept *constructive* criticism and profit by it is equally important. It means you are willing to learn and grow.

How well you are personally adjusted shows in many other ways. You demonstrate *dependability* and *accuracy* by reporting to duty on time and completing your assignment carefully. Your *readiness* to help your co-workers shows your respect for them and the place you share together on the nursing team. You demonstrate your understanding of human relationships when you are *empathetic*, *patient*, and *tactful* with others.

PATIENT RELATIONSHIPS

A good health assistant shows empathy for the patient by being eager to serve and by using a gentle touch.

Patients come in all sizes and shapes, young, Figure 8-1A, old, and in between. Some have major, complicated illnesses, Figure 8-1B, while others have physical problems that may be helped with rest and medication, Figure 8-1C. Some patients are in the health facility to begin their lives; others will end their lives there.

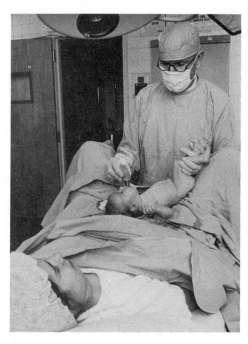

A. Some patients are just beginning their lives.

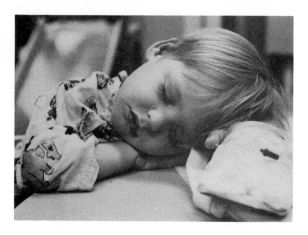

B. Some patients, like this leukemic child, have devastating illnesses.

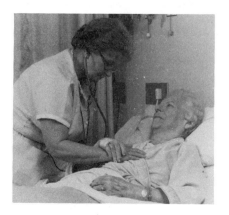

C. Some patients are older, needing rest and medication.

FIGURE 8-1.   Patients are people of all ages.

Every patient entering a health care facility presents a unique set of problems and concerns to the staff. These problems and concerns are perceived by the patient as being of the utmost importance. As you compare the conditions of many patients in your own mind, however, it might seem that one has more serious problems than another. Since no patient shares your knowledge he will not know this, so never forget that, to the patient, his or her problems *are* the most important.

Meeting the Patient's Needs

Patients are composites of their life experiences which are now complicated with illness. Their social, spiritual, and physical needs must continue to be met even though they are in a different, more confined setting. The restriction imposed by illness limits, to a great degree, their ability to satisfy these needs through the normal channels. This is naturally frustrating and puts great strain on the patient's ability to establish and maintain good, interpersonal relationships.

Fear, pain, and unrealistic perceptions of activities around them, unknown future potentials, worries about family, and the unavailability of social support systems may even cause some patients to become irritable, complaining, and uncooperative.

Meeting the Family's Needs

Families and friends are very concerned when one of their loved ones is no longer readily available to them and, indeed, may have a life-threat-

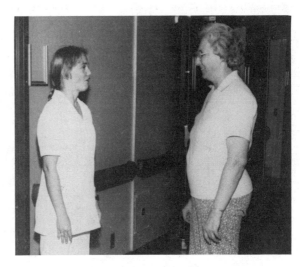

FIGURE 8-2. A helpful, cheerful attitude can be very reassuring to concerned visitors.

ening illness. This puts stress in their lives too; they need to be reassured, Figure 8-2. Their anxiety sometimes makes them demanding and, at times, uncooperative.

Some of these same factors, as well as those of insecurity, fatigue, and personal conflict, might spill over to influence relationships between co-workers as well.

The nursing assistant who understands human behavior makes allowances for these stresses and realizes that ill people, co-workers, and families under stress are sensitive and not always on their best behavior. This is why sensitivity and awareness of the needs of others is most important at this time. It is in these situations that patience and tact are most essential. Sometimes just quietly listening to another or rephrasing the way you are communicating can change an entire interaction. Try to be aware not only of the words used but of the body language exhibited, Figure 8-3. Look for clues such as the tone of a voice or the movement of hands that reveals, as with words, much about the inner feelings of another. Keep

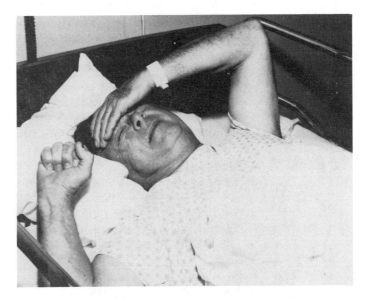

FIGURE 8-3. Be alert to body language as you observe your patient. *(Photo reproduced courtesy of Eli Lilly and Co.)*

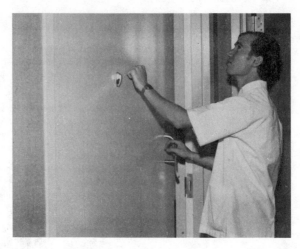

FIGURE 8-4.   The call light should be answered promptly.

always in mind that people are three-dimensional. They are spiritual, physical, and social human beings.

PATIENT RIGHTS

Even though they are hospitalized, patients continue to have certain basic rights.

Patients have the right to know that orders will be followed accurately and procedures will be carried out efficiently. If you are ever in doubt about how to proceed, don't hesitate to ask. If an error does occur, report it immediately.

Patients need to know that they will be properly identified so that treatments not intended for them will not be mistakenly carried out or given.

They need to feel secure that their needs will be recognized and given prompt attention; that you will recognize them as persons—not by condition—but by name. Mrs. Robinson is not "the gallbladder in Room 228," she is Mrs. Robinson!

You add to this sense of security every time you call them by name, check their nameband before carrying out a procedure, or when you promptly answer their call bell, Figure 8-4.

The American Hospital Association has developed a "Patient Bill of Rights," Figure 8-5. In some facilities, this document is presented to the patient on admission. In others, it is clearly posted in every unit.

STAFF RELATIONSHIPS

You are part of a staff of people, all of whom share a single goal: to help the patient. This single purpose welds you together into a unit which

The American Hospital Association presents a Patient's Bill of Rights with the expectation that observance of these rights will contribute to more effective patient care and greater satisfaction for the patient, his physician, and the hospital organization. Further, the Association presents these rights in the expectation that they will be supported by the hospital on behalf of its patients, as an integral part of the healing process. It is recognized that a personal relationship between the physician and the patient is essential for the provision of proper medical care. The traditional physician-patient relationship takes on a new dimension when care is rendered within an organizational structure. Legal precedent has established that the institution itself also has a responsibility to the patient. It is in recognition of these factors that these rights are affirmed.

FIGURE 8-5.   A patient's bill of rights

1. The patient has the right to considerate and respectful care.

2. The patient has the right to obtain from his physician complete current information concerning his diagnosis, treatment, and prognosis in terms the patient can be reasonably expected to understand. When it is not medically advisable to give such information to the patient, the information should be made available to an appropriate person in his behalf. He has the right to know by name, the physician responsible for coordinating his care.

3. The patient has the right to receive from his physician information necessary to give informed consent prior to the start of any procedure and/or treatment. Except in emergencies, such information for informed consent should include but not necessarily be limited to the specific procedure and/or treatment, the medically significant risks involved, and the probable duration of incapacitation. Where medically significant alternatives for care or treatment exist, or when the patient requests information concerning medical alternatives, the patient has the right to such information. The patient also has the right to know the name of the person responsible for the procedures and/or treatment.

4. The patient has the right to refuse treatment to the extent permitted by law, and to be informed of the medical consequences of his action.

5. The patient has the right to every consideration of his privacy concerning his own medical care program. Case discussion, consultation, examination, and treatment are confidential and should be conducted discreetly. Those not directly involved in his care must have the permission of the patient to be present.

6. The patient has the right to expect that all communications and records pertaining to his care should be treated as confidential.

7. The patient has the right to expect that within its capacity a hospital must make reasonable response to the request of a patient for services. The hospital must provide evaluation, service, and/or referral as indicated by the urgency of the case. When medically permissible a patient may be transferred to another facility only after he has received complete information and explanation concerning the needs for and alternatives to such a transfer. The institution to which the patient is to be transferred must first have accepted the patient for transfer.

8. The patient has the right to obtain information as to any relationship of his hospital to other health care and educational institutions insofar as his care is concerned. The patient has the right to obtain information as to the existence of any professional relationships among individuals, by name, who are treating him.

9. The patient has the right to be advised if the hospital proposes to engage in or perform human experimentation affecting his care or treatment. The patient has the right to refuse to participate in such research projects.

10. The patient has the right to expect reasonable continuity of care. He has the right to know in advance what appointment times and physicians are available and where. The patient has the right to expect that the hospital will provide a mechanism whereby he is informed by his physician or a delegate of the physician of the patient's continuing health care requirements following discharge.

11. The patient has the right to examine and receive an explanation of his bill regardless of source of payment.

12. The patient has the right to know what hospital rules and regulations apply to his conduct as a patient.

No catalogue of rights can guarantee for the patient the kind of treatment he has a right to expect. A hospital has many functions to perform, including the prevention and treatment of disease, the education of both health professionals and patients, and the conduct of clinical research. All these activities must be conducted with an overriding concern for the patient, and, above all, the recognition of his dignity as a human being. Success in achieving this recognition assures success in the defense of the rights of the patient.

Approved by the
House of Delegates
of the
American Hospital Association
February 6, 1973

FIGURE 8-5. (Continued)

must work smoothly if your goal is to be accomplished. Good interpersonal relationships will make your working times both harmonious and fruitful.

Each of you has a specific role to fulfill and jobs to carry out. Do not overstep your authority or attempt to criticize others. Listen to instructions from your supervisor carefully and phrase questions about your assignment in such a way that your supervisor knows you are looking for clarification—not challenging authority. Remember that your tone of voice can often change the message that you are trying to convey.

Be prompt in carrying out orders and report any work you are unable to finish.

Co-workers can often help one another when a task is particularly difficult or physically taxing, such as lifting a heavy patient, moving equipment, or simply when another member of the team gets behind in their work. Be ready to offer help to others and accept help when you need it.

A cheerful, positive attitude is as important for staff members' relationships as it is in establishing rapport with patients. The same dignity and courtesy that you extend to patients should be extended to every staff member.

Always keep your common goal in mind. Recognize co-workers as important members of the total team and staff interpersonal relationships will flourish.

Summary

Good interpersonal relationships with patients, visitors, and co-workers help the health care assistant to be effective. Tactful approaches help to establish good relationships. Personal adjustment is made easier if the assistant understands and obeys hospital policies and procedures. Patients, co-workers, and visitors must be treated with dignity.

SUGGESTED ACTIVITIES

1. Role play the following situations:
   a. An assistant enters the room of a patient.
   b. Another assistant asks you to assist her in lifting a heavy patient.
   c. A patient requests that you mail a letter for him, and you are very busy.
   d. A patient asks you to arrange her flowers when she is able to do so.

2. Discuss tactful ways an assistant might handle the following situations:
   a. A visitor asks why the patient isn't allowed out of bed.
   b. The patient wishes to know how high her temperature is this morning.
   c. The patient complains because she was awakened early and is very tired.
   d. The patient complains of the lack of care given by another assistant.

VOCABULARY

Learn the meaning and the correct spelling of the following words.

accuracy	interpersonal relationships	readiness
dependability	patience	sympathy
empathy	rapport	tact

UNIT REVIEW

A. Brief Answer.

1. Are people always on their best behavior when they are in the hospital? Explain your answer in one or two sentences.

B. Clinical Situations. Briefly describe how a health care assistant should react to the following situations.
1. A visitor demands extra chairs around a patient's bed.

2. A patient expresses fear of falling from the hospital bed.

3. A co-worker unjustly accuses you of not carrying your share of the responsibility.

C. Completion.
1. Interpersonal relationships means _____.
2. A good example of a satisfactory relationship between two people is _____
_____.
3. Hospital rules and policies are written for the protection of _____.

Unit 9 Death and Dying

OBJECTIVES

As a result of this unit, you will be able to:

- Describe the signs of approaching death.
- Describe the spiritual preparations for death practiced in the various religious denominations.
- Demonstrate the procedure for postmortem care.

Death is the final stage of life. It may come suddenly, without warning, or it may follow a protracted period. It sometimes strikes the young but it always awaits the old. As a nursing care assistant, you will be providing continuing care throughout the dying period and into the after-death period *(postmortem)*. Accepting the idea that death is the natural result of the life process may help you respond to your patient's needs more generously.

In the period before death, the patient with a *terminal* diagnosis needs and receives the same care as the patient who is expected to recover. Attention is paid to physical as well as emotional needs.

The whole concept of death and dying is handled differently by different people, Figure 9-1. Some patients may have had time to psychologically prepare for their death; some may actually look forward to relief from the pain and the emotional burden of a long illness. Other patients may be fearful or angry and demonstrate moods which swing from outright denial to depression. If there is adequate time and support, patients can be helped to reach a more accepting frame of mind.

THE ROLE OF THE HEALTH CARE ASSISTANT

You, the nursing care assistant, spend much time with the patient and have a unique opportunity to be a source of strength and comfort. You should be quietly sympathetic without showing emotion, and carry out your duties in a quiet, efficient way. This type of behavior instills confidence in both patient and family, Figure 9-2. Developing the proper attitude and approach for this type of situation is not easy. It will come with experience.

The response of the assistant is consistent and guided by the attitude of the patient. Because this attitude may change from day to day, you must be open and receptive. Make sure you inform the nurse of incidents related to the patient which reflect his moods and needs.

Each person's idea of death and the hereafter differs. Your own feelings about death and dying influence your ability to care for the dying patient. Honestly explore your feelings by talking about them with others until you can resolve any conflicts you may have, Figure 9-3. Your acceptance of death as a natural occurrence will enable you to meet patient needs in a realistic manner.

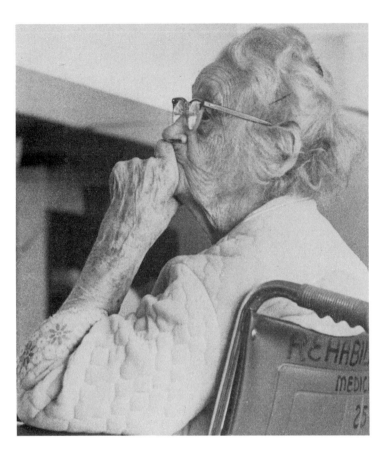

FIGURE 9-1. Patients with a terminal diagnosis handle the information in different ways.

PHYSICAL CHANGES

As death approaches, body functions slow down. The patient loses general voluntary and involuntary muscle control. The jaw tends to drop, and breathing becomes irregular and shallow. Special mouth care is essential. (See the Procedure in Unit 18.) Involuntary voiding and defecation may also occur. As circulation slows, the extremities become cold, the pulse becomes rapid and progressively weaker, and the skin pales. The eyes stare and do not respond to light.

The patient may not be responsive, but this does not mean that he can no longer hear. You must be careful in what you say, because hearing

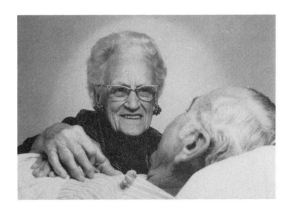

FIGURE 9-2. The support of family and friends is vital during the dying period. Liberal visiting hours are encouraged.

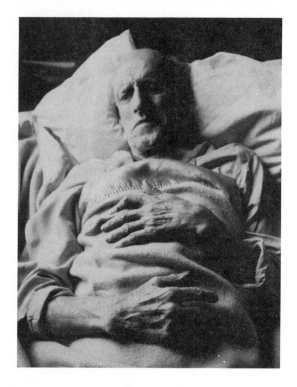

FIGURE 9-3. Until you resolve your conflicting feelings about dying, you cannot successfully help your patient through his difficult period of adjustment.

is one of the last senses to be lost. When breathing stops and the pulse is no longer felt, you should call the nurse who will summon the physician. The physician then examines the patient and fixes the time of death. Under no circumstance should the nursing assistant inform the family. This is the responsibility of the doctor or head nurse, Figure 9-4.

EMOTIONAL PREPARATION FOR DEATH

Health workers have the unique privilege of helping patients prepare for death, of providing support during the final hours, and of helping the family face the crisis. The knowledge of impending death comes to the patient directly from the doctor or indirectly from the staff. A diagnosis of terminal illness is very difficult to conceal from the patient. Forced cheerfulness and evasiveness are just as revealing as other changes in staff be-

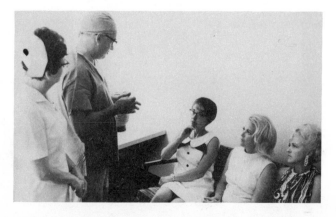

FIGURE 9-4. Information about the patient's condition is given to the family by the doctor or nurse.

havior. Fewer visits to the patient's room and shorter periods of patient contact are apt to occur when the staff has knowledge that is not shared by the patient.

You must recognize that most terminally ill patients do eventually come to realize and accept that death is part of their near future. Each patient reacts to this realization in a unique way. How many feelings the patient wishes to share and with whom are very personal decisions. Be available to listen but do not force the issue.

Upon being told of the terminal diagnosis, the patient will proceed through several stages of emotional adjustment. Dr. Elizabeth Kübler Ross has identified five stages of grief. They are denial, anger, bargaining, depression, and acceptance.

Denial begins when the person is made aware that he or she is going to die. He may not accept this information as truth, but may instead deny it. Statements such as, "This isn't happening to me," or "I'm too young to die" may indicate that the patient is in the denial stage.

The stage of *anger* comes when the patient is no longer able to deny the fact that he is going to die. The patient may blame those around him, including those who are giving him care, for his illness. Added stresses, however small, are likely to upset the patient who is in the anger stage. Statements such as, "It's all your fault. I should never have come to this hospital," are typical of a patient in the anger stage.

During the *bargaining* stage of the grief process, the patient attempts to bargain for more time to live. He may ask to be allowed to go home to finish a task before he dies, or he may make private "deals" with God: "If you will let me live another two months, I promise I will try to be a better person." Basically, the patient in this stage is saying, "I know I'm going to die, and I'm ready to die, but not just yet."

Depression is the fourth stage identified in the grief process. During this stage, the patient comes to a full realization that he will die soon. He is saddened by the thought that he will no longer be with family and friends, and by the fact that he may not have accomplished some goals that he had set for himself. He may also express regrets about not having gone somewhere or done something—"I always promised my wife that we would go to Europe, and now we'll never go."

STAGES OF GRIEF	RESPONSE OF THE HEALTH CARE ASSISTANT
Denial	Reflect patient's statements, but try not to confirm or deny the fact that he is dying.
	EX: "The lab tests can't be right . . . I don't have cancer."
	"It must have been difficult for you to learn the results of your tests."
Anger	Understand the source of the patient's anger; provide understanding and support; listen; try to meet reasonable needs and demands quickly.
Bargaining	If it is possible to meet the patient's requests, do so; listen attentively.
Depression	Avoid cliches that dismiss the patient's depression ("It could be worse—you could be in more pain."); be caring and supportive; let the patient know that it is ok for him to be depressed.
Acceptance	Do not assume that, because the patient has accepted his death, he is unafraid, or that he doesn't need emotional support; listen attentively and be supportive and caring.

FIGURE 9-5. The patient may exhibit various emotional responses to dying. The health care assistant should be caring and supportive of the patient as he sorts out his feelings.

Acceptance is the stage during which a patient understands and accepts the fact that he is going to die. During this stage, he may strive to complete unfinished business. Having accepted his eventual death, he may also try to help those around him to deal with it.

Initially, the patient may react to the situation by denying the truth. The patient may refuse all opportunities to discuss his or her illness with the staff or with the family. Interpersonal relationships with family and staff may be greatly strained. You must accept the patient's behavior with understanding, interpret the patient's very real needs for the family, and support the family in meeting their own needs. One patient may become defeated, full of despair, actively expressing a loss of hope. Another may reach out, trying to verbalize feelings and thoughts of an uncertain future. None of the reaction states are predictable, falling into one rigid pattern or another. Despair and anxiety may give way to moments of active hostility or periods of searching, groping questions. If there is adequate time and support, some patients may be able to move psychologically through each stage to a point of acceptance of their illness and death.

Not all patients progress through these stages in sequential order nor does movement from one level to the next mean that the previous level will no longer be experienced. For example, a patient who displays anger one day may be full of optimism and denial the next. The staff must be aware of the possible psychological positions and be able to identify the patient's current reactions. Frequently, denial comes first, followed by anger and despair. Frustrated by feelings of helplessness, the person lashes out at those who are nearby. If each of these stages is expressed with some degree of success, the person is then able to move on to a level of grieving, for one's self and for loved ones. When all five stages have been passed, it is believed that the patient is better able to accept the termination of life.

Sacrament of the Sick

When a patient's condition is critical, the doctor will place his name officially on the *critical list*. Then the family and the chaplain will be notified.

If a Catholic patient appears to be in danger of dying, the priest must be called for the *Anointing of the Sick*. It is preferable that the family be present and leave the room only while the confession is heard. The practicing Catholic and his family consider it a privilege to have the opportunity for confession while the patient is still in possession of his faculties. Many patients recover completely, but this hope should not prevent the reception of this sacrament. The priest will decide after discussing it with the family.

While most of the other religions do not have specific rituals such as the last rites, providing privacy for the patient and family is very important. Privacy does not mean leaving the patient and family entirely alone. Continue to provide your assigned care of the patient in a quiet, dignified manner.

A bible or spiritual reading of the patient's faith, if requested, may be of some spiritual help through this crisis. Dying is a lonely business. Privacy, but not total solitude, should be the guiding rule.

POSTMORTEM CARE

The patient's body should be treated with respect at all times. Before death occurs, the limbs should be straightened and the head elevated on a pillow. The body should be cleaned by gently washing it with warm water; discharges must be washed off and wiped away.

Care of the body after death is called postmortem care. This may be your responsibility. Treat the body with the same dignity you would a living person. *Check the hospital procedure manual before proceeding with postmortem care.* One procedure for postmortem care is described next.

Procedure
GIVING POSTMORTEM CARE

1. Wash hands and assemble the following equipment:
   - Shroud or clean sheet
   - Basin with warm water
   - Washcloth
   - Towels
   - Identification cards (3)
   - Cotton
   - Bandages
   - Pads as needed
2. Remove all appliances, tubing, and used articles.
3. Work quickly and quietly; maintain an attitude of respect. If it is necessary to speak, do so only in relation to the procedure.
4. Place the body on the back, head and shoulders elevated. Close the eyes by grasping eyelashes. Replace dentures in patient's mouth. The jaw may need to be secured with light bandaging. Pad beneath the bandage. Tight bandaging or undue pressure from the hands may leave marks, so handle the body gently.
5. Bathe as necessary. Remove any soiled dressings and replace with clean ones.
6. Pad between the ankles and knees with cotton. Tie lightly.
7. Pad the anal area in case of drainage.
8. Put the shroud on the patient.
9. Collect all belongings. Wrap and label. Valuables remain in hospital safe until signed for by a relative.
10. Fill out the identification cards and fasten
    a. One on the body
    b. One on the patient's clothing and valuables (securely wrapped)
    c. One on the compartment in the morgue
11. Close doors and empty corridor of patients and visitors. With assistance, place body on gurney. Cover with sheet and take to the morgue.

Summary

Assisting with terminal and postmortem care is a difficult but essential part of nursing duties. It requires a high degree of sensitivity, understanding, and tact. Both the patient and his family require support during this trying period. Care must be taken to provide for the individual religious preferences and practices of the patient and his family. The procedure for postmortem care must be carried out with efficiency and dignity.

SUGGESTED ACTIVITIES

1. Investigate and discuss the special considerations given to the dying patient and his family.
2. Invite various religious leaders to discuss spiritual needs of the terminal patient.
3. In small groups, explore your feelings about dying and death.
4. Using a mannequin, practice giving postmortem care to the patient who has just died.
5. Role play with other members of the class the part of an assistant aide and three family members who have just lost a loved one.
6. Read *On Death and Dying* or *Live Until You Die*, by Elizabeth Kübler-Ross.

VOCABULARY Learn the meaning and correct spelling of the following words.

Anointing of the Sick denial terminal
critical list postmortem

UNIT REVIEW

A. Brief Answer.

1. What should you do before moving the body to the morgue to prevent upsetting other patients?

B. Clinical Situations. Briefly describe how a health care assistant should react to the following situations.

1. Your terminal patient who had been crying earlier, suddenly appeared cheerful and talked about a trip he was planning next year.

2. The patient expresses a desire to see his clergy.

C. Completion.

1. When the patient's condition is critical, the _____ places the patient's name on the critical list.
2. Anointing of the Sick is requested for the patient of _____ belief.
3. As death approaches, body functions _____.
4. Time of death is determined by the _____.
5. Care must be taken when talking in the room of a dying patient because
_____.
6. Three identification cards are completed at the time of death. They are secured on the _____, the _____, and the _____.

Section Three
Self-evaluation

A. Identify the age group with its characteristic by matching Column I and Column II. (Each may be used more than once.)

Column I

1. Gradual loss of vitality and stamina. Sight and hearing become less acute
2. Beginning realization of own mortality
3. Rapid growth and system stabilization
4. Careers and families established
5. Period of gradual losses
6. Associated with final career advancement
7. Physical status gradually fails, and dependency increases
8. Control gained over elimination
9. Desire for independence and security make this a turbulent period
10. Period of beginning physical sexual changes.

Column II

a. infancy
b. preschool
c. school age
d. preadolescent
e. adolescent
f. adulthood
g. middle age
h. later maturity
i. old age

B. Choose the right answer by encircling the proper letter.

11. Communications are transmitted in
    a. words.
    b. facial expression.
    c. body language.
    d. All of the above.
12. A key to successful relationships is to remember
    a. all patients react to stress the same way.
    b. words alone communicate feelings and thought.
    c. people always say exactly what they mean.
    d. each person is unique.
13. The spiritual needs of people
    a. are less when they are sick.
    b. may be disregarded because physical needs come first.
    c. are usually greater when they are sick.
    d. do not change when they are sick.
14. If a patient expresses a desire for a visit from the clergy you should
    a. call your rabbi.
    b. let your team leader know.
    c. encourage her by telling her she is going to get better and doesn't really need a clergyman.
    d. call her clergy for her.
15. Factors influencing patient appetites include
    a. inactivity.
    b. hospital odors.
    c. pain.
    d. All of the above.
16. Breathing needs can be aided by
    a. keeping patients flat.
    b. supporting patients in an orthopneic position.
    c. withholding oxygen.
    d. making the patient ambulate more.
17. Your patient is having trouble sleeping. You may help by
    a. giving medication for pain.

      b. allowing the patient to talk with you.

      c. disconnecting the IV.

      d. giving the patient a full meal.

18. When you report on duty on time and prepared, you demonstrate your

      a. sympathy.   c. cooperation.

      b. tact.   d. dependability.

19. Patients consider their problems

      a. less important than your own concerns.

      b. equally important to the problems of roommates.

      c. most important.

      d. less important than the concerns of other staff members.

20. The patient's Bill of Rights includes the right to know

      a. orders will be properly carried out.

      b. privacy will be preserved.

      c. needs will be recognized and met.

      d. All of the above.

21. When learning of a terminal diagnosis the first response of the patient usually is

      a. anger.   c. depression.

      b. denial.   d. acceptance.

22. Signs that death is approaching include

      a. loss of general control.

      b. breathing becomes irregular and shallow.

      c. extremities become cold as circulation slows down.

      d. All of the above.

23. When a patient is in final stages of life

      a. leave him alone.

      b. you do not have to be careful what you say.

      c. visit frequently.

      d. mouth care is no longer needed.

24. When giving postmortem care

      a. remove dentures.

      b. leave equipment in the room.

      c. bathe as necessary.

      d. place the body in a natural sitting position.

25. Anointing of the sick is

      a. a religious procedure.

      b. the oiling of the sick body.

      c. part of morning care.

      d. administered only in Catholic hospitals.

Section Four
Infection Control and Safety Measures

Unit 10 Basic Medical Asepsis

OBJECTIVES

As a result of this unit, you will be able to:

- Name the most common microbes and identify their shapes and characteristics.
- Relate specific microbes to the disease conditions they cause.
- Explain how disease may be caused by bacteria and other microbes.
- List ways disease is spread and controlled.
- Demonstrate the procedure for handwashing.

We are surrounded by a world of tiny, living beings which we cannot see and who make their presence known solely by their effect. This is much the same way that the wind, which we cannot see either, makes us aware of its effect on the trees which bend and sway.

These tiny beings are organisms which can be seen only with a microscope, Figure 10-1. They are everywhere: on our skin, in our mouth, and in and on the food we eat. "Micro" means small and because these organisms are so tiny, they are called *microorganisms* or *microbes*.

Many of these microbes are very useful to us. They help in the manufacture of cheeses and leather and even in the baking of cakes. Other microbes called *pathogens* cause disease. Pathogen is the medical term for germs. It is these microbes that will be discussed.

CHARACTERISTICS OF MICROBES

Characteristics are special features. For example, the color of a person's hair is one of his characteristics. It helps to distinguish him from other people. Microbes also have distinguishing characteristics. Sometimes it is their shape; sometimes it is the way they grow in a test tube, or the special requirements they need to live. Microorganisms can often be grown (cultivated) on a nutrient material so they can be further studied. Adding colored dyes *(staining)* helps certain characteristics show more clearly. Understanding the characteristics of microbes and their growth requirements enables us to control their growth, reproduction and spread.

Protozoa

Protozoa are simple, one-celled organisms. They cause such diseases as diarrhea, malaria, and inflammation of the brain, Figure 10-2.

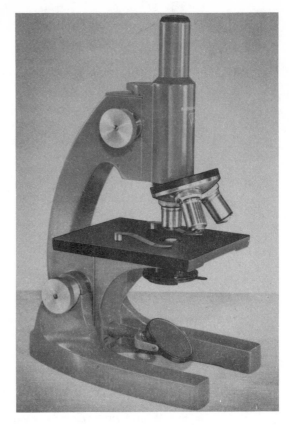

FIGURE 10-1.   The microscope magnifies microbes so that we can see them. *(Photo courtesy of Bausch and Lomb Optical Company)*

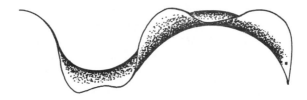

FIGURE 10-2.   This protozoan causes African sleeping sickness.

Bacteria

Bacteria are simple, one-celled organisms. They are named according to their shapes. The round bacteria are called *cocci*, the rod-shaped ones are called *bacilli*, and the corkscrew, or spiral-shaped, ones are called *spirilla*, Figures 10-3, 10-4, and 10-5.

When these organisms grow, they tend to group themselves into communities called *colonies*. If a small part of a colony is examined under a microscope, we see that bacteria are often in pairs, clusters, or chains.

These groupings have been given names: *diplo;* pairs, *staphylo;* clusters, and *strepto;* chains. Round microorganisms grouped together in chains are called streptococci. A very important member of this family is the *Streptococcus hemolyticus* that causes septic sore throats and rheumatic fever. The staphylococcus is the cause of many infections such as abscesses and boils, and these organisms are found in clusters.

A microorganism involved in gonorrhea is the *Neisseria gonorrheae* which is a round organism found in pairs.

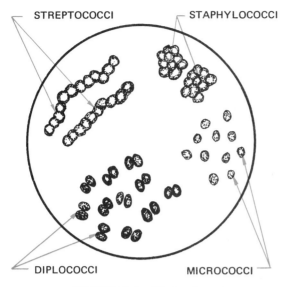

FIGURE 10-3.   Kinds of cocci

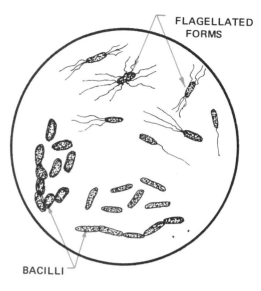

FIGURE 10-4.   Kinds of bacilli

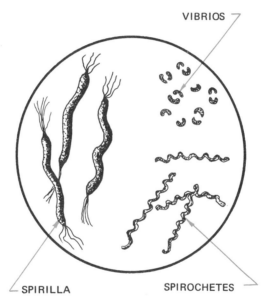

FIGURE 10-5.   Spirilla forms

Viruses

Viruses are even smaller than bacteria. We are not sure whether they are living organisms or chemicals. We class them as microorganisms because they can increase their numbers (something a chemical cannot do) and because they cause disease in somewhat the same ways as protozoa and bacteria.

FAVORABLE CONDITIONS FOR GROWTH

Most of the germs that cause disease in humans grow best at body temperature. They grow best where light is limited, and where there is moisture and food for nourishment. Yet microbes have even been found in hot sulfur springs and in the cold depths of the ocean. From these discoveries, one can readily see that microorganisms of one kind or another are everywhere.

Aerobic Organisms

Some microorganisms live best where there is plenty of oxygen available; surfaces such as the skin are ideal. These are called *aerobic*. A common member of this group is the aerobic *Staphylococcus aureus*. These organisms are round, grouped in clusters, look yellow (aureus) when growing, and require oxygen to live. They are responsible for many infections we see developing in hospital patients. An infection which develops after hospitalization is *hospital-acquired* and is called a *nosocomial infection*. Nosocomial infections can be very serious and even life-threatening. In addition, a hospital-acquired infection can greatly increase the length of hospital stay and expense.

Anaerobic Organisms

Anaerobic organisms grow best where there is little oxygen. Many in this group are important in breaking down waste products in the human digestive tract, others may cause disease. The anaerobic tetanus bacillus is a good example of the latter.

The bacilli are found in the soil where there is little free oxygen. They gain entrance into the body most frequently through a deep puncture wound. As the edges of such a wound close over, the oxygen is closed out and the bacillus grows. These organisms also grow best when their particular kind of nourishment is present. Dead tissue is ideal food for this organism, and there is always some tissue in a wound which has been destroyed by the injury. Growing in a wound, the tetanus bacillus causes the disease tetanus, or *lockjaw*.

Because this organism is found in the soil, special care must be given to dirty wounds. Frequently they will be washed out with hydrogen peroxide which, when exposed to the air, releases oxygen. The presence of this oxygen discourages the growth of the tetanus bacillus since, as you remember, this organism doesn't grow well in oxygen. A *hyperbaric chamber* is used to deliver oxygen under pressure to the tissues of a patient with an anaerobic infection, Figure 10-6.

Organisms which live on dead matter or tissue are called *saprophytes*; organisms which live on living matter or tissue are called *parasites*. The tet-

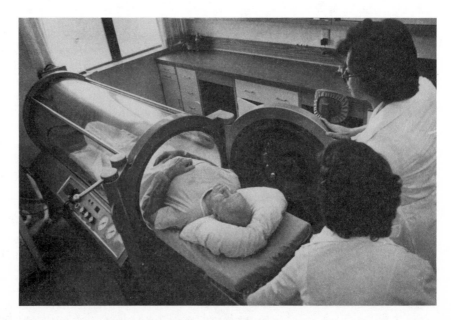

FIGURE 10-6. Anaerobic organisms do not grow well in high concentrations of oxygen as found in the hyperbaric chamber.

anus bacillus, then, can be called a saprophyte. *Staphylococcus aureus* is an example of a parasite.

HOW PATHOGENS AFFECT THE BODY

Microbes act in different ways to produce disease in the human body. Some pathogens attack and destroy the cells they invade. For example, the microscopic protozoan which causes malaria invades the red blood cells and begins to grow. Eventually the red blood cells are split open, and the person experiences chills followed by fever.

Other microbes, such as tetanus organisms, produce poisons called *toxins* which travel to the central nervous system where they cause damage. Still others compete with the host tissue they are in for the available nourishment. The host cells die of starvation.

In some cases, the very presence of the organism causes the body to react violently. This is known as an *allergic reaction*, or sensitivity. We are all familiar with the runny nose and watery eyes that occur without fever. It is believed that often these symptoms are due to the presence of a microbe or other substance, such as pollen or dust, to which the individual is sensitive.

In the beginning of the unit you learned that microbes are everywhere. This might make you wonder why we are not ill all of the time. There are two major reasons: (1) many microbes inhabit the body which are not harmful. Some are even helpful in maintaining health. For example, some of the microbes live in our intestinal tract and help produce vitamins B and K which are essential to our lives; and (2) there are several factors which influence the development of an infection: the general health of the individual, the numbers and strength of the organisms, and the presence or absence of favorable conditions for growth.

Very old or very young persons, those who are poorly nourished or in generally poor health are more susceptible to infections. Large numbers of organisms or even a few of those that are very strong (aggressive) can cause serious illness. Emotional stress and fatigue also play a role in the progress of an infectious disease.

BODY DEFENSES

The body has natural, external defenses against the invasion of pathogens. The intact skin acts as a mechanical barrier. Some of the skin chemicals: called *secretions*, kill or inhibit microbial growth.

The body also has many internal defenses, such as fever and inflammation, along with many special cells—phagocytes—whose sole purpose is to defend the body against microbes and other foreign invaders.

Our respiratory, digestive, and reproductive tracts are lined with a special tissue called *mucous membrane*. The mucus is sticky and traps foreign materials before they can get deep into the body and cause damage. Then, microscopic hairs: called *cilia*, propel the mucus and the trapped foreign invaders out of the body. Coughing and sneezing also help to remove foreign materials from the respiratory tract.

In the stomach there is hydrochloric acid, a very strong chemical, which is harmful to most microbes. Even the tears have special bacteria-killing chemicals (bacteriocidal) to protect the eyes.

SPECIAL MICROBIAL FORMS

Some organisms have the ability to become *spores* when the environment is not right for their growth, Figure 10-7. These spores are similar to

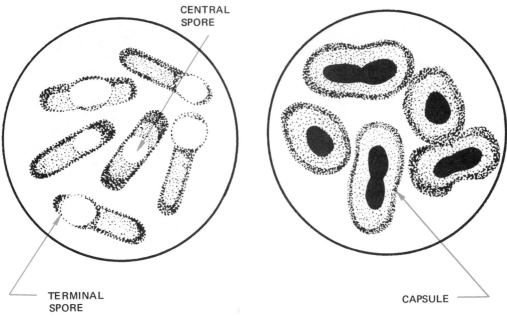

FIGURE 10-7.   Bacteria with spores   **FIGURE 10-8.**   Bacteria with capsules

a bear which goes into hibernation when his environment becomes unsuitable. The tetanus organism is capable of forming spores which remain in the soil for long periods of time. When they gain entrance into the body, and conditions are once more favorable, they become active. Spores are more difficult to destroy than active forms of organisms. Special care must be taken to destroy those microbes which may be on articles and equipment in the health care facility.

Some kinds of bacteria have capsules, or coverings, which make it difficult for them to be destroyed, Figure 10-8. Others have small, whiplike structures called flagella which help them to move, as seen previously in Figure 10-4.

NORMAL FLORA

The organisms that are normally found on the body surfaces (*normal flora*) include pathogens. Infection does not occur, however, until they gain entrance into the body. They even act to control the overabundant growth of one another. Sometimes, when drugs such as antibiotics are given for an infection, the organisms causing the infection die, leaving others to flourish and cause a different kind of infection.

In order to cause disease, organisms must gain entrance into the body through *special routes*. For example, a person might swallow tetanus organisms and not become ill. These same organisms, gaining entrance through a puncture wound in the skin, would cause lockjaw. The organism had gained entrance through its special route, in this case the skin. As another example, typhoid organisms rubbed into the skin cannot cause typhoid fever. This same organism can cause typhoid fever if it is swallowed.

TRANSMISSION OF DISEASE

Diseases caused by microorganisms may be spread in two ways: (1) directly; germs are spread from person to person by sneezing or coughing, Figure 10-9, drainage from wounds, or excreta, and (2) indirectly; germs

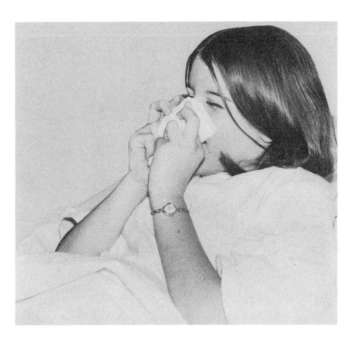

FIGURE 10-9. The common cold, a viral infection, is easily transmitted by sneezing.

may be spread by an object which a sick person has touched which is then handled by another person.

Fomes are substances that absorb and transmit infectious material. These objects with germs on them, fomites, are said to be *contaminated*. Since germs are so small that you cannot see them, dishes, toys, and other things that come in contact with an infected person can easily carry pathogens.

Remember that fomites are only one way infectious disease organisms can be spread. Coughing and sneezing make many germs airborne and easily transmitted to others. Body excretions and secretions, such as feces (solid waste), urine (liquid waste), saliva, and blood carrying infectious germs can be a source of infection. Infectious microbes can even be transmitted from a pregnant woman to an unborn child.

Infectious diseases are spread whenever there are infectious organisms which can enter the body of a susceptible person.

DISEASE PREVENTION

Medical Asepsis

Medical asepsis is the term used to describe procedures followed to keep germs from being spread from one person to another. It includes (1) handwashing, thorough cleaning of articles that come in contact with the patient: called sterilization and disinfection, and (2) complete separation of the patient and his possessions from others. The second technique is called isolation.

HANDWASHING. Handwashing is the single most important technique which, when properly carried out, prevents the spread of germs from patient to patient or between patients and health care staff. This technique should be carried out before and after using the bathroom, handling a bedpan, handling food, feeding a patient, and caring for each patient. Warm water makes good lather and is less damaging to the skin than hot water. **CAUTION:** Do not lean against the sink or allow the uniform to touch the sink. It is essential that each person use the same technique, following it exactly.

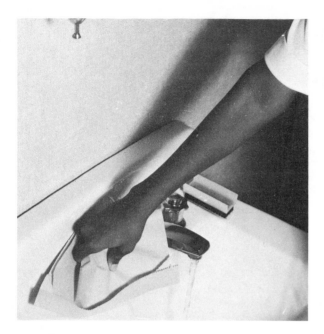

A. A dry, clean paper towel should be used to turn the faucet on and off.

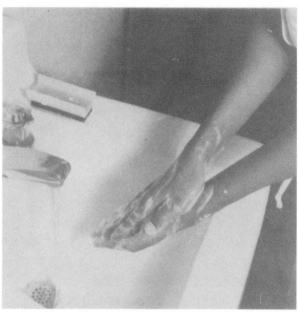

B. Fingertips should be pointed down while washing hands.

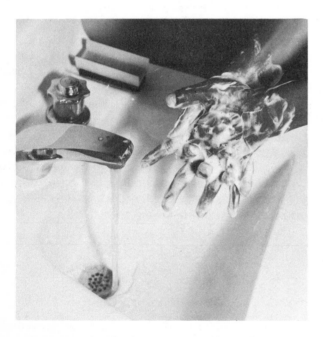

C. Interlace the fingers to clean between the fingers.

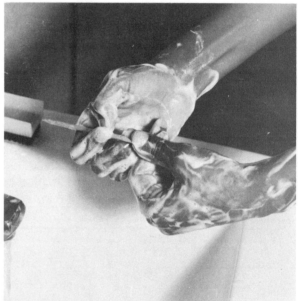

D. Using the blunt end of an orange stick to clean under the fingernails.

FIGURE 10-10.   Handwashing procedure. *(From Simmers, Diversified Health Occupations, 1983, Delmar Publishers Inc.)*

Procedure

HANDWASHING

1. Assemble the following equipment and move to a sink:
   - Soap
   - Waste can
   - Paper towels
2. Turn the faucet on with a dry paper towel held between the hand and the faucet, Figure 10-10A. Warm water is the best.

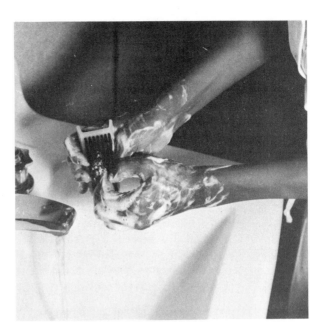

E. Using a hand brush to clean under the fingernails.

FIGURE 10-10.   (Continued)

3. Wet hands with the fingertips pointed downward. **CAUTION:** Do not allow water to run up forearms. Keep hands pointed down at all times so water runs off fingertips, Figure 10-10B.
4. Pick up the soap, rinse, and lather the hands well. Rinse soap and replace in soap dish. (The soap may also be held in hands during the procedure.)
5. Rub the hands together in a circular motion for approximately 1 to 2 minutes and, by interlacing fingers, clean between the fingers, Figure 10-10C. Rinse and repeat. Clean the fingernails with the blunt edge of an orange stick or a handbrush, Figure 10-10D and E.
6. Rinse the hands, fingertips down, and dry them thoroughly.
7. Turn off the faucet with another clean paper towel.
8. Drop the paper towel in the waste can.

Surgical Asepsis

Surgical asepsis is the special term used to describe the procedures followed to destroy organisms before they enter the body. This special technique is carried out in the operating room when the patient's natural defenses are lowered by the surgical incision in the body. Everything coming in contact with the patient must be sterile, that is, free of all organisms that might have been present on an article.

If it is suspected there might be any organisms present, or if that article has been touched by an unsterile item, that article must be considered contaminated. All instruments, dressings, gowns, gloves, and linen used in surgery must be sterile. Sterile technique is employed in the medical setting when handling sterile instruments, changing dressings or carrying out sterile procedures.

Many of these procedures are considered to be of an advanced nature, and so have been moved to Unit 39. They are:

- Opening a Sterile Package.
- Transferring Forceps in Solution.
- Donning Sterile Gloves.

The procedures are to be carried out only after adequate practice and supervision and only in accord with specific hospital policy regarding *who* is allowed to do them.

For that reason, and even if you are not allowed to complete the procedures, it is important you realize the various important aspects of them. A brief discussion of them has been included here.

STERILE TECHNIQUES

Sterile technique is an exacting procedure. *There can be no mistakes.* For this reason, usually only very specially trained people are given this responsibility. There will be times that you might be called upon to assist someone as they perform these duties. You will need to develop an awareness of correct technique and be ready to assist without fear of contamination.

The term *sterile field* refers to an area of sterile equipment and materials. This may be a table covered with a sterilized sheet or a sterile towel placed on an over-bed table. Only the center of the towel is actually used and equipment is kept two inches in from the edges all around as an added precaution.

Never reach or pass anything that is unsterile over a sterile field when you are assisting. Go around or hold the article away from the side. The logic is simply that you might drop the unsterile article on to the field or touch the field. In either case, the field would be contaminated and the entire set-up would have to be discarded.

Care of Contaminated Articles

Some contaminated articles such as tissues or dressings must be completely destroyed. They should be tightly wrapped and burned. In fact, many hospitals are using as much disposable equipment as possible. Other articles such as equipment are expensive and must be cleaned and reused. To make them safe for reuse they must be *disinfected* or *sterilized*.

Disinfection involves destroying the pathogens, usually with chemicals. It is important that all articles to be disinfected are washed, dried, and then left to soak the required length of time (usually 20 minutes) in chemicals. All parts of the article must come in contact with the disinfectant. Tubes being disinfected should be filled with the disinfectant. Instruments should be opened up or taken apart and then submerged in the disinfectant.

Sterilization is the destruction of all microbes, even the nonpathogens. Usually heat in some form is used to sterilize. Some articles may have to be boiled for 20 to 30 minutes to be sterilized. Others may be sterilized in steam in a machine called an *autoclave*. The autoclave works something like a pressure cooker. Special tape is used to secure coverings on articles to be sterilized in the autoclave, Figure 10-11A. The tape changes color during the process, giving evidence of the sterilization, Figure 10-11B. When the article could be harmed by heat, special gas autoclaves are used. Thermometers are sometimes sterilized in this manner.

Opening a Sterile Package

Sterile equipment such as gloves, dressings, instruments, swabs and throat sticks are double wrapped in cloth or paper and sealed. Most will have a seal which changes color to indicate that the sterilizing process has

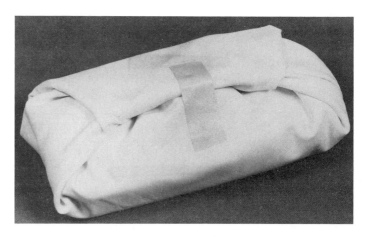

A. Autoclave steam indicator tape before sterilization

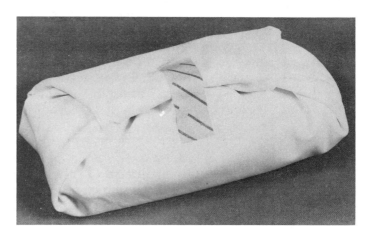

B. Autoclave steam indicator tape after sterilization *(Photos reproduced courtesy of 3M Company)*

FIGURE 10-11.

been completed. Commercially-prepared products will be sealed. If the color code has not changed or a seal does not look intact, do not consider it sterile. If you have any question, do not take a chance. Touch only the outside of the package. Remember, only sterile surfaces may contact sterile surfaces.

Transfer forceps, which are instruments used to pick up sterile equipment, are sometimes soaked in a disinfectant solution and are used almost like sterile fingers. If you are trained to use these forceps, remember—your hand touches only the non-sterile handle; the soaked, disinfected tips are used to arrange sterile equipment and supplies.

Sometimes, transfer forceps are double wrapped, and must be opened like any sterile package. Once the package is safely opened, it forms a sterile field. The forceps are lifted by the handle, being careful not to touch the tips to anything not sterile.

Gloving

Gloves are sterilized in double layered packages of cloth or paper. They are arranged so that when opened, the gloves will be on the proper side for gloving. The palms will be up with thumbs pointing to outer edge and the wrist will be cuffed and folded over. Disposable gloves are included in many prepackaged trays for various procedures such as giving an enema or in many other aspects of personal care.

The inside of the glove which comes in contact with the skin, once touched, is considered contaminated. In putting on gloves, the most important principle to remember is that glove surfaces must only touch glove while skin surfaces many only touch skin surfaces.

Summary

Microscopic organisms that cause disease are pathogens, commonly called germs. Germs differ from one another in the way they look, cause disease, and grow. Germs enter and leave the body by special routes, transmitting disease by both direct and indirect means. The spread of disease can be controlled by proper medical or surgical asepsis, which destroys or removes the pathogens, and by practicing good sterile technique.

SUGGESTED ACTIVITIES

1. Examine slides of bacteria projected on a screen. Identify each type you examine. Draw a picture of each type you examine.

2. In class discussion, explain how each of the following measures helps to prevent the spread of disease.
   a. Washing dishes with hot water and detergent and rinsing them well.
   b. Covering the mouth and nose when sneezing or coughing.
   c. Handwashing after using the bathroom.
   d. Handwashing before eating.

VOCABULARY

Certain words in this unit are new but are often heard and used in the field of medicine. They have been listed below. Their spelling and meaning are important. Make a list of the words and definitions for future reference.

aerobic	disinfect	mucous membrane
allergic reaction	fomites	spirilla
anaerobic	hyperbaric chamber	spore
autoclave	medical asepsis	staining
bacilli	microbes	staphylo-
bacteria	microorganisms	sterile field
cocci	parasites	sterilize
colony	pathogens	strepto-
contamination	protozoa	toxin
diplo-	saprophyte	virus

UNIT REVIEW

A. Brief Answer.

1. What is a fomite? Name 6 objects that can act as fomites.

2. What is the difference between the shape of cocci and bacilli?

3. Why do bacteria form spores?

4. How may articles be disinfected?

B. **Clinical Situations.** Briefly describe how a health care assistant should react to the following situations.

1. You have been asked to disinfect some plastic tubing.

2. You found a package of sponges and the autoclave tape had not changed color.

3. You have been assigned to disinfect a metal instrument.

4. You emptied one patient's bedpan and you were ready to move on to the next patient's room to take vital signs.

C. **Identification**

1. Indicate which of the following bacteria are (a) bacilli, (b) cocci, or (c) spirochete by placing a, b, or c in the space under each drawing.

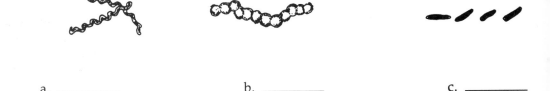

a. _____   b. _____   c. _____

Unit 11 Preparation of the Isolation Unit

OUTLINE

Isolation Technique
Reverse Isolation Technique
PROCEDURE: *Preparing the Isolation Unit*
PROCEDURE: *Donning Clean Mask, Gown, and Gloves*
PROCEDURE: *Removing Contaminated Gown, Gloves, and Mask*
PROCEDURE: *Transferring Nondisposable Equipment Outside the Isolation Unit*
PROCEDURE: *Collecting a Specimen in the Isolation Unit*
PROCEDURE: *Care of Laundry in the Isolation Unit*
PROCEDURE: *Transporting the Patient in Isolation*

OBJECTIVES

As a result of this unit, you will be able to:

- Prepare an isolation unit.
- Put on a clean mask and gown.
- Remove a contaminated mask and gown.
- Transfer food and expendable items in the isolation unit.
- Demonstrate the procedure for transporting a patient from the isolation unit.

Disease may be transferred from one person to another either directly or indirectly. These diseases are called *communicable*. Some diseases are transmitted more easily than others, so special precautions must be taken to prevent their spread.

Common ways communicable diseases may be spread are through upper respiratory secretions, such as droplets from the nose and mouth. Other diseases are spread through solid body wastes and are called *enteric*. Still others can be spread through draining wounds or infected materials such as blood on needles.

Each mode of transmission requires special precautions to prevent the spread of germs from the infected person to others.

The Center for Disease Control (CDC) in Atlanta, Georgia has established guidelines for diseases which are communicable and spread in each way. Color coding is used to help health personnel rapidly identify the type of transmission and the appropriate isolation precautions, Figure 11-1.

COLOR CODING	
Red	Respiratory
Brown	Enteric
White	Blood
Green	Skin/Wound
Yellow	Strict General Isolation
Blue	Reverse Isolation

FIGURE 11-1. Color codes help members of the health care team determine appropriate isolation techniques.

ISOLATION TECHNIQUE

Anything which comes in contact with the patient is considered contaminated and must be treated in the same special way. *Isolation technique* is the name given to the method of caring for patients with easily transmitted diseases. It is essential that every person use exactly the same technique.

The isolation area may be a unit or a single room. A room with adjoining sink and toilet facilities is best. Some hospitals have special areas used only for the care of isolation patients.

Handwashing and the use of a covering gown is basic to the practice of the isolation technique. Wearing a gown prevents self-contamination and contamination of the uniform. A clean gown must be put on before entering an isolation room and discarded in the contaminated laundry bag before you leave. At times a mask is also required. Masks are effective for only 30 minutes and must cover both nose and mouth.

Frequently-used equipment remains in the patient's unit. Special handling is required for all articles or specimens that leave isolation. Two persons, one inside the isolation unit and the other outside the unit, are needed to carry out the procedure, which is called *double-bagging.* Uncontaminated persons and objects are commonly called "clean." Contaminated persons and objects are commonly called "dirty."

REVERSE ISOLATION TECHNIQUE

There are occasions when an individual needs to be protected from the microorganisms naturally found in the environment and on other people. The patient may have suffered extensive burns or may be receiving treatments that lower the body's natural resistance to infection.

Reverse isolation technique requires that the environment, the patient, and all objects coming in contact with the patient must be either sterile or at least as free from microorganisms as possible.

Patients in reverse isolation may be cared for in private rooms or special reverse isolation units. The preparation of the patient unit is more extensive than for regular isolation. It requires several days during which the room is cleaned and disinfected, checked for the presence of microorganisms, and supplied with disinfected furniture and equipment. During the patient's stay, the unit is cleaned and disinfected daily. Samples from the environment are collected and tested for microorganisms which can cause contamination. This technique is known as *culturing.*

Shampoos, frequent bathing with surgical soaps, and the administration of antibiotics decrease the normal number of organisms found on the patient's body. All equipment, including eating utensils, are sterilized before use, and only sterile linen comes in contact with the patient. Those caring for the patient must wash their hands, using surgical technique, and put on sterile gowns, gloves, caps, and masks before entering the room.

In some hospitals where patients have very little or no resistance to infection because of birth defects, special medical treatments, or disease, the reverse isolation procedure is extremely complex. Only specially prepared professional nurses carry out the technique and care for these immunosuppressed patients.

Procedure

PREPARING THE ISOLATION UNIT

Outside the Door
1. Place a "Barrier," "Isolation," or "Precaution" sign on the door. Some hospitals use signs that are color-coded in accordance with the CDC's guidelines, Figure 11-2. Other health care facilities use a modified form of these precaution notices, Figure 11-3.
2. Place a bedside table or cart beside the door and supply with:
   - Isolation gowns, caps, masks and gloves if ordered
   - Paper and plastic bags
   - Large laundry bags specially marked as "Isolation" (Red plastic bags are often used)

Inside the Room
1. Line wastepaper basket with a plastic bag.
2. Supply a laundry hamper and a laundry bag, frequently made of a gelatinous material which dissolves in very hot water.

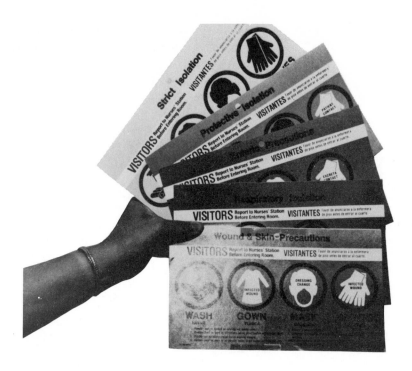

FIGURE 11-2.   Signs indicating specific precautions are posted outside the isolation room.

INFECTIOUS DISEASE PRECAUTIONS

ROOM _____
DATE _____
INITIATED BY _____

MODE OF TRANSMISSION

☐ DRAINAGE/SECRETIONS   ☐ URINE

☐ BLOOD/SERA/MUCOSA   ☐ SPUTUM (Droplet)

☐ FECAL/ORAL   ☐ SPUTUM (Airborne)
****

☐ Private Room Necessary   ☐ Gown—Necessary When
  ☐ Door Must Be Closed   ☐ Entering the Room
                                          ☐ In Contact with the
☐ Wash Hands Before and After Patient   Patient
  Contact
                                        ☐ Gloves—Necessary When
☐ Isolation Cart from Central   ☐ Entering the Room
                                          ☐ In Contact with the
☐ Disposable Food Service   Patient

☐ Needle & Syringe Precautions   ☐ Mask—Necessary When
                                          ☐ Entering the Room
☐ Red Bag All Trash   ☐ In Close Contact with
                                              Patient
☐ Yellow Bag All Linens
                                        Other Instructions _____
☐ Disinfect Equipment Before Leaving the
  Room   _____

☐ Terminal Cleaning Per HSKG.   _____

                                        _____

                                        _____

FIGURE 11-3.   Modified precaution alert. This may be posted outside the patient's unit and is recorded in the nursing care plan.

3. Put antiseptic solution dispenser over sink.
4. Check the supply of paper towels and liquid soap in a foot-operated dispenser.
5. Place a basin of disinfectant solution for soaking contaminated articles near the sink.

Procedure

DONNING CLEAN MASK, GOWN, AND GLOVES

1. Remove rings and secure them inside uniform pocket.
2. Remove watch and place it in a plastic bag or on a clean paper towel to be carried into the room with you.
3. Wash hands.
4. Adjust mask over nose and mouth and tie securely.
5. Put on gown, by slipping arms into sleeves, Figure 11-4A.
6. Slip fingers under inside of neckband and grasp ties in the back, Figure 11-4B. Secure in bowknot. Only the inside of the gown and the neck and mask ties are considered "clean" areas.
7. Reach behind and overlap the edges of the gown over so that your uniform is completely covered. Secure waist ties in a bowknot, Figure 11-4C.
8. Put on gloves, if required (see Procedure in Unit 39).

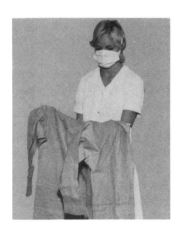
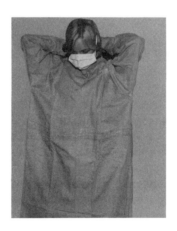
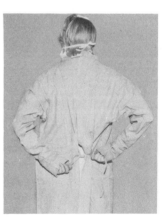

A   B   C

A. After tying on the mask, put on the gown outside the isolation unit. Be careful not to touch the outside of the gown while putting arms in sleeves.

B. Slip fingers inside of the neckband and tie gown.

C. Fold the back of the gown edges so that the entire uniform is covered. Tie the gown.

FIGURE 11-4.

Procedure

REMOVING CONTAMINATED GOWN, GLOVES, AND MASK

1. Remove gloves, turning inside out and dispose in receptacle.
2. Undo waist ties and loosen gown at waist.
3. Turn faucets on with a clean paper towel. Discard towel in wastepaper basket.
4. Wash hands carefully (see Procedure, Unit 10). Dry with paper towels. Using paper towel to operate dispenser, wet hands with antiseptic and rub together. Air dry.
5. With a dry paper towel, turn off faucets. Hands are now considered clean.

6. Undo mask. Holding by ties only, deposit in proper container.
7. Undo neck ties, loosen gown at shoulders.
8. Slip the fingers of the right hand inside the left cuff without touching the outside of the gown. Pull gown down over the left hand.
9. Pull the gown down over the right hand with the gown-covered left hand.
10. Fold gown with contaminated side inward. Roll and deposit in laundry bag or waste container, if disposable.
11. Rewash hands using same technique.
12. Remove watch from clean side of paper towel. Touch only clean side of paper towel and deposit it in the wastepaper basket.
13. Open door with clean paper towel. Prop door open with foot and drop paper in wastepaper basket.

It is understood that the preceding two procedures will be followed each time the nursing care assistant enters or leaves the isolation unit. It should be further understood that even if a procedure involving the isolation unit does not require you to don a gown, gloves, and mask, thorough hand-washing must take place before and after the procedure.

Procedure

TRANSFERRING FOOD AND DISPOSABLE EQUIPMENT OUTSIDE THE ISOLATION UNIT

1. Two people assist in the transfer. One person is inside the unit, and a "clean" person is outside.
2. Leftover liquids and food from the patient's meal are disposed of in the toilet. Be careful not to splash. Hard food such as bones should be wrapped in plastic. Check hospital policy for guidelines regarding disposal of food.
3. Door is opened with paper towel and propped with foot.
4. Clean person on outside holds cuffed plastic bag over hands to receive tray.
5. Clean person secures top of plastic bag tightly.
6. Clean person places an isolation label on bag before sending it to kitchen area.
7. *Disposable* or *expendable* (throwaway) items such as dishes may be put in the waste container in the room.
10. Dressings should be sealed in a plastic bag and then deposited in a cuffed bag held by the outside person, Figure 11-5.

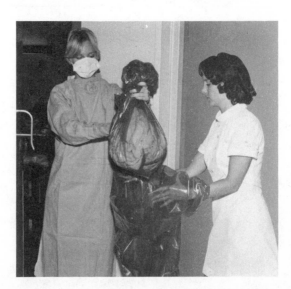

FIGURE 11-5.   Double-bagging technique showing cuff of bag protecting the clean nurse's hands.

11. The person outside the unit secures the second bag. The bag is then sent to the appropriate departments (laundry, kitchen, central supply, maintenance) where the items will be cared for according to department procedures.

Procedure

TRANSFERRING NONDISPOSABLE EQUIPMENT OUTSIDE THE ISOLATION UNIT

1. Equipment that must be reused (*nonexpendable*) may be double bagged in paper labeled "isolation" and sent to the central service for sterilization.
2. Some equipment may also be washed and soaked in a disinfectant solution in the room for a prescribed length of time before being sent for sterilization.

Procedure

COLLECTING A SPECIMEN IN THE ISOLATION UNIT

1. Bring a clean specimen container and cover into the unit and place on a clean paper towel.
2. Place specimen into container without touching the container.
3. After caring for the receptacle in which specimen was collected, wash your hands thoroughly.
4. Cover specimen and label. Double bag specimen as with equipment. Attach requisition with clip. The person outside the room will then take it to the laboratory.

Procedure

CARE OF LAUNDRY IN THE ISOLATION UNIT

1. Bring clean linen to unit as needed.
2. When laundry hamper is one-half to two-thirds full, the top is closed by the person inside the unit. A clean person cuffs and holds the specially marked laundry bag outside the room and receives the laundry bag.
3. The cover of the outside bag is securely tied and the linen deposited in accord with hospital policy. Many hospitals today use a plastic type outer bag which dissolves in the washer, freeing the linen. This eliminates the need for personnel to handle the linen after it leaves the isolation unit.

Procedure

TRANSPORTING THE PATIENT IN ISOLATION

1. Notify the department that the patient from isolation is on the way.
2. Cover the wheelchair or stretcher with clean sheets and wheel it into the room.
3. Identify the patient and tell him what you plan to do and how he can assist you.
4. Put on gown and assist the patient into the wheelchair or onto the stretcher.
5. Mask the patient, if necessary.
6. Wrap the patient in a sheet and instruct him not to touch the wheelchair or stretcher.
7. Remove your gown as you leave the unit, following proper technique.
8. Upon return from the other department, return the patient to the door of the unit. Put on a gown and take the patient into the isolation unit. Assist the patient into bed.

9. Remove the sheet from the stretcher or wheelchair and deposit in soiled linen hamper.
10. Wash hands before removing the wheelchair from the room.

Summary

When patients have diseases that are easily transmitted to others, special techniques must be used. The patient is placed in isolation, and everyone coming in contact with the patient must practice strict isolation techniques. The special technique of reverse isolation is used to protect the patient from infectious hazards in the environment.

SUGGESTED ACTIVITIES

1. Investigate the specific isolation procedure for your hospital.
2. Discuss conditions that might require isolation and conditions that might require reverse isolation.
3. Practice putting on isolation attire and removing without contaminating your uniform.
4. Practice double-bagging linen.

VOCABULARY

Learn the meaning and correct spelling of the following words:

communicable   enteric disease   immunosuppressed patient
culture   expendable   isolation technique
double-bagging   nonexpendable   reverse isolation technique

UNIT REVIEW

A. Brief Answer. Answer the following questions.
1. What is the purpose of wearing a mask and gown in the isolation unit?

2. What articles are placed outside the isolation unit?

B. Clinical Situations. Briefly describe how a health care assistant should react to the following situations.
1. You saw the color coding red on an isolation unit.

2. You were assigned to function as the "clean" person on an isolation unit.

3. You were responsible for caring for nondisposable equipment from an isolation unit.

C. Completion. Complete the following sentences.
1. The purpose of isolation is _____.
2. Anything within the regular isolation unit is considered _____.
3. A "clean area" is usually set up _____.

4. The procedure of covering a contaminated article with two bags requires _____ person(s) and is called _____.
5. A gown should be used _____ time(s) only.
6. The purpose of reverse isolation is to protect the _____.
7. In reverse isolation all articles entering the unit must be _____.
8. The clean area in reverse isolation is _____ the unit.

Unit 12 Environmental Control and Safety Measures

OBJECTIVES

As a result of this unit, you will be able to:

- Keep the patient's unit clean and orderly.
- Clean and care for the basic equipment used for patient.
- List safety measures used in a patient's unit.

The hospital bed is the patient's home while he is sick; his room becomes his world and he has control over neither. Cheerful and pleasant surroundings give the patient more of a sense of well-being; consistent attention to safety factors help foster feelings of security in this foreign environment and *both* aid in speeding recovery.

THE PATIENT ENVIRONMENT

The basic patient unit consists of a hospital bed with rails, bedside table, chair, reading lamp, and overbed table. This equipment may be located in a single or private room, double-, or multiple-bed room. Rooms with two beds are called semiprivate. Rooms with more beds are referred to as *wards*, and each bed is numbered, Figure 12-1. The equipment from one unit should not be used by other patients.

Hospital Beds

Hospital beds differ in the way in which they operate. Some are electrically controlled while others are operated by the turning of cranks. Most hospital beds may be raised to the high horizontal position so that there is less strain for those giving care. All hospital beds break in the middle so that the head may be raised, Figure 12-2, permitting the patient to be supported in a sitting position. They also break behind the knees to increase physical comfort for the bedridden patient.

Siderails, which are used to keep the patient from falling, can be attached to the bed or they may be separate. Check to make sure the rails are raised and securely attached before leaving the patient. Beds should always be left in the lowest horizontal position when siderails are down. Siderails should be up at night since patients may become disoriented in dim light and unfamiliar surroundings. Be sure, if restraints are being used, that they are never tied to the siderails and that tubes such as IV lines or catheters are always free of the siderails. Raising and lowering the siderails could put undue stress on such tubes.

Temperature, Air Circulation, and Light

Keep in mind the patient's condition, his personal preference and the needs of the other patients in the room as you maintain the temperature, light and the circulation of air in the room.

The temperature of the room is best kept at about 70 degrees F. A

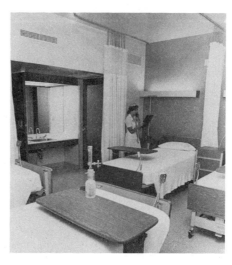

FIGURE 12-1. This four-bed unit is called a ward. Note the curtains which are used to separate care units and to provide privacy.

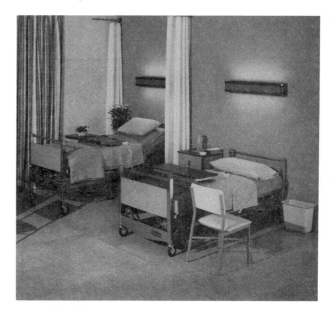

FIGURE 12-2. This semi-private room includes all the necessary furniture and equipment. The far bed demonstrates how beds may be positioned. (Note the high horizontal position and the elevated backrest.) *(Photo courtesy of Simmons Co.)*

lower temperature may cause chilling and a higher temperature may make the patient uncomfortable. Windows opened at the top and bottom insure adequate movement of air and help to control the temperature. Screens or curtains may be used to shield patients from drafts. In the newer hospitals, rooms are automatically air conditioned.

Rooms are equipped with ceiling lights which illuminate the entire room and individual unit lights to illuminate a single patient bed. Additional spotlights can be brought from the utility room when needed to provide extra light for delicate procedures. The best lighting is indirect since glare causes fatigue. Be sure to return these extra lights as soon as you are finished because added clutter in a room is hazardous. Use as much light as needed to safely carry out your job but be careful to shield other patients as much as possible.

Patients often find it difficult to sleep if lights are too bright. There

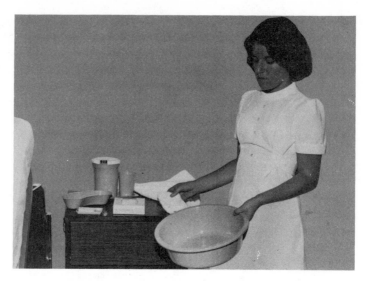

FIGURE 12-3.   Checking bedside equipment.

should be only enough light at night to enable the staff to work safely. Be sure to turn ceiling lights off when leaving the room.

Cleanliness, Noise Reduction, and Equipment

You are responsible for the cleanliness, quiet, and order of the units to which you are assigned. Since noise and clutter are very disturbing to someone who is ill, you can make a very real contribution in this regard and increase the patient's peace of mind. Make sure you speak quietly. Wheels of equipment should be well oiled to prevent squeaking. Avoid banging equipment and trays against other surfaces. Keep the area neat as you work and check its overall appearance before you leave.

The health care assistant is responsible for keeping the patient supplied with fresh water, disposable drinking cups, tissues, and straws. The assistant must make sure that all necessary equipment such as the wash basin, emesis basin, bedpan, urinal, soap, and towels are always available, clean, and in good condition, Figure 12-3.

CLEANING AND CARE OF BASIC EQUIPMENT. The daily or *concurrent cleaning* of equipment is an important part of your job that contributes to the safety of your patient. Damp dusting will cut down on the amount of dust which, you will remember, helps to spread germs. *Stretchers* and wheelchairs used to transport patients are usually made of materials that can be kept clean with soap and water. Bedside equipment and *IV standards* can be cleaned in this way also.

You will recall that IV standards are poles, usually made of stainless steel that can be attached to the bed or which stand freely on the floor. They are used to hang bags or bottles of fluids which are given to patients through tubes in their veins—called IVs, or intravenous lines.

When a patient leaves the hospital, the room must be thoroughly cleaned. In some hospitals this *terminal cleaning* will be part of your responsibility. In other hospitals, the housekeeping department will have this responsibility. The procedure for terminal cleaning follows.

Procedure
TERMINAL CLEANING OF PATIENT UNIT

1. Assemble the following equipment:
   - Basin of warm water
   - Soap
   - Brush
   - Laundry hamper
   - Newspaper for waste
   - Scouring powder

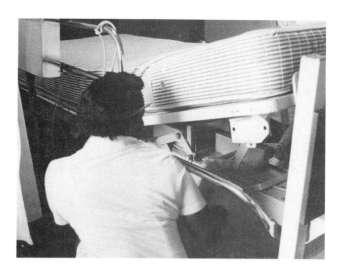

FIGURE 12-4. Terminal cleaning is done after the patient is discharged.

- Cleaning cloths
- Disinfectant solution
- Stretcher
- Radiator brush

2. Remove any special equipment. Be sure it is clean and returned to the proper area.
3. Remove all disposable material from bedside table and wrap in newspaper to be burned. Do not discard anything which may be claimed by the patient or by members of his family.
4. Remove all basic equipment from bedside stand. Wash with hot water and detergent. Sterilize equipment according to hospital policy. If disposable, clean the equipment and send home with patient or place in waste receptacle.
5. Strip bed and discard linen in laundry hamper. Place pillows on chair.
6. Take rubber drawsheet, if used, to utility room and wash with soap, water, and disinfectant solution. Allow to dry thoroughly. Some facilities put plastic drawsheets in the laundry.
7. Move stretcher beside the bed. With help, lift mattress from bed to stretcher.
8. Dry dust the coils of the bedsprings, using the long-handled radiator brush.
9. Using a cleaning cloth and disinfectant solution, proceed as follows:
   a. Wash plastic cover on mattress with a damp cloth and damp dust pillow surface.
   b. Wash framework of bed, including the bedsprings, Figure 12-4. Remove parts for thorough cleaning.
   c. Wash bedside table inside and out. Leave drawers open to air.
   d. Wash bedside chair after placing pillows on mattress.
   e. Wash lamp and call bell cord.
10. Damp dust all surfaces of mattress and pillows.
11. Place clean equipment in stand and stock bedside table according to hospital policy.
12. Air bed as long as possible to be sure all moisture has evaporated.
13. Replace mattress.
14. Make a closed bed (see Procedure in Unit 15). (Some hospitals place a gown under the pillow.)
15. Place bedside table on right side of bed at head. Place chair at foot on same side. Place overbed table across from chair. Leave unit orderly.
16. Wash hands. Return cleaning supplies.

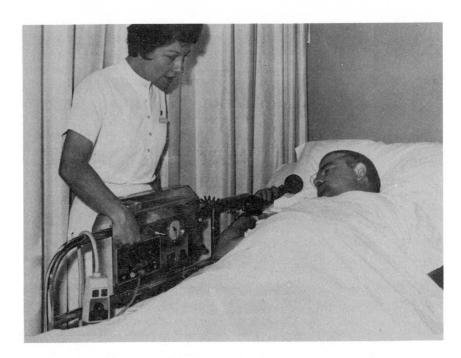

FIGURE 12-5. A careful explanation of the signal panel makes the patient feel more secure.

SAFETY MEASURES

Safety is the responsibility of everyone and must be an integral part of everything you do to or for the patient. This concern covers not only the patient, but extends to the safety of the unit and the entire environment. Accidents involving patients and staff can be greatly reduced if simple measures are followed.

The signal cord is the patient's means of letting someone know he is in need, and it must always function and be left within easy reach. The patient should be carefully instructed in the use of the signal cord and should be informed of where the emergency button is located in each bathroom, Figure 12-5.

Equipment and Its Disposal

You must see to it that equipment is kept in safe condition, Figure 12-6. Any needed repairs should be reported promptly. Frayed wires, loose

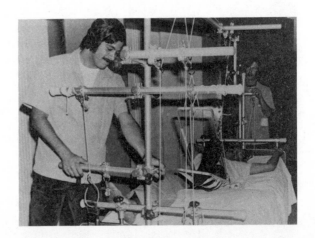

FIGURE 12-6. All equipment must be checked for security.

wheels, faulty electrical plugs, latches which do not hook, and siderails that do not fasten correctly are among those hazards that must be reported.

Disposal of equipment into proper containers will prevent many serious accidents. Most facilities dispose of "sharps," such as needles and blades, in special containers.

Never handle broken bits of glass with your hands. Larger pieces can be picked up with forceps. Small pieces can be picked up by moistening several thicknesses of paper towel and gently bringing the edges together so that your fingers do not touch the fragments.

Always know what you are handling and the proper method for its disposal.

Preventing Falls

Patients often misjudge the distance from the bed to the floor and fall as they attempt to get out of bed. For this reason, the bed should be in its lowest horizontal position when care is complete and you leave the patient. Siderails must be up and securely attached.

Tripping and falling accidents among ambulatory patients are common. For this reason, protruding objects, such as the wheels of a bed and crank handles, should be turned inward to prevent injuries. When special equipment, such as IV standards are no longer needed, they should be cleaned properly and taken from the room. They can cause accidents also.

Blankets, which may be used to cover patients who are sitting up, should not be permitted to touch the floor. This will prevent the patient from slipping on the blanket and falling, and it also keeps the blanket from being *contaminated*.

Any material that is spilled should be quickly cleaned up.

Rails along corridor walls provide added security for *ambulatory* (up and about) patients, Figure 12-7.

Basic Guidelines for Moving or Transferring Patients

Lowering the bed before assisting patients out of bed generally eliminates the need for a footstool. If a footstool is required, however, keep it out of the line of traffic within the room. Also, be sure to place one of your

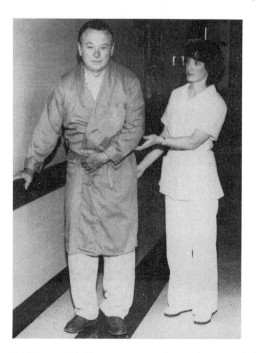

FIGURE 12-7. Corridor rails offer support and security to ambulatory patients.

feet firmly on top of it to keep it from slipping, or hook your foot behind one leg of the stool.

Procedures for lifting, moving, and transporting patients are covered in detail in Unit 14. As a general rule, when assisting a patient in any transfer, make sure the wheels of both the bed and transfer vehicle, such as the stretcher or wheelchair, are locked. Brace chairs as patients rise or sit to prevent slipping. Hook one of your feet behind the front leg of the chair as your patient is being seated.

There are many other things you can do to prevent accidents as you carry out your duties. Always walk to the right in corridors, and stay to the right when transporting patients in *gurneys* (stretchers or litters) and wheelchairs. Be especially careful at intersections, going up or down ramps, or when moving in narrow passageways. Although you may feel pressured to move quickly at times, always walk, never run. Horseplay is never appropriate.

Fire Safety

Learn the location of fire doors, escape routes, and fire extinguishers on your unit and, if you do not know how to use them, ask for a demonstration. Review the procedure you are to follow in case of emergencies such as a fire. Role play the emergency procedure until you are familiar with it.

Remember, too, that electrical appliances and open flames are prohibited when oxygen is in use, Figure 12-8.

IN CASE OF FIRE. If a fire occurs, safety of the patient is paramount. Sound the alarm by using the call board which connects the patient to the switchboard; manual alarms may also be activated. Give the location and the nature of the fire. Then move the patients out of the area as quickly as possible. Bed patients are moved in their beds. Ambulatory patients need to be escorted and directed to safe areas.

Be prepared to follow instructions when a nurse or someone in authority assumes control but in the meantime, carry out the safety policies of your facility.

Once the patients are safe, check to be sure oxygen is shut off and electrical equipment is disconnected. Shut doors and fire doors if they are part of the safety equipment, Figure 12-9. Be sure to keep all exits acces-

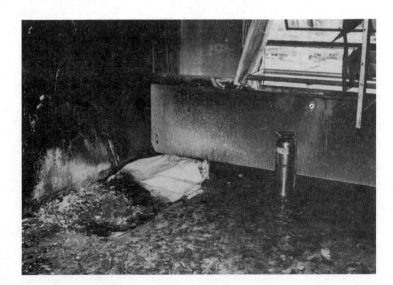

FIGURE 12-8.   Flames spread quickly from a spark, completely destroying this unit. (*Photo courtesy of United Press International*)

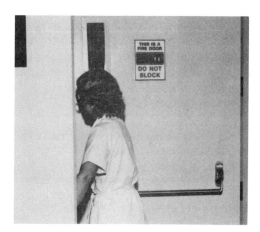

FIGURE 12-9. Move patients to safety and then shut fire doors.

sible. If you have been trained in the use of a fire extinguisher, it may be used on small fires.

In all situations, get patients to safety, follow hospital policy and keep calm.

Emergencies

In any emergency, keep calm. Assess the situation, signal for help, and never leave the patient alone. When help arrives, listen carefully to the nurse or other health care professional, and closely follow the directions given. Make safety rules and hazard prevention a growing part of your awareness. As part of your training, you may receive instruction in basic first aid and cardiopulmonary resuscitation, CPR.

Summary

The nursing staff is responsible for maintaining a safe, comfortable environment for the patient. The bed and unit is the patient's home during his hospital stay. All equipment must be readily available and kept in clean operating condition. Safety is the business of everyone. Knowing the rules assures your full participation. The cleanliness of the unit must be maintained on a daily basis and the unit completely cleaned before being used by a new patient.

SUGGESTED ACTIVITIES

1. Discuss the operation of specific types of beds in your hospital.

2. Practice changing the position of the hospital bed. Remember to turn wheels and cranks inward when you are finished.

3. Practice terminal cleaning of a unit.

4. Discuss ways you can help keep a patient's unit clean and orderly.

5. Make a list of situations in which the patient should have privacy provided.

6. Make a list of the basic equipment kept in each patient's unit.

7. Discuss the location and operation of safety equipment such as fire extinguishers.

8. Determine the numbering system for beds in your health care facility.

VOCABULARY Learn the meaning and correct spelling of the following words.

ambulatory patient	gurney	stretcher
contaminate	IV standard	terminal cleaning
concurrent cleaning	litter	ward

UNIT REVIEW **A. Clinical Situations.** Briefly describe how a health care assistant should react to the following situations.

1. An emergency, such as a patient falling out of bed, occurs.

2. There are broken pieces of glass on the floor.

3. You have to carry out a delicate procedure such as shaving a patient and the light seems inadequate.

B. Completion. Complete the following sentences.

1. The basic patient unit consists of:
    a.
    b.
    c.
    d.
    e.
2. Four ways the assistant can help prevent accidents are:
    a.
    b.
    c.
    d.
3. Before entering a patient's room the assistant should _____.
4. Concurrent cleaning takes place _____.
5. Terminal cleaning takes place _____.
6. Another name for a stretcher is a _____.

Section Four
Self-evaluation

A. Define the following words:
  1. protozoa _____
  2. bacteria _____
  3. contamination _____
  4. fomites _____
  5. autoclave _____

B. Match Column I with Column II on microorganisms.

Column I	Column II
_____ 6. disease-causing organisms	a. staphylococcus
_____ 7. arranged in pairs	b. saprophytes
_____ 8. grow best in little oxygen	c. pathogens
_____ 9. grow on dead materials	d. toxins
_____ 10. sensitivity	e. spores
_____ 11. arranged in chains	f. streptococcus
_____ 12. hard-to-destroy forms	g. allergy
_____ 13. poisons	h. diplococcus
_____ 14. grow on living organisms	i. aerobic
_____ 15. arranged in clusters	j. parasites
	k. anaerobic
	l. vegetative

C. Choose the phrase which best completes each of the following sentences by encircling the proper letter
  16. Using proper hand washing technique, you should
    a. rinse with finger tips pointed up.
    b. use very hot water.
    c. not include the fingernails at this time.
    d. turn faucets on and off with a paper towel.
  17. If the seal on a commercially prepared sterile package of gauze is broken you will
    a. consider the package contaminated.
    b. use it anyway since the contents look clean.
    c. know the condition of the seal is not important.
    d. know that the seal has to be broken before use anyway.
  18. The CDC
    a. is a state agency.
    b. establishes guidelines for disease control.
    c. stands for the communicable disease committee.
    d. stands for current disease comments.
  19. When a patient is in isolation
    a. equipment can be moved in and out without special precautions.
    b. frequently-used equipment remains in the patient unit.
    c. one person can move equipment safely in and out of the unit.
    d. contaminated equipment is labelled "clean."
  20. Reverse isolation technique
    a. is used when the patient has a communicable disease.
    b. requires less extensive preparation than regular isolation.
    c. is used when patients have little resistance to disease.
    d. requires sterilization of all articles leaving the room.

21. When isolation technique is being used, a sign will be placed on the door which might read
    a. stop.
    b. keep clear.
    c. free area.
    d. barrier.

D. Complete the following statements correctly.
22. Pathogens cause disease when they gain entrance into the body by their _____.
25. One very important way to control the spread of bacteria is by proper _____.
24. The special way of caring for patients with easily transferrable diseases is called _____.

25. Disease spread through feces are called _____.

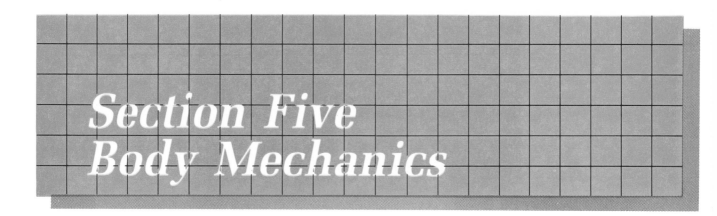

Section Five
Body Mechanics

Unit 13 Principles of Body Mechanics

OBJECTIVES

As a result of this unit, you will be able to:

- Define body mechanics.
- List the basic rules for proper body mechanics.
- List the reasons for changing the patient's position frequently.

Your body is like a well-organized machine. Each part is designed to do a special job: your eyes to see, your ears to hear, and your muscles to help you move. Some muscles help give your body shape and form. Others are attached to bones in such a way that it is possible for you to move or lift heavy objects. Muscle groups can do their best when used properly. Using the right muscles to do the job is called proper *body mechanics*.

BODY MECHANICS FOR THE HEALTH CARE ASSISTANT

Much of your work will require physical effort. Moving patients, carrying equipment, and pushing wheelchairs require muscle power. You will be less tired and less likely to strain yourself if you know how to use your body properly.

Good body mechanics start with proper posture. Correct posture is important in all positions, not only when you are standing. Correct posture makes lifting, pulling, and pushing easier, Figure 13-1.

Posture

Good posture does not mean being stiff. It means that there is a good balance between your muscle groups. Your back or spine is like a *flexible* (bendable) rod with a crossbar near the top and another near the bottom. The arms are attached to the top bar and the legs to the bottom bar. Strong muscles attach the arms and legs to the back. The muscles of the spine itself are small, and were not meant to lift heavy loads. Their main job is to bend the back in different directions and to hold the back steady, like an anchor, while the muscles of the legs and shoulders do the heavy work. To avoid straining your back muscles, you should bend from the hips and knees when moving an object and hold an object close to you when carrying it.

Good standing posture begins by straightening the back and pulling

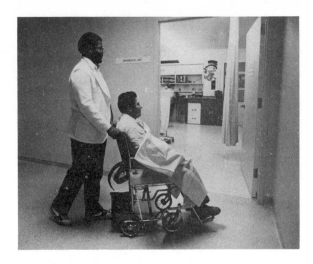

FIGURE 13-1. Notice the posture of the health assistant as this patient is transported by wheelchair.

in the abdominal "tummy" muscles. The arms are at the sides; the feet are slightly separated (about 12 inches) and flat on the floor, Figure 13-2. Keeping your feet separated makes you steadier.

Lifting

There are six basic rules to remember that will help your muscles work for you.

1. Keep your back steady.

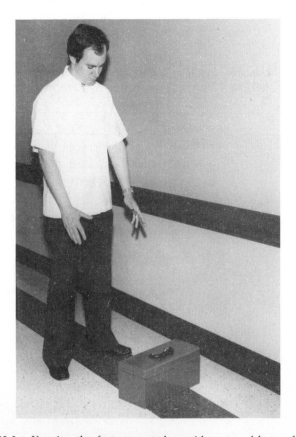

FIGURE 13-2. Keeping the feet separated provides a good base of support.

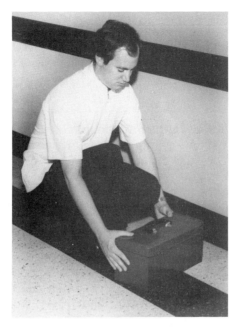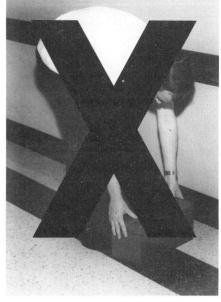

A. The correct way to maintain balance when picking up an object is to bend from the hips and knees.

B. The incorrect, and possibly injurious, way to pick up an object is to bend from the waist.

FIGURE 13-3.

2. Bend from the hips and knees to get close to the object; do not bend from the waist, Figure 13-3A and B.
3. Keep feet separated to provide a good base of support.
4. Use the weight of your body to help to push or pull the object.
5. Use strongest muscles to do the job.
6. Avoid twisting your body as you work and bend for long periods of time.

Always ask for help if you feel the patient or object is too heavy to move by yourself. Do not take chances. Various mechanical devices are available to assist in moving the helpless or heavy patient. The health assistant using one of the mechanical lifts must make sure that the support slings are smoothly positioned under the patient and that all parts of the equipment are safe and in working order.

BODY MECHANICS FOR THE PATIENT

Body mechanics for the patient who is ambulatory are very similar to those of the health care team. While they are probably doing no lifting, whether heavy or not, their good posture habits should not be allowed to be neglected.

For the bedridden patient, however, body mechanics is something very different, dealing mainly with good alignment while in bed, and frequent, regular changes of position.

Body Alignment

Proper *alignment* of the patient's body must be constantly kept in mind. Pillows of different sizes can be used to support the patient in good position and help relieve strain.

When the head of the bed is elevated, patients have a tendency to slide toward the foot of the bed. Assistance may be needed to regain proper positioning. In addition, patients who are *incapacitated* may need special assistance (see Unit 32).

Turning sheets (half sheets or draw sheets) may be used to help lift patients who are heavy or otherwise unable to help themselves.

Changes in Position

Frequent change in position is important for several reasons. Staying in one position for long periods causes muscles to tighten. Sometimes this tightening results in a shortening of muscles called *contractures*. Patients with contractures suffer disability and deformity. They are not able to use their muscles properly.

Another very important reason for frequent position change is to prevent the formation of *decubitus ulcers* or bedsores. Being in one position for long periods of time interferes with the circulation of the blood. Pressure areas develop. Soon, because the nourishment brought by the blood has been stopped, the skin breaks and ulcers develop. Bedsores are very serious and can be largely prevented by conscientious nursing care and frequent change of position. When a patient is unconscious or unable to change his own position, turning every hour is frequently ordered.

Perspiration allowed to accumulate between skin surfaces tends to irritate the skin and cause additional tissue breakdown. Placing a bath blanket or pillow between areas such as the legs helps to prevent this.

Summary

Proper use of muscles reduces fatigue and strain. Nursing tasks are easier when proper body mechanics are followed. Techniques of good body mechanics must be employed in all activities. The largest muscle masses should be used when heavy lifting is done. Use of proper body mechanics helps to prevent serious injuries, in addition to making any job easier.

Care must be taken to keep the patient in good alignment at all times. Frequent changes of position help to prevent deformities from contractures and the development of decubiti. It also aids general body functions and comfort.

SUGGESTED ACTIVITIES

1. Practice proper body mechanics when:
   - standing
   - sitting
   - bending
   - walking

2. Practice lifting small articles alone.

3. Practice lifting large articles with assistance.

VOCABULARY

Learn the meaning and correct spelling of the following words.

alignment	contracture	flexible
body mechanics	decubitus ulcer	

UNIT REVIEW

A. Brief Answer.

1. List three reasons a patient's position should be changed frequently.

2. List any three of the six basic rules for body mechanics.

B. **Clinical Situations.** Briefly describe how a health care assistant should react to the following situations.
   1. There was no one readily available in the X-ray department when you arrived with a patient who had to be moved.

   2. Your patient has slipped down to the bottom of the bed.

   3. You have a heavy patient to lift onto a stretcher.

Unit 14 Moving, Lifting, and Transporting Patients

OBJECTIVES

As a result of this unit, you will be able to:

- Describe and demonstrate the proper procedure for turning a patient.
- Describe and demonstrate the correct procedure for helping a patient sit up or move up in bed.
- Describe and demonstrate the correct procedure for helping a patient into a chair or wheelchair.
- Describe and demonstrate the proper procedure for lifting a patient using a mechanical device.
- Describe and demonstrate the correct procedure for transferring a patient from bed to stretcher.
- Describe and demonstrate the proper procedure for transporting a patient by wheelchair or stretcher.
- Describe and demonstrate proper procedure for log rolling the patient.

MOVING AND LIFTING PATIENTS

Lifting, moving, and transporting patients is a major responsibility of the health care assistant. Proper body mechanics and observance of safety rules will protect both you and your patients from injury. *Always* determine whether help is needed to lift or move a patient before proceeding with your assignment. Never be afraid to ask for help since, by exercising caution, you are also preventing potentially serious injuries.

If a patient has an IV or other tubes in place, be sure to avoid placing any stress on them. If necessary, have someone help to support them as the patient is being moved. Never let the IV tubing drop below the bed level or let drainage equipment be lifted above the drainage site.

Portable oxygen units on wheels and portable IV standards are available. At times, two people will be needed to safely transport the patient and any equipment in use.

The following procedures should be followed when you are lifting, moving, or transporting patients. As you practice these procedures, keep in mind the six basic rules of good body mechanics that were discussed in Unit 13.

As with all prior procedures, certain things must be done before the beginning and at the completion of the procedure itself. They *may not vary.*

- Wash your hands thoroughly, following the procedure described in Unit 10.
- When the procedure is complete, wash your hands again, and report the completion of the procedure to your supervisor.

So much handwashing may seem to be unnecessary because of the short length of time that you are with the patient. Just remember though (1) that your hands can transmit germs and (2) that patients already weakened by disease have a much lower susceptibility to germs.

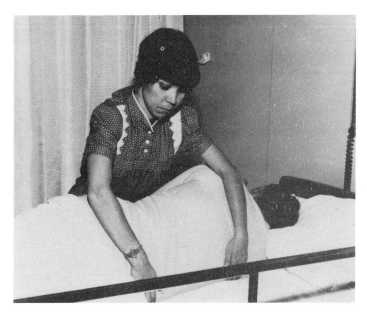

FIGURE 14-1. As the patient is turned toward you, slip your hands to the back for support.

Procedure

TURNING THE PATIENT TOWARD YOU

1. Wash hands.
2. Identify patient and explain what you plan to do.
3. Lock the bed and elevate to working height.
4. Cross the patient's far leg over the leg that is nearest to you.
5. Place hand nearest the head of the bed on the patient's far shoulder. Place your other hand on the hips on the far side, Figure 14-1. You should brace yourself against the side of the bed.
6. Roll the patient toward you—slowly, gently, and smoothly. Help patient bring upper leg toward you and bend comfortably.
7. Put up siderail. Be sure it is secure.
8. Go to the opposite side of the bed.
9. Place hands under the patient's shoulders and then hips. Pull toward the center of the bed. This helps the patient maintain the *sidelying* position.
10. Make sure the patient's body is properly aligned and safely positioned.
11. If patient is unable to move self, position legs and support with pillows. If the patient has an *indwelling* catheter, make sure the tubing is not between his legs in order to prevent undue stress on it.
12. A pillow may be placed behind the patient's back. Secure it by pushing the near side under the patient to form a roll.
13. Wash hands and report completion of the procedure to your supervisor.

Procedure

TURNING THE PATIENT AWAY FROM YOU

1. Wash hands.
2. Identify patient and explain what you plan to do.
3. Lock the bed and put up the siderail on the opposite side of the bed. Raise bed to working horizontal height.
4. Have patient bend knees, if able. Cross the arms on the chest.
5. Place arm nearest head of the bed under patient's head and shoulders and the other hand and forearm under the small of his back. Bend your body at hips and knees. Keep your back straight. Pull the patient toward you.

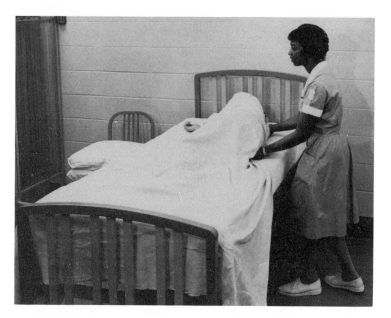

FIGURE 14-2. Turning the patient away from you (Remember that the opposite siderail must be up.)

6. Place forearms under patient's hips and pull them toward you.
7. Move patient's ankles and knees toward you by placing one hand under the ankles and one under the knees.
8. Cross patient's nearer leg over other leg at ankles.
9. Roll patient away from you, slowly and carefully, by placing one hand under the patient's shoulder and one hand under the hips, Figure 14-2.
10. Place hands under the patient's head and shoulders and draw them back toward the center of the bed.
11. Move patient's hips to the center of the bed as in step 5.
12. Place a pillow for support behind the patient's back.
13. Make sure that patient's body is in good position. Support upper leg with pillow.
14. Replace siderail on near side of bed and return bed to lowest height. Note: A turning sheet (folded large sheet or half sheet) may be placed under the heavy or helpless patient to make moving easier. It must extend from above the shoulders to below the hips to be effective.
15. Wash hands and report completion of the procedure to your supervisor.

Procedure

ASSISTING THE PATIENT TO SIT UP IN BED

1. Wash hands.
2. Identify the patient and explain what you plan to do.
3. Lock the bed. Be sure bed is lowered all the way.
4. Face the head of the bed; keep your outer leg forward. Turn your head away from the patient's face.
5. Lock near arms (patient and assistant), Figure 14-3.
6. Support the patient with other arm by making a cradle for the head and the shoulders.
7. Bring the patient to sitting position. Adjust bed position and pillows for support and comfort.
8. Wash hands and report completion of the procedure to your supervisor.

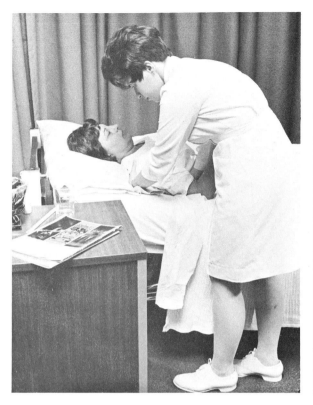
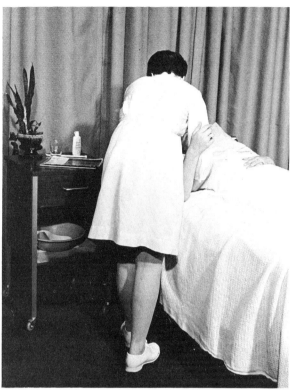

FIGURE 14-3. Assisting the patient to sit up

Procedure

ASSISTING THE PATIENT TO MOVE TO THE HEAD OF THE BED

1. Wash hands.
2. Identify patient and explain what you are planning to do and how the patient may assist.
3. Lock wheels of bed. Raise bed to high, horizontal position and lower siderail on side nearest to you.
4. Remove the pillow and place on chair, or place it at the head of the bed, on its edge, for safety.
5. Face the head of the bed, positioning the foot that is farthest away from the edge of the bed approximately twelve inches in front of the other foot.
6. Place arm nearest head of the bed under the patient's head and shoulders and lock other arm with patient's arm.
7. Instruct patient to bend knees and press in with heels as you lift shoulders and move patient smoothly toward the head of bed on a count of three, Figure 14-4. An alternate method is as follows:
   a. Place pillow at the head of the bed on its edge.
   b. Have patient grasp head of bed with hands.
   c. Slip your hands under patient's back and buttocks.
   d. Have patient press in with heels and assist the patient to raise his hips and move to the head of the bed.
8. Replace pillow under the patient's head and make patient comfortable.
9. Lower bed and raise siderail.
10. Leave unit tidy.
11. Wash hands and report completion of task to nurse.

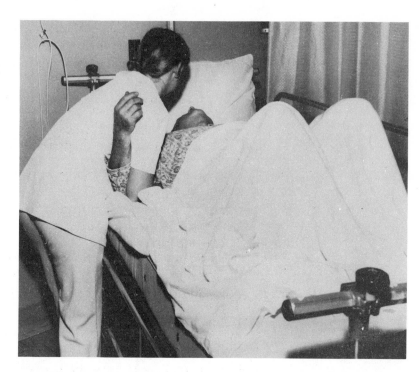

FIGURE 14-4.   Assisting the patient to move to the head of the bed.

Procedure

**MOVING A
HELPLESS PATIENT
TO THE HEAD OF
THE BED**

1. Wash hands.
2. Ask a co-worker to assist from opposite side of bed, Figure 14-5.
3. Identify patient and explain what you plan to do. *Do this even if the patient seems unresponsive.*

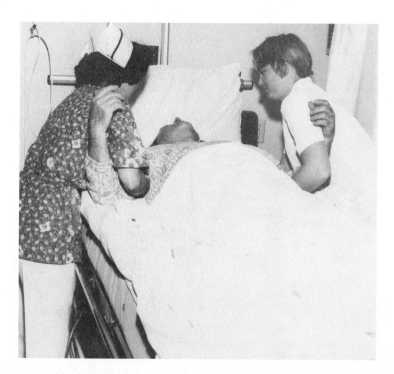

FIGURE 14-5.   When the patient is unable to assist, two persons can support and move him to the head of the bed.

4. Lock wheels of the bed. Raise bed to high horizontal position and lower siderails.
5. Remove pillow and place on chair, or place it at the head of the bed, on its edge, for safety.
6. Raise top bedding and expose draw sheet. Loosen both sides of draw sheet.
7. Roll edges close to both sides of patient's body.
8. Face the head of the bed, grasping the roll with the hand closest to patient, Figure 14-6.
9. Position your feet twelve inches apart with the foot that is farthest from bed edge forward.
10. Place free hand and arm under patient's neck and shoulders, cradling head from both sides.
11. Bend your hips slightly.
12. Together, on a count of three, raise the patient's hips and back with the draw sheet, while supporting head and shoulders. Move the patient smoothly toward the head of the bed.
13. Replace pillow under the patient's head.
14. Tighten and tuck in draw sheet.
15. Check the patient for proper body alignment.
16. Adjust bedding.
17. Raise siderails and lower bed.
18. Leave unit tidy.
19. Wash hands and report completion of task to nurse. Record, if necessary.

(All repositionings and turnings of patients should be recorded on the patient's chart.) Note: Do not leave the patient lying on his back for prolonged periods of time unless turning is contraindicated.

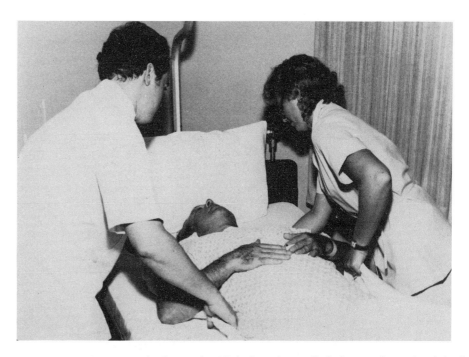

FIGURE 14-6. Keep your back straight. With drawsheet rolled close to the patient's body, lift and move smoothly to the head of the bed.

Procedure

ASSISTING THE PATIENT INTO A CHAIR OR WHEELCHAIR

1. Wash hands.
2. Identify the patient and explain what you plan to do and how to help. Have the patient's slippers and robe close by.
3. Screen the unit to provide privacy.
4. Cover the chair or wheelchair with a cotton blanket.
5. Place chair or wheelchair near the head of bed facing the foot of the bed; lock the wheelchair and raise foot peddles. (Note: Whenever possible, position chair or wheelchair so that it is secure against a wall or solid furniture to ensure that it will not slide backward.)
6. Lock bed and elevate head. Lower the bed to lowest horizontal position.
7. Drape patient with a bath blanket and fanfold bedding to foot of bed.
8. Assist the patient to a sitting by placing your arm (the one closest to the head of the bed) around the patient's shoulders. Place your other arm under the patient's knees and *pivot* (rotate) the patient toward the

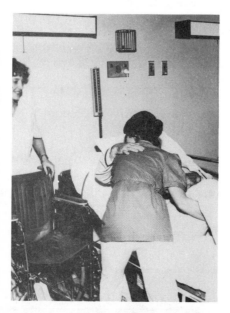
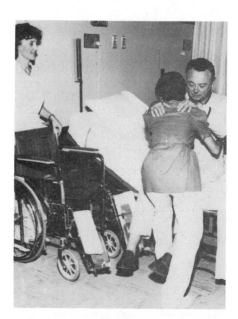
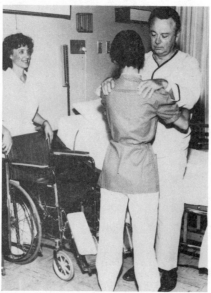
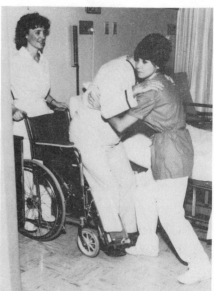

FIGURE 14-7. Assisting the patient from bed to wheelchair. Note that the assistant maintains a broad base of support as she helps the patient move.

side of the bed slowly and smoothly. Remain facing the patient to prevent a fall, Figure 14-7.

9. Assist the patient in putting on robe and slippers.
10. Still facing the patient, check to be sure he or she is ready to stand.
11. Have patient place feet on floor or footstool with both hands on your shoulders. Place your hands on either side of the patient's underarms. Raise patient slightly and help to slide off edge of bed gradually to a standing position. If using a footstool, have patient step to the floor.
12. Keeping hands in same position, help patient to turn slowly until the patient's back is toward the chair.
13. Have another person hold chair or move to side of patient, placing one foot behind front leg of chair. Lower patient gradually to a sitting position in chair, bending at your hips and knees. Keep your back straight. Arrange robe or blanket smoothly. If the patient is in a wheelchair, place both feet on the footrests and lock the wheelchair securely.
14. Cover patient with bath blanket. Stay with the patient until you are sure there are no adverse side effects. Report anything unusual to supervising nurse.
15. Leave signal cord and drinking water in reach. Make sure bed and unit are tidy.
16. Wash hands and report completion of task to your supervisor.

Procedure

ASSISTING THE PATIENT INTO BED FROM A CHAIR OR WHEELCHAIR

1. Wash hands. Identify the patient and explain what you plan to do.
2. Screen the unit for privacy.
3. Check to see that the bed is in the lowest horizontal position and that the wheels are locked. Raise head of bed, fanfold bedding to the foot, and raise opposite siderail.
4. Position chair or wheelchair at foot of the bed. Lock wheels of wheelchair and lift foot peddles.
5. Have patient place feet flat on floor.
6. Remove bath blanket, fold, and return to bedside stand.
7. Stand in front of the patient. Keep your back straight and your base of support broad.
8. Place your hands on either side of the patient's chest. Have patient place his hands on your shoulders. Assist patient to stand.
9. Pivot the patient toward the bed slowly and smoothly. Assist patient to sit on edge of bed.
10. Remove robe and slippers.
11. Place one arm around the patient's shoulders and one arm under the patient's legs and swing the patient's legs onto the bed.
12. Lower head of bed and assist patient to move into center of bed.
13. Draw top bedding over patient. Remake, if necessary.
14. Make patient comfortable with signal cord within reach.
15. Wash hands.
16. Report completion of your assignment.

Procedure

LIFTING A PATIENT USING A MECHANICAL LIFT

1. Wash hands and assemble equipment. If possible, obtain assistance from a co-worker.
2. Check the slings and straps for frayed areas or poorly closing clasps.
3. Take lift to patient's bedside and screen unit. Identify the patient and explain what you plan to do. Place wheelchair or chair at right angles to foot of bed, facing the head.
4. Lock the bed and roll patient toward you.

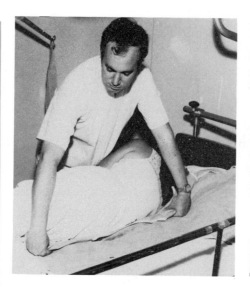

A. Roll the patient toward you and place the sling under her body.

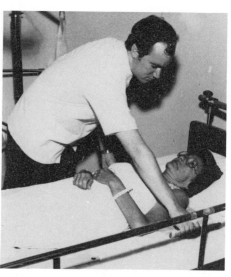

B. Make sure top of sling is positioned under the shoulders.

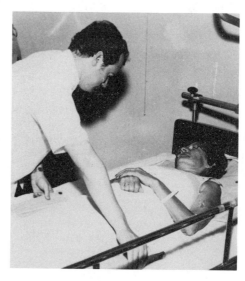

C. Position sling smoothly under hips.

FIGURE 14-8.

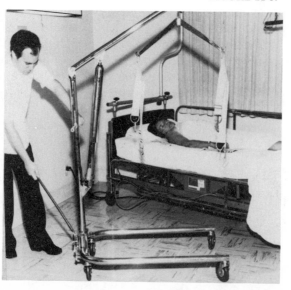

FIGURE 14-9.   Grasp the shifter handle in one hand and place the opposite hand on the steering handle on the mast for balance. Stay close to the bed.

5. Position slings beneath the body behind shoulders and buttocks, Figure 14-8. Be sure the sling is smooth.
6. Roll patient back onto the sling and position properly.
7. Attach *suspension* straps to sling. Check fasteners for security.
8. Position lift frame over bed with base legs in maximum open position and lock, Figure 14-9.
9. Elevate head of the bed and bring patient to a semi-sitting position.
10. Attach suspension straps to frame. Position patient's arms inside straps.
11. Secure restraint straps if needed.
12. Talking to the patient, slowly lift the patient free of the bed, Figure 14-10.
13. Guide the lift away from the bed.
14. Position patient close to the chair or wheelchair (with wheels locked).
15. Slowly lower patient into chair or wheelchair. Pay particular attention to the position of the patient's feet.

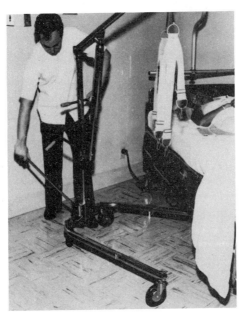

A. Move the handle to your right to release the lock pin then bring the handle toward you in a complete half circle. Lock legs in full open position.

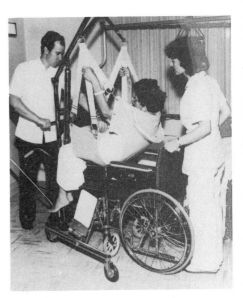

B. Hook straps from inside to out.

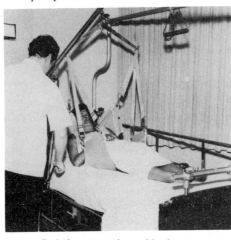

C. Lift patient free of bed.

D. Swing patient into wheelchair.

FIGURE 14-10.

16. Unhook the suspension straps and remove lift.
17. If the patient is to remain up for a period of time in the chair, make sure he is comfortable and secured in the chair before leaving him.
18. Wash hands.
19. A record of the procedure is then made on the patient's chart.

Procedure

TRANSFERRING A CONSCIOUS PATIENT FROM BED TO STRETCHER

1. Wash hands.
2. Screen unit and elevate bed to level of stretcher.
3. Move stretcher against and parallel to bed. Lock both the stretcher and the bed, Figure 14-11.
4. Identify the patient and tell what you plan to do and how you can be assisted.
5. Cover patient with bath blanket and fanfold bedding to the foot of the bed.
6. With one person beside the stretcher and the other person on the opposite side of the bed, assist the patient to move onto the stretcher. If only one person is available, raise the opposite siderail and stand beside the stretcher to brace it.
7. At the completion of your portion of the task, wash your hands and report to your supervisor.

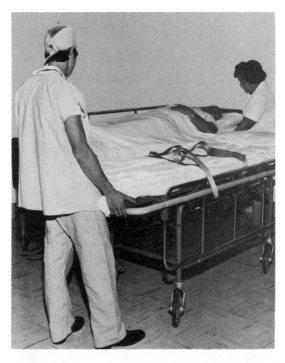

FIGURE 14-11.   Assistants helping to transfer the patient from the bed to the stretcher.

Procedure

TRANSFERRING A CONSCIOUS PATIENT FROM STRETCHER TO BED

1. Wash hands. Identify patient and explain what you plan to do.
2. Lock wheels of bed and raise to horizontal position equal to height of stretcher. Fanfold bedding to foot of bed.
3. Be sure there is another person to help.
4. Push stretcher close to bed and lock wheels.
5. Position one assistant next to stretcher and another assistant against the opposite side of bed.

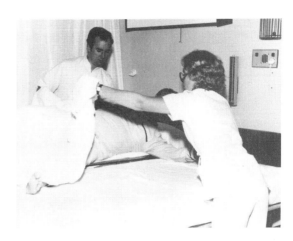

FIGURE 14-12. The conscious patient can assist in transferring into bed.

6. Loosen stretcher restraints and blanket covering patient.
7. If patient is able to move, hold covering loosely and assist patient to slide from stretcher to bed.
8. If a turning or drawsheet is used, roll sheet to edges of the patient's body. Place one arm under the patient's shoulders while grasping turning sheet with the other.
9. At an agreed upon signal, lift the turning sheet and slide the patient onto the bed.
10. Move stretcher out of the way.
11. Assist patient to a comfortable position in the center of the bed.
12. Pull top bedding up over patient and slip bath blanket from underneath.
13. Return bed to lowest horizontal position. Adjust side rails in up position.
14. Place signal cord within reach. Wash hands.
15. Report return of patient to the nurse.

Procedure

TRANSFERRING AN UNCONSCIOUS PATIENT FROM STRETCHER TO BED

1. Wash hands. Identify patient.
2. Lock wheels of bed and raise to horizontal position equal to height of stretcher. Fanfold bedding to the foot of the bed.
3. Enlist help from two other assistants.
4. Position one assistant next to opposite side of bed and one at the foot of the stretcher. The third person will be positioned on opposite side of stretcher.
5. Position stretcher against bed, lock wheels, and lower siderails of stretcher.
6. Loosen stretcher restraints and bath blanket covering patient.
7. Roll turning sheet close to patient's body.
8. Assistant on opposite side of bed uses both hands to grasp turning sheet, lift and draw patient onto bed.
9. Assistant at foot of bed lifts feet and legs.
10. Assistant opposite stretcher places one arm for support under head and shoulders of patient and, with the other hand, grasps the turning sheet to guide the patient. All assistants must coordinate their activities and move together as a signal is given.
11. Move stretcher out of the way.
12. Using the turning sheet, position patient in bed.

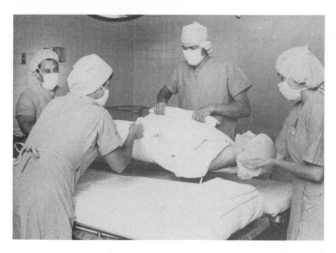

FIGURE 14-13. Note the proper way to transfer the unconscious patient from stretcher to bed using a lift sheet. Note that the head, neck, shoulders, and body are all properly supported.

13. Pull top bedding up over patient and slip bath blanket from underneath.
14. Adjust siderails in up position.
15. Return bed to lowest horizontal position. Wash hands.
16. Report the return of the patient to the nurse.

Procedure

TRANSFERRING AN UNCONSCIOUS PATIENT FROM BED TO STRETCHER

1. Wash hands.
2. Request help of three other assistants.
3. Take stretcher to patient's bedside.
4. Identify patient.
5. Lock wheels of bed and raise to horizontal position equal to stretcher height.
6. Position one assistant next to opposite side of bed and one at the foot of the bed. The third assistant will be positioned on opposite side of stretcher after stretcher is positioned. The fourth person stands at the head of the stretcher.

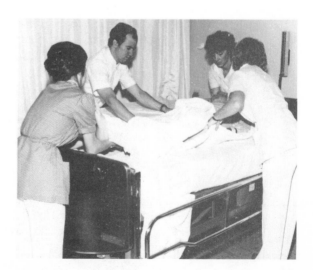

FIGURE 14-14. Transferring the unconscious patient from bed to stretcher. Note that one person supports the patient's head, neck, and shoulders.

7. Lower siderails and position stretcher close to bed. Lock stretcher wheels.
8. Loosen turning sheet and roll against patient.
9. At a prespecified signal all assistants act together as follows:
   - Assistant at foot of bed lifts feet and legs.
   - Assistant on opposite side of bed lifts and guides the patient's body with turning sheet.
   - Assistant opposite stretcher grasps the turning sheet with both hands, raises and draws patient onto stretcher.
   - Assistant at head of stretcher cradles patient's head and neck with hands under shoulders, arms together.
10. Patient is centered on stretcher and covered with bath blanket.
11. Secure stretcher restraint and raise side rails of stretcher.
12. Transport patient as directed.
13. Clean and return equipment.
14. Wash hands.
15. Report completion of task to the nurse.

Procedure

LOG ROLLING THE PATIENT

1. Wash hands.
2. Ask another assistant to help.
3. Identify patient and explain what you plan to do.
4. Screen unit.
5. Elevate bed to waist high horizontal position and lock wheels. Siderails should be securely raised.
6. Lower siderail on side opposite to which patient will be turned. Both assistants should be on the same side of the bed.
7. Move the patient as a unit toward you.
8. Place a pillow lengthwise between the patient's legs. Fold his arms over his chest.
9. Raise the siderail and check for security.
10. Go to the opposite side of bed and lower the siderail.
11. Turning the patient to his side may be done by:
    a. using a turning sheet which has been previously placed under the patient.
       - Reach over patient, grasping and rolling the turning sheet toward the patient.
       - One assistant should be positioned beside the patient to keep shoulders and hips straight.
       - Second assistant should be positioned to keep thighs and lower legs straight.
    b. If a turning sheet is not in position, the first assistant should position hands on far shoulder and hips.
       - Second assistant positions hands on far thigh and lower leg.
12. At a specified signal, the patient is drawn toward both assistants in a single movement keeping spine, head, and legs in straight position.
13. Additional pillows are placed behind the patient to maintain the position. A small pillow or folded bath blanket may be permitted under the head and neck. Leave pillow between the legs and position small pillows or folded towels to support the arms.
14. Check patient for comfort, alignment, and support. Leave call signal within reach.
15. Raise siderail and lower bed. Unscreen unit.
16. Wash hands and report completion of your task to the nurse.

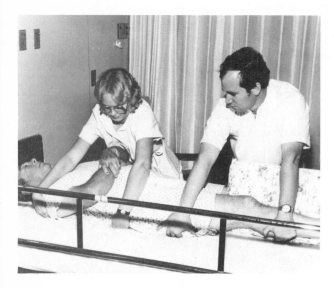

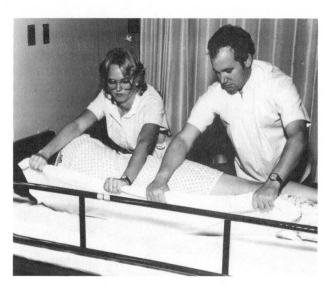

A. Place a pillow between the legs. Positioning hands on shoulders, hips, and legs, turn the patient as a single unit.

B. Log rolling a patient with a draw sheet

FIGURE 14-15.   Log rolling a patient using two methods.

TRANSPORTING PATIENTS

You may be assigned to transport patients from their unit to some other hospital department. For example, patients may need to have tests done or receive treatments which cannot be performed in their rooms. On occasion, the entire bed will be used for transport but, more often than not, transportation will be by wheelchair or stretcher.

Procedure

TRANSPORTING A PATIENT BY WHEELCHAIR

1. Wash hands.
2. Identify patient and explain what you plan to do.
3. Screen unit.
4. Position wheelchair beside bed at right angles to foot, facing the head of the bed.
5. Lock wheelchair wheels and raise foot plate.
6. Place bath blanket opened on the wheelchair to cover patient once seated.
7. Follow procedure for assisting patient into a wheelchair, page 132.
8. Once seated, cover the patient with bath blanket. Be sure it does not drag on the floor.
9. Position patient's feet on foot rests.
10. Unlock wheels of chair.
11. Guide chair from behind.
12. Carry out the following precautions:
    a. Stay to the right of corridors.
    b. Be careful when approaching intersecting hallways.
    c. Back down slanted ramps.
    d. Back into and out of elevators and doorways, turning head to assure clearance. Figure 14-15A and B shows both the correct and incorrect ways to do this.
13. Transport patient to assigned area. Do not leave patient alone. Wait until another health care worker assumes responsibility for the patient's care.
14. Unless instructed to wait, return to the unit.
15. Wash hands.

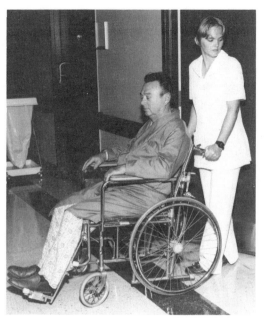

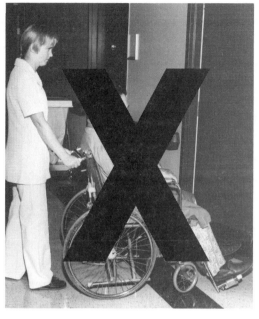

A. Correct method. Always back into doorways and elevators when transporting a patient by wheelchair.

B. Incorrect method. Note the incorrect movement of the patient in a wheelchair toward a closed door.

FIGURE 14-16.

16. Report completion of task to nurse.
    Record:
    • Date and time
    • Destination
    • Transported by wheelchair

Procedure

TRANSPORTING A PATIENT BY STRETCHER

1. Wash hands.
2. Identify patient and explain what you plan to do.
3. Screen unit.
4. Lock wheels of bed. Raise horizontal height to same level as stretcher. Lower siderails on one side.
5. Cover patient with bath blanket, fan folding bedding to foot of bed.
6. Position stretcher against bed and lock wheels.
7. Assist patient to move onto stretcher, keeping covered with bath blanket. To assist the helpless patient, see procedure, page 138.
8. Secure strap over patient's legs and raise both siderails.
9. Assume a position at the patient's head and push the stretcher.
    a. Stay to the right of corridors.
    b. Back down slanted ramps and through doorways, Figure 14-17.
    c. Be careful when approaching intersections.
    d. Back into elevators.
10. Transport patient to assigned area. Do not leave patient alone. Wait until another health care worker assumes responsibility for the patient's care.
11. Unless instructed to wait, return to the unit.
12. Wash hands.

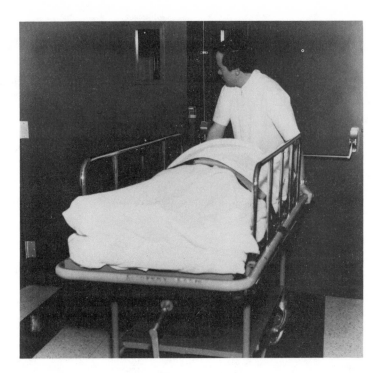

FIGURE 14-17. Note the careful approach toward a doorway when transporting a patient by stretcher (gurney).

13. Report completion of task to nurse.
      Record:
         • Date and time
         • Destination
         • Transported by stretcher.

Summary

Great care must be taken when lifting and moving patients to ensure that neither you nor your patient will be injured in the process. The principles of good body mechanics must be considered when positioning patients.

SUGGESTED ACTIVITIES

1. Practice turning patients toward and away from you.

2. Practice assisting patients to a sitting position.

3. Practice assisting patients out of bed.

4. Practice transporting patients by wheelchair and stretcher.

VOCABULARY

Learn the meaning and correct spelling of the following words.

contraindicated	indwelling catheter	sidelying
drawsheet	mechanical lift	suspension
gurney	pivot	turning sheet

UNIT REVIEW

A. Brief Answer.

1. What are two things you should always do before turning a patient in bed?

2. How do you prevent the patient from being injured when he is being rolled away from you?

3. After positioning a patient, what should you check for?

4. List three safety precautions to observe when using a mechanical lift.

5. List four precautions to keep in mind when transporting a patient by wheelchair or stretcher.

B. Clinical Situations. Briefly describe how a health care assistant should react to the following situations.
   1. You have a very heavy patient to lift.

   2. An unconscious patient arrives at the unit by stretcher and must be transferred to the bed.

Section Five
Self-evaluation

A. Choose the phrase which best completes each of the following by encircling the proper letter.
1. Proper body mechanics include
   a. keeping knees and hips straight as you bend.
   b. keeping your back flexed.
   c. twisting your body as you work.
   d. using the strongest muscles to do the job.
2. When turning a patient in bed, remember to
   a. unlock the bed.
   b. roll the patient toward you.
   c. place your hand under the patient's near shoulder.
   d. All of the above.
3. In assisting the patient to sit up in bed, remember to
   a. keep your feet close together.
   b. keep your face close to the patient's face.
   c. lock arms with the patient.
   d. lock hands with the patient.
4. In assisting a patient to move to the head of the bed, you should
   a. unlock the bedwheels.
   b. add a pillow under the patient's head.
   c. face the head of the bed.
   d. place the foot farthest away from the bed edge behind the other foot.
5. If you are alone and assisting a patient to move to the head of the bed
   a. lower the bed.
   b. raise the head of the bed.
   c. have patient grasp head of bed.
   d. ask the patient to keep his knees straight.
6. When moving a helpless patient to the head of the bed
   a. ask a co-worker to assist.
   b. lower bed to lowest possible horizontal position.
   c. tighten lower bedding.
   d. position feet close together.
7. When assisting a patient into a wheelchair
   a. place chair at end of bed.   c. lock bed and chair wheels.
   b. lower foot pedals.   d. raise bed.
8. When lifting a patient using a mechanical lift
   a. check the slings and straps for safety.
   b. place the chair so that it faces the bed.
   c. unlock the wheels.
   d. position lift frame over bed with base legs close together.
9. To transfer a conscious patient alone from bed to stretcher
   a. unlock bed wheels.
   b. place stretcher parallel against bed.
   c. stand beside bed.
   d. lower both siderails.
10. When transporting a patient by wheelchair
   a. keep foot plates up.   c. do not allow bath blanket to drag.
   b. guide chair from the side.   d. keep wheels of chair locked.

144

11. When transporting any patient
    a. keep to the left of corridors.
    b. be careful approaching intersections.
    c. head down slanted ramps.
    d. move forward into elevators.
12. When transporting using a gurney
    a. leave siderails down.
    b. secure straps.
    c. keep wheels locked.
    d. keep to left of corridors.
13. Good standing posture includes
    a. feet close together.
    b. arms out straight.
    c. feet separated.
    d. abdominal muscles relaxed.
14. One basic rule of good body mechanics is
    a. keep feet close together.
    b. bend from the hips and knees.
    c. twist body as you work.
    d. keep your back relaxed.
15. Another basic rule of good body mechanics is
    a. use the weight of your body to help move objects.
    b. stand an arm's length away from the object being moved.
    c. keep feet close together.
    d. bend from your waist.
16. When a patient has an IV in place and must be moved remember
    a. avoid stress on tubes.
    b. tubes are flexible and can be twisted without harm.
    c. it is all right to allow the tube to drop below the infusion site.
    d. No answer applies.
17. If the patient being moved has a drainage tube in place
    a. slight stress creates no problem.
    b. also not allow drainage container to drop below drainage site.
    c. never allow the drainage container to be raised above drainage site
    d. All answers apply.
18. Staying in one position for too long periods leads to
    a. improved circulation.
    b. contractures.
    c. more flexible joints.
    d. greater comfort.
19. When carrying an object
    a. hold it with extended arms.
    b. use your back muscles.
    c. hold it close to the body.
    d. keep knees straight and tensed.
20. Proper alignment can be maintained with
    a. turning sheets.
    b. draw sheets.
    c. pillows.
    d. cradles.
21. When using a turning sheet
    a. roll it closely to patient's side.
    b. move one side at a time.
    c. it should extend just under the shoulders.
    d. it should extend just under the hips.

B. Match Column I with Column II.

Column I		Column II
22. contractures		a. bendable
23. alignment		b. position
24. decubitus ulcer		c. muscle shortening
25. flexible		d. bedsore
		e. rigid
		f. muscle relaxation

Unit 15 Bedmaking

OBJECTIVES

As a result of this unit, you will be able to:

- List the different types of beds and their uses.
- Operate each type of bed.
- Make an unoccupied and an occupied bed.

The patient's room, to say nothing of his bed, is his home while he is hospitalized. A well-made bed offers both comfort and safety. It is an extremely important contribution to the well-being of the patient.

OPERATION AND USES OF HOSPITAL BEDS

The types of beds and the methods used in their operation may vary in different hospitals, but the basic principles of bedmaking are the same. A Gatch bed is generally in use; the stationary one is about 26 inches high. Modern hospitals are equipped with beds which may be operated manually or electrically. These beds may be raised to the desired height for bedside nursing or may be lowered to 13 inches to accomodate the out-of-bed patient, Figure 15-1.

The Circle® bed and the Stryker frame are special kinds of beds which are used when patients cannot be turned within the bed, Figures 15-2 and 15-3.

Patients with severe burns or spinal injuries are examples of those who are often placed in a Circle® bed. When it is necessary for the patient's position to be changed, the frame is fastened on top of the patient and the entire bed is rotated forward. After the rotation the patient is on his abdomen.

Correct operation of any bed is important to the safety of the patient, so be sure you know how to operate the bed before you try. Always seek assistance and instruction from the nurse or another health care professional when using these beds to turn a patient.

BEDMAKING

The Closed Bed

The closed bed is made following the discharge of the patient and after terminal cleaning. It remains closed until a new patient is to be ad-

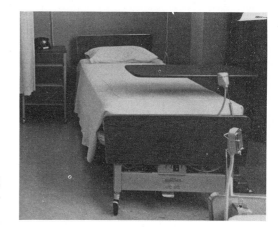

FIGURE 15-1. A typical hospital bed which can be adjusted for height and position.

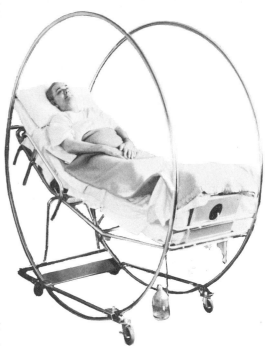

FIGURE 15-2. The Circle® bed

1. POSTERIOR FRAME
2. ANTERIOR FRAME
3. OVERHEAD BAR
4. SLIDING UTILITY TRAY
5. MIDDLE SECTION WHICH CAN BE REMOVED (NOT VISIBLE)
6. PADDED CANVAS STRAP WHICH SUPPORTS FOREHEAD WHEN PATIENT IS LYING ON THE ABDOMEN

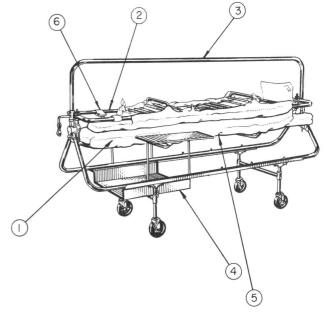

FIGURE 15-3. The Stryker turning frame

mitted. Details are important. The bed will be properly made and comfortable for the patient if you give attention to the following details:

- The bottom sheet must be free from wrinkles and carefully tucked in at the corners.
- The top covers must be neatly adjusted and firmly tucked under the mattress at the foot of the bed. The spread must be properly placed.

Procedure

MAKING A CLOSED BED

1. Wash hands and assemble the following equipment:
   - 2 pillowcases
   - Pillow
   - Spread
   - Blankets as needed
   - 2 large sheets (90″ × 108″)
   - Cotton drawsheet or half sheet*
   - Plastic or rubber drawsheet*
   - Mattress pad and cover

*Note: Newer hospital mattresses which are treated with plastic do not require a moisture-proof sheet or cotton half sheet (drawsheet). In selected cases, the half sheet is used as a lifter to assist in moving the patient or to simply keep the bottom sheet clean. Some hospitals are using fitted bottom sheets. If this is so, substitute a fitted sheet for one of the large 90″ × 108″ sheets.

2. Elevate the bed to a comfortable height. Lock bed wheels so the bed will not roll and place chair at the side of the bed.
3. Arrange linen on chair in order in which it is to be used.
4. Position mattress at the head of the bed by grasping mattress handles (or the edge of the mattress, if no handles are present).
5. Place mattress cover on mattress and adjust it smoothly for corners. You will work entirely from one side of the bed until that side is completed. Then go to the other side of the bed. This conserves time and energy.
6. Place mattress pad even with the top of the mattress and unfold.
7. Place on the bed and unfold the bottom sheet, right side up, wide hem at the top. The small hem should be brought to the foot of the mattress, Figure 15-4. Center fold should be at the center of the bed.
8. Tuck 12 to 18 inches of sheet smoothly over the top of the mattress.
9. Make a mitered corner, Figure 15-5A to E. The square corner, preferred by some hospitals, is made in a similar way to the mitered corner.
10. Tuck in the sheet on one side, keeping the sheet straight. Work from the head to the foot of the bed. If using a fitted sheet, adjust it over

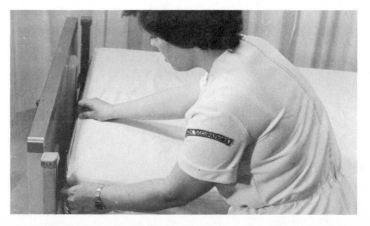

FIGURE 15-4. Position the small hem of the bottom sheet even with the foot of the mattress. (*From Simmers,* Diversified Health Occupations, *1983, Delmar Publishers Inc.*)

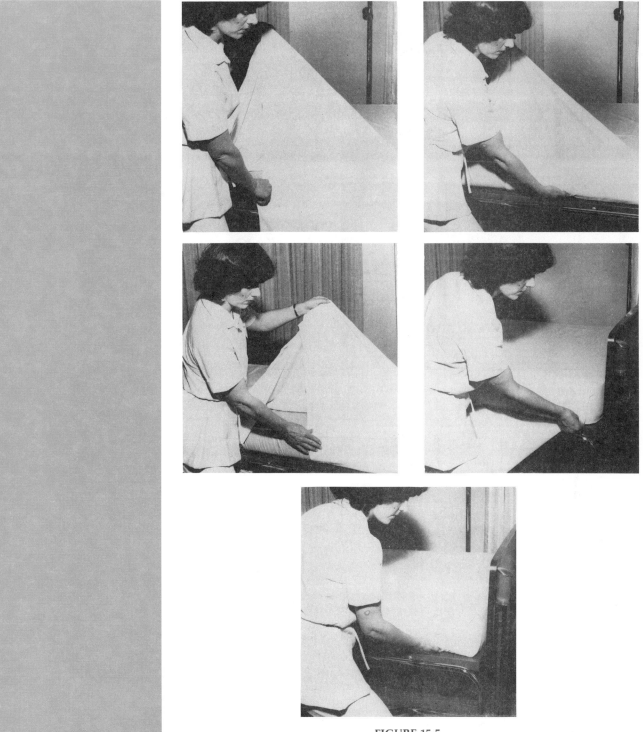

FIGURE 15-5.

A. To make a mitered corner, pick up the sheet hanging at the side of the bed about 12 inches from the bed, forming a triangle.

B. Tuck the lower portion under the mattress.

C. Holding fold with one hand, bring triangle down.

D. Hold the sheet firmly and tuck under the mattress all the way to the foot of the bed.

E. Square the corner, but allow the sheet to rest untucked on bed. Grasp edge of sheet and gently loosen until top triangle is squared and is even with the head of the bed mattress. Tuck folded part of the sheet under the mattress.

the head and bottom ends of mattress (see Figure 15-6A and B for examples of proper and improper placement).

11. If used, place the plastic drawsheet and half sheet with upper edge about 14 inches from head of mattress and tuck under one side. Be sure the half sheet covers the plastic sheet.

12. Place the top sheet, wrong side up, hem even with the upper edge of the mattress, Figure 15-7, and center fold in the center of the bed.

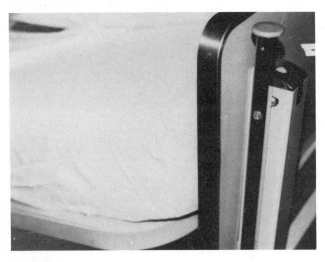

A. Proper placement of fitted bottom sheet. Be sure it is tucked under the corner smoothly.

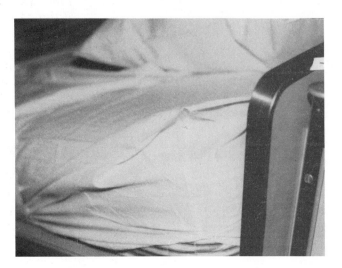

B. Improper placement of fitted bottom sheet.

FIGURE 15-6.

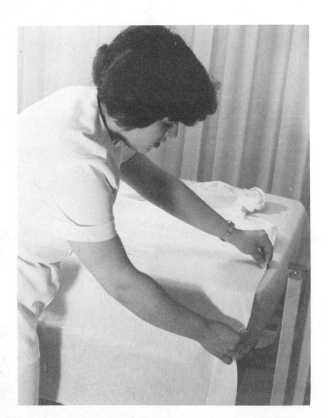

FIGURE 15-7.   Position the top sheet on the bed, wrong side up, with the wide hem even with the top edge of the mattress. (*From Simmers, Diversified Health Occupations, 1983, Delmar Publishers Inc.*)

13. Spread the blanket over the top sheet and foot of mattress. Keep blanket centered.
14. Tuck top sheet and blanket under mattress at the foot of the bed as far as the center only and make a box corner.
15. Place spread with top hem even with head of mattress. Unfold to foot of bed.
16. Tuck spread under mattress at the foot of bed and make mitered corner.
17. Go to other side of the bed. Fanfold the top covers to the center of the bed in order to work with lower sheets and pad.
18. Tuck bottom sheet under head of mattress and make mitered corner. Working from top to bottom, smooth out all wrinkles and tighten these sheets as much as possible to provide comfort. (Adjust fitted bottom sheet smoothly and securely around mattress corners.)
19. Grasp protective drawsheet, if used, and cotton drawsheet in the center. Tuck these sheets under the mattress.
20. Tuck in top sheet and blanket at foot of bed and make mitered corner.
21. Fold top sheet back over blanket, making an 8-inch cuff.
22. Tuck in spread at foot of bed and make a mitered corner. Bring top of spread to head of mattress.
23. Insert pillow into pillow case in the following way.
    a. Place hands in the clean case, freeing the corners.
    b. Grasp the center of the end seam with hand outside the case and turn case back over hand.
    c. Grasp the pillow through the case at the center of one end. Pull case over pillow with free hand.
    d. Adjust the corners of the pillow to fit in the corners of the case.
24. Place pillow at head of bed with open end away from the door.
25. Lower bed to lowest horizontal position. Replace bedside table parallel to bed. Place chair in assigned location. Place overbed table over the foot of the bed opposite the chair. Place signal cord or call panel within easy reach of the patient.
26. Wash hands.

The Open Bed

The open bed is like a sign saying "welcome" to the patient, Figure 15-8. It indicates that the arrival has been made known to the assistant and

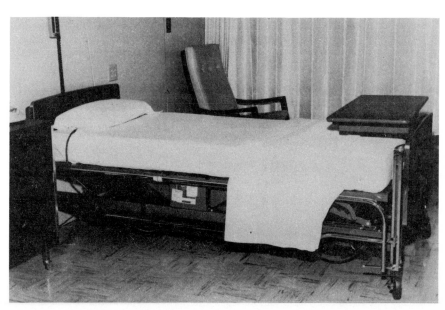

FIGURE 15-8. Note completed open bed with draw-sheet in proper position.

that the unit has been prepared. The closed bed is opened by *fanfolding* the top bedclothes either halfway, or along the entire length of the bed down to the foot. Toepleats should be made in the foot of the bed in accord with the procedure for the occupied bed.

Procedure **OPENING THE CLOSED BED**	1. Wash hands. 2. Raise bed to comfortable working height in the horizontal position. 3. Loosen top bedding and make toepleats at foot of bed. 4. Facing head of bed, grasp top sheet and spread and fan fold to foot of bed. 5. Return bed to lowest horizontal position and overbed table over foot of bed. 6. Place call bed under the pillow or within easy reach. 7. Check bedside stand for standard equipment and linen. Replace any missing equipment or linen. 8. Leave unit tidy and in order. Wash hands.

The Occupied Bed

Unless the patient is permitted out of bed by doctor's order, the bed is made with the patient in it. The patient frequently enjoys this refreshing procedure if the assistant is skillful. Making the bed follows the bed bath, while the patient is covered with a bath blanket, but it may be done any time it would add to the comfort of the patient.

Procedure **MAKING AN OCCUPIED BED**	1. Wash hands and assemble the following equipment: • Cotton drawsheet or turning sheet for selected patients • 2 large sheets (or fitted bottom sheet) • 2 pillowcases • Laundry hamper 2. Identify the patient and explain what you plan to do. 3. Place bedside chair at the foot of the bed. 4. Arrange linen on chair in the order in which it is to be used. 5. Screen the unit for privacy. 6. Bed should be flat with wheels locked unless otherwise indicated. Raise to working horizontal height. 7. Loosen the bedclothes on all sides by lifting the edge of the mattress with one hand and drawing bedclothes out with the other. Never shake the linen because this spreads germs. Adjust mattress to head of bed, Figure 15-9.

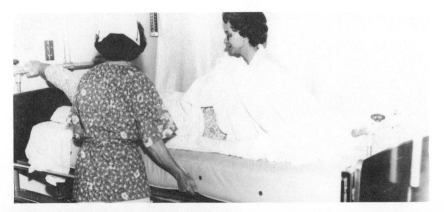

FIGURE 15-9. The patient grasps the head of the bed and pushes in with heels while two caregivers pull mattress to the head of the bed.

8. Remove top covers except for top sheet, one at a time. Fold to bottom and pick up in center. Place over the back of chair.

9. Place the clean sheet or bath blanket over top sheet. Have the patient hold the top edge of the clean sheet if he is able. If the patient is unable to help, tuck the sheet beneath the patient's shoulder.

10. Slide the soiled sheet out, from top to bottom. Discard in hamper.

11. Ask the patient to move to the side of the bed toward you; assisting if necessary. Move one pillow with the patient and remove the other pillow. Pull up the siderail. (Alternatively, you may ask the patient to turn toward the opposite side of the bed, holding onto the raised side rail. You would then fanfold the sheet, as in step #12, but there would be no need to go to the other side of the bed.)

12. Go to the other side of the bed. Fanfold the soiled cotton drawsheet, if used, and bottom sheet close to the patient, Figure 15-10.

13. Straighten mattress pad. If bottom sheet is to be changed, place a clean sheet on the bed so that the narrow hem comes to the edge of the mattress at the foot and the lengthwise center fold of the sheet is at the center of the bed. Fanfold opposite side of sheet close to patient.

14. Tuck top of sheet under the head of the mattress.

15. Make a mitered corner.

16. Tuck side of sheet under mattress, working toward the foot of the bed.

17. Position fresh turning sheet. If drawsheet is used, position and tuck it under the mattress.

18. Ask or assist patient to roll toward you, over the fanfolded linen. Move the pillow with the patient. Raise side rails.

19. Go to the other side of the bed. Lower side rail. Remove the soiled linen by rolling the edges inward and place in hamper. Keep soiled linen away from your uniform.

20. Pull the clean bottom sheet into place and tuck it under the mattress at the head of the bed. Make a mitered corner.

21. Pull gently to eliminate wrinkles. Then tuck the side of the sheet under

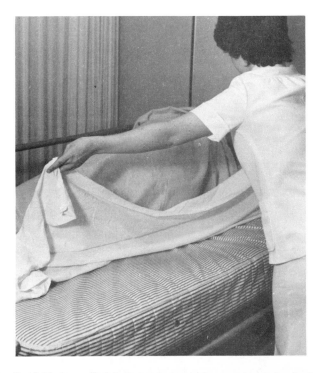

FIGURE 15-10. Fanfold the soiled bottom sheet to the center of the bed as close to the patient as possible. (*From Simmers*, Diversified Health Occupations, *Delmar Publishers Inc.*)

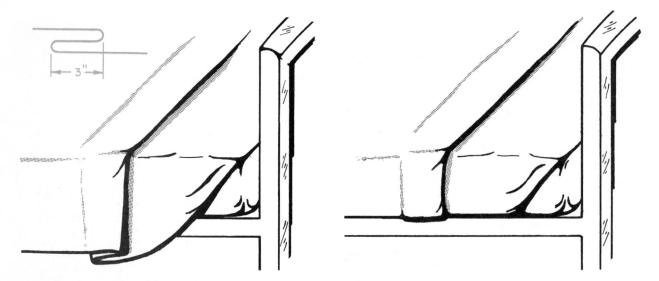

FIGURE 15-11. Making a toepleat. Before tucking in the mitered corner, make a 3-inch fold toward the foot of the bed (left). Complete the mitered corner (right).

     the mattress, working from top to bottom.
22. Pull the drawsheet into place and tuck firmly under the mattress.
23. Complete the bed as an unoccupied bed, making *toepleats* in top sheet and blanket. Toepleats provide room so that pressure is not exerted on the patient's toes. One procedure for making toepleats is described in Figure 15-11. Some patients prefer not to have the blanket, topsheet or spread tucked in.
24. Assist the patient to turn on his back. Place clean pillowcase on pillow not being used. Replace pillow. Change other pillow case.
25. Adjust bed position for the patient's comfort. Be sure siderails are up and secure. Lower bed to lowest horizontal height.
26. Place signal cord within patient's reach. Replace bedside table and chair. Remove hamper. Wash hands.
27. Let the nurse know you have completed the task.

The Surgical Bed

     The surgical bed provides a safe warm environment to receive the postsurgical patient. It must be made in such a way that movement from gurney to bed is made with maximum safety and with a minimum of effort. For this reason the bed should be left open and at stretcher height. All equipment needed to monitor vital signs and to supervise recovery should be in place and ready for use.

Procedure

MAKING THE SURGICAL BED

1. Wash hands.
2. In addition to those articles required for a basic bed, assemble one extra drawsheet and one protective (rubber) drawsheet.
3. Lock bed. Strip and discard used linen.
4. Make bottom foundation bed as instructed earlier in this unit. (Steps 1–11 in Making the Occupied Bed. Repeat on opposite side of bed.)
5. Place protective drawsheet over head of mattress drawsheet and cover with cotton drawsheet. Miter corners and tuck in on sides.
6. Place top sheet, blanket, and spread in usual manner. Do not tuck in.
7. Fold linen back at foot of bed even with edge of mattress.
8. Fanfold upper covers of top linen to far side of bed.

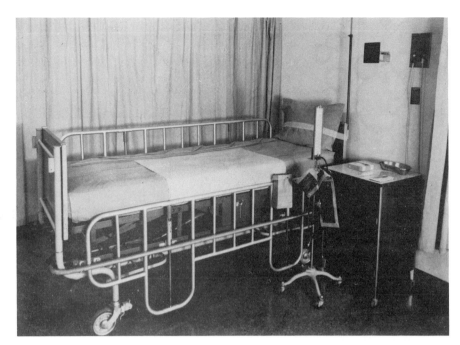

FIGURE 15-12. The surgical bed

9. Tie waterproof pillow to head of bed with gauze bandaging or place according to hospital policy, Figure 15-12.
10. Leave bed at same height as stretcher.
11. Wash hands and report completion of this task to the nurse.

| Summary | Proper bedmaking is an important part of a health assistant's work. A drawsheet or a turning sheet may be used depending upon the individual patient's need. Some facilities are using fitted bottom sheets. The procedure may be modified to accommodate this difference. A skillfully made bed provides comfort and safety for the patient. |

SUGGESTED ACTIVITIES

1. Practice operating the beds that are found in your hospital. Be sure you know how to adjust siderails for safety.

2. Practice making closed, open, occupied, and surgical beds.

VOCABULARY   Learn the meaning and correct spelling of the following words.

box (square) corner   fanfold   Stryker frame
Circle® electric bed   mitered corner   turning sheet
closed bed   open bed   toepleats
drawsheet   siderails

UNIT REVIEW   **A. Brief Answer.** Answer the following questions.

1. Why should the wheels of the bed be locked before the assistant starts to work on the bed?

2. Why should one side of the bed be made at a time?

3. Why are the sheets unfolded rather than shaken out?

4. How should the pillow be placed on the bed?

5. What is the purpose of the open bed?

6. What is the purpose of the surgical bed?

7. Why is it important to screen the patient unit before beginning to make an occupied bed?

8. What must be the position of the bed and siderails of the occupied bed before leaving?

9. What is the purpose of toepleats?

10. What is the proper position for the overbed table when the bed is closed or unoccupied?

11. When is the closed bed made?

B. **Clinical Situations.** Briefly describe how a health care assistant should react to the following situations.
   1. You finish making the occupied bed and you notice the bed is at the working horizontal height.

   2. You were assigned to give care to a patient in a bed with which you are not familiar.

Unit 16 Admission, Transfer, and Discharge

OBJECTIVES

As a result of this unit, you will be able to:

- Demonstrate the procedure for admitting a patient to the hospital unit.
- Demonstrate the procedure for transferring a patient.
- Demonstrate the procedure for discharging a patient.

Although the nurse is responsible for carrying out hospital procedure and physician's orders regarding all admissions, transfers, and discharges, the assistant usually carries out the routine procedures associated with admission, transfer, and discharge. Very often auxiliary personnel and personnel from the admissions office will accompany the patient to the ward, Figure 16-1.

Since changes in weight are a frequent indicator of the patient's condition, a baseline measurement is usually obtained on admission. Measurements of weight and height must be accurately made and recorded according to hospital policy, because medications may be ordered according to the patient's size. Measurements may be recorded in feet and inches or in centimeters; weight measurements as pounds or kilograms.

The upright scale is found in most hospitals and is used for ambulatory patients, Figure 16-2. In-bed scales are also available for weighing patients who must remain in bed.

When a patient is transferred, all details must be taken care of according to hospital policy, to ensure that there is no interruption in treatment or loss of time as a result of failing to register the transfer. The assistant may accompany the discharged patient to the hospital exit.

ADMISSION

When a patient is admitted to a hospital, the necessity for the admission process is usually a cause of concern to the patient, his family, and his friends. The first impression created is very important, and because the assistant is one of the first staff members to see the patient, the value of the assistant's courtesy, confidence, and efficiency cannot be overestimated, Figure 16-3.

When a patient is ready for admission, it is well to ask if the patient requires a gurney or wheelchair to reach the unit. Ask if any special equipment such as oxygen or a fracture bed is needed and whether there are any special instructions.

Part of the patient's chart usually goes to the unit. You will be responsible for its care. Observe the patient carefully, listening for complaints as you escort and assist the patient to the room and to bed. Initial observations are very important since they become the basis of comparison for future observations.

If it is necessary to ask visitors to leave, this must be done in a kindly

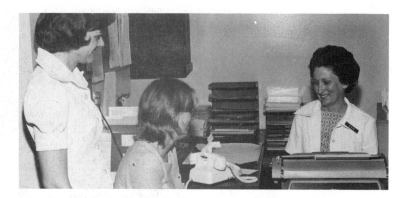

FIGURE 16-1.   After the admission procedure, the health care assistant may be called to escort the patient. Courtesy is extended at all times.

manner since they are most anxious to remain and see the patient settled and comfortable. Show them where they may wait. Let them know approximately how long they will have to wait and the availability of coffee and smoking areas. Your courtesy toward them will go a long way in establishing peace of mind for them and the patient.

Procedure

ADMITTING THE PATIENT

1. Wash hands and assemble the following equipment:
   - Equipment for urine specimen
   - Equipment for taking temperature
   - Pad and pencil
   - Patient's chart
   - Stethoscope

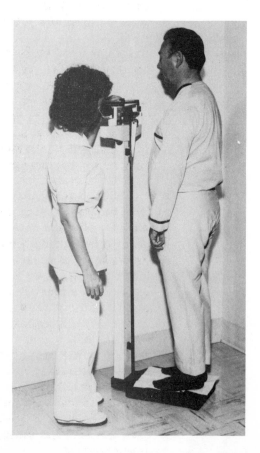

FIGURE 16-2.   Weighing the patient on the upright scale.

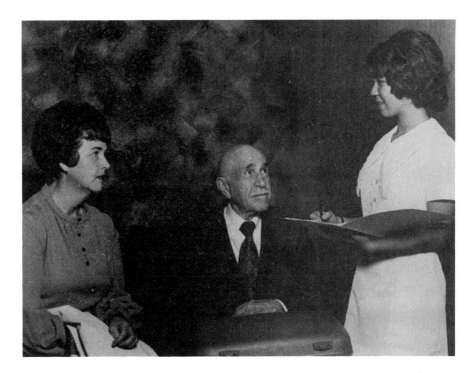

FIGURE 16-3.   The health assistant can do much to put both patient and family at ease.

- Blood pressure cuff
- Watch with second hand

2. Prepare the unit for the patient by making sure that all necessary equipment and furniture are in their proper places. Check the unit for adequate lighting and provide ventilation. Open the bed and make a toe-pleat.

3. Identify the patient both by asking the name and by checking the identification bracelet. Introduce yourself and take the patient and family to the unit. Do not appear to rush the patient. Be courteous and helpful to patient and family.

4. Ask the patient to be seated. Ask the family to go to the lounge or lobby while the patient is getting ready for bed. Introduce the patient to the other patients in the room. Explain the signal system and the standard hospital regulations. Insofar as it is permitted, explain what will happen in the next hour.

5. Screen the unit.

6. Help the patient to undress and put on a hospital gown or nightclothes from home. Care for clothing according to hospital policy.

7. Check the patient's weight and height (see next procedure).

8. Help patient get into bed. Adjust siderails as needed.

9. If the patient is wearing any jewelry or has valuables which were not left at the cashier's office, make a list of them and ask the patient to sign it; this protects the hospital. The relatives should also sign the list and take the valuables home or you should put them in the hospital safe.

10. Tell the patient that a urine specimen is necessary and offer the bedpan or urinal. Assist the patient as necessary. Allow him to use the bathroom, if ambulatory.

11. Pour the specimen from the bedpan to the specimen bottle and put on the cap. Be sure to label the specimen correctly. (See Unit 21.)

12. Take temperature, pulse, respiration, and blood pressure (see Units 22 through 24).

13. An admission form is usually completed at this time. Vital information includes allergies, medications being taken, and food preferences and dislikes.
14. Position the patient as ordered. Place the signal cord within reach and instruct him again in its use. Give fresh drinking water only if permitted. Remove the screen. Tell relatives they may visit the patient.
15. Orient the patient and relatives to the unit by explaining visiting hours and mealtimes, as well as how to use the phone.
16. Clean and replace equipment according to hospital policy.
17. A record of the information that was taken will be made according to hospital policy on the patient's chart.
18. Wash hands.

Procedure

WEIGHING AND MEASURING THE PATIENT

1. Escort the patient to the scales.
2. Place a paper towel on the platform of the scale.
3. Be sure the weights are to the extreme left and the balance bar hangs free. The lower bar (large indicator) is *calibrated* in *increments* of 50 pounds. The upper bar (small indicator) is calibrated in increments of single pounds. The even numbered pounds are marked with numbers. The long line between even numbers indicates the odd number pounds. Each small line indicates one quarter of a pound.
4. Assist the patient to remove his shoes and help him step up onto the scale platform. The balance bar will rise to top of the bar guide.
5. Move the large weight to the closest estimated patient weight, but not more than the patient weighs.
6. Move the small weight to the right until the balance bar hangs free half way between the upper and lower bar guide.
7. Add the two figures and record the total as the patient's weight in pounds or kilograms according to hospital policy. For example: The weight shown in Figure 16-4 is determined as follows:

Large indicator	150 pounds	
Small indicator	4 pounds	
Total	154 pounds	

or

154 ÷ 2.2 = 70 kilograms

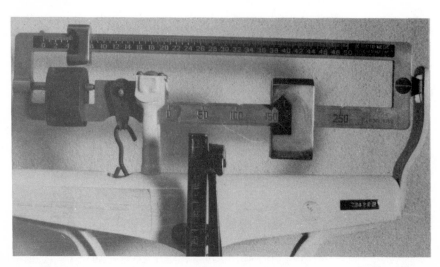

FIGURE 16-4. The weight shown by the small indicator is added to the weight shown by the large indicator in order to determine the patient's weight.

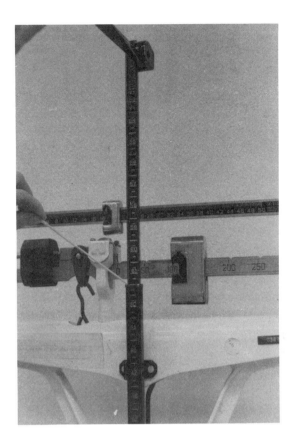

FIGURE 16-5. The patient's height is read at the movable point of the ruler. Note: Do not press down on the patient's head with the ruler.

8. While the patient stands on the platform, facing away from it, raise the height bar until it rests levelly on the patient's head.
9. The reading is made at the movable point of the ruler, Figure 16-5.
10. Note the number of inches indicated. Record this information according to hospital policy in inches, feet and inches, or centimeters. Remember, there are 12 inches to 1 foot and that 2.5 centimeters equal 1 inch. For example: The height shown in figure 16-5 is 62 inches. This may be recorded as 62 inches; 5 feet 2 inches (62 ÷ 12 = 5 feet 2 inches) or as 155 centimeters (62 inches × 2.5).
11. Assist the patient to put on his shoes and return to the room.
12. Make a record of the height and weight in the admission notes.

TRANSFER

It may be necessary for the patient to be moved to another unit, Figure 16-6. Preparations for the transfer will be handled by the nurse, but you may be asked to assist. A positive attitude on your part is important whether it is the patient's own preference, or because a change in the patient's condition makes it necessary. In the latter case it may be that the patient does not fully understand the reasons for the transfer.

After the new unit has been notified and is prepared for the transfer, all of the patient's belongings are gathered together. Medicines, charts, and other personal information are taken to the new unit with the patient. Sometimes the entire bed is moved. Be sure to take the patient's chart and any medications to the new location and deliver them to the nurse. Never leave them unattended.

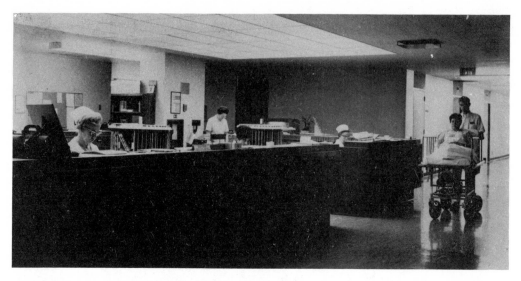

FIGURE 16-6. This patient and her belongings are being transferred from one wing to another.

Make sure that the patient is comfortable in his new environment before you return to your own unit. A notation is made on the patient's chart which includes the time of transfer, the location of the new unit, and any special observations you have made about the patient's reaction.

Procedure
TRANSFERRING THE PATIENT

1. Wash hands and assemble the following:
   - Patient's chart
   - Nursing care plan
   - Medications
   - Paper bag
2. Determine the unit to which the patient will be transferred. Check to see that it is ready.
3. Learn from team leader the method of transfer and get necessary vehicle (wheelchair, stretcher, or patient's own bed).
4. Check to see if any equipment is to be transferred with patient.
5. Take equipment to bedside.
6. Identify patient and explain what you plan to do. Screen unit for privacy.
7. Gather all patient's belongings together. Place expendables in paper bag to transport with you. Check against clothes list.
8. Assist patient to put on robe and slippers, if permitted. Assist patient into wheelchair or stretcher, as directed. The entire bed is often used so make sure siderails are up during transport.
9. Transport patient and belongings to new unit. Use all precautions related to safe transport.
10. Introduce patient to staff and proceed to patients room.
11. Assist staff in helping patient into bed. Assist in putting away patient's belongings and helping patient to become settled.
12. Give any transferred medications, nursing care plan, and chart to new team leader.
13. Before leaving unit, chart the following:
    - Date and time
    - Procedure: Transfer per wheelchair, stretcher, or bed
    - Name unit of transfer
    - Patient reaction
14. Return to original unit and report completion of task.

DISCHARGE

The discharge of a patient requires the written order of the physician. If a patient indicates an intention of leaving without an order, report it to your supervisor immediately. The nurse will make the necessary arrangements. Hospitals have special policies which must be followed in these cases.

The patient should be spared any fatigue or unnecessary delay when being routinely discharged. Check to see that the physician has written an order for discharge before preparing the patient. Gather all the patient's belongings and assist in packing if necessary. Most patients who are well enough to be discharged prefer to assemble their own things. Make sure, however, to check the closet and bedside table. Disposable equipment is often sent home with the patient. If this is the policy in your facility be sure that the equipment is clean.

Check with the nurse for any medications or other treatment-related equipment that should be sent home with the patient. *Never* allow a patient to leave the health care agency unassisted.

Procedure

DISCHARGING THE PATIENT

1. Check to be sure the physician has ordered the patient to be discharged.
2. Wash hands. Go to the unit, taking a wheelchair there if necessary.
3. Tell the patient what you plan to do.
4. Screen the unit.
5. Help the patient to dress if necessary.
6. Collect the patient's personal belongings and help check them against the admission list. Pack if necessary. Check valuables against list according to hospital policy. Make sure that all of the patient's belongings have been removed from the closet and bedside stand. Check to see if medications or other equipment are to go home with patient.
7. Tell the patient or a member of his family how to collect valuables from the hospital safe if they were put there.
8. Help patient into wheelchair if necessary.
9. Take patient to the discharge entrance of the hospital, Figure 16-7. Help patient into the car.

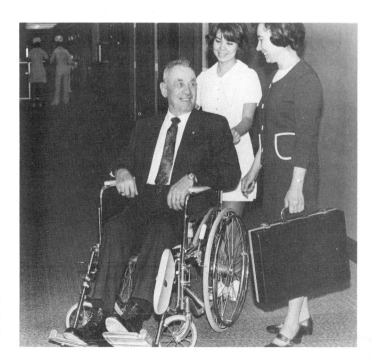

FIGURE 16-7. Discharging the patient. Remember that the health care assistant accompanying the patient is responsible for the safety of the patient until the patient is in the car.

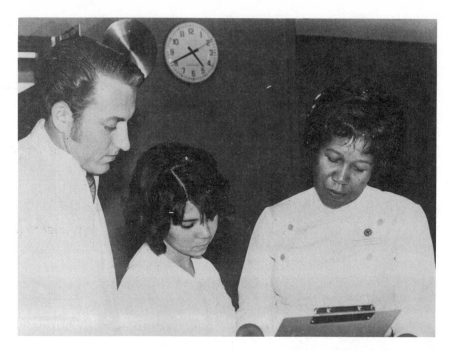

FIGURE 16-8.   The time of discharge must be recorded on the patient's chart.

10. Return wheelchair if used. Strip hospital unit. Clean and replace equipment used in care of patient according to hospital policy. Ventilate the unit. Wash hands.
11. A record of discharge will be made in accord with hospital policy, Figure 16-8. Record usually includes date, time, and method of transport.

Summary

The health assistant assists the nurse in the admission, discharge, and transfer of patients. You can do much to ease the feelings of fear and anxiety that patients and their families feel at this time. Being courteous, unrushed, and observant are important ways in which you can help.

SUGGESTED ACTIVITIES

1. Investigate the procedures for the admission, transfer, and discharge of patients at your hospital or health facility.

2. With the aid of a classmate role playing the patient, practice admitting, transferring, and discharging.

3. Practice weighing and measuring patients.

UNIT REVIEW

A. **Brief Answer.** Answer the following questions.
   1. Why is it important for the assistant to observe the patient carefully upon admission?

   2. How is the unit prepared for the new patient?

3. How do you care for the patient's valuables upon admission?

4. What materials are transferred to the new unit with the patient?

5. What should you do if a patient wants to leave the hospital without a doctor's order?

6. Record the following weights and heights in metric measurement:
   a. 154 pounds = _____ kg
   b. 132 pounds = _____ kg
   c. 6 feet = _____ cm
   d. 5 feet 4 inches = _____ cm

B. **Clinical Situations.** Briefly describe how a health care assistant should react to the following situations.
   1. Your patient tells you he intends to leave the health care agency without his doctor's permission.

   2. Your patient has just been discharged.

Section Six
Self-evaluation

Choose the phrase which best completes each of the following sentences by encircling the proper letter.

1. When making an occupied bed, remember
   a. the unit need not be screened.
   b. toepleats may be omitted.
   c. one side of the bottom is made at a time.
   d. one complete side of the bed is made at a time.

2. During the patient's bed bath
   a. the patient is completely uncovered.
   b. the water is changed to maintain warmth.
   c. the unit is not screened.
   d. the top linen remains in place.

3. If a patient tells you he plans to leave the hospital without his doctor's permission, you had best
   a. notify the supervising nurse at once.
   b. discuss the problem with other assistants.
   c. try to talk him out of it.
   d. call his family and tell them of his plans.

4. When admitting a patient, remember
   a. allow the patient to keep large amounts of money at the bedside.
   b. tell the family to leave because you have work to do.
   c. be courteous and helpful to both the patient and his family.
   d. None of the above.

5. During the admission procedure, you will
   a. collect a urine specimen.
   b. take vital signs.
   c. help patient undress and get into bed.
   d. All of the above.

6. What type of bed is made after a patient is discharged?
   a. Open bed
   b. Surgical bed
   c. Closed bed
   d. Circle bed

7. An open bed is made by
   a. fan folding the top bedclothes to the foot of the bed.
   b. adding an extra pillow.
   c. leaving the top bedding off.
   d. padding the bottom linen.

8. When gathering linen to make a bed
   a. put spread on the top of the pile.
   b. include a bathblanket.
   c. include a drawsheet.
   d. put linen in order of use.

9. When making an unoccupied bed
   a. make entire bottom of bed first.
   b. change the pillow slip first.
   c. make one entire side first.
   d. place the bottom sheet even with the head of the mattress.

10. Pillow cases should
    a. face the open doorway.
    b. face away from the open doorway.
    c. face in any direction since it doesn't matter.
    d. face the foot of the bed.

11. Before leaving the patient after making an occupied bed be sure
    a. the bed is in the highest horizontal position.
    b. the top bedding has been tucked in with a square corner.
    c. the head of the bed is elevated.
    d. the siderails are up.
12. The surgical bed is prepared for the
    a. preoperative patient.
    b. postoperative patient.
    c. the patient in the recovery room.
    d. the patient who is newly admitted.
13. Charting related to admission should include
    a. date.
    b. time.
    c. pertinent observations.
    d. All of the above.
14. Charting related to discharge should include
    a. presence of visitors.
    b. method of transport.
    c. report of a final urine specimen.
    d. response of other patients.
15. After discharge
    a. return wheelchair if used.
    b. strip unit.
    c. clean and replace all used equipment.
    d. All of the above.
16. When a patient is admitted, you should
    a. determine the proper transportation.
    b. check on the need for special equipment.
    c. observe the patient carefully.
    d. All of the above.
17. When asking visitors to leave
    a. tell them abruptly they can't stay.
    b. let them know how long you will be.
    c. don't take the time to tell them about smoking areas.
    d. All of the above apply.
18. When discharging a patient
    a. allow them to walk from the unit to the outside.
    b. throw all disposables away.
    c. call the doctor to check his order.
    d. gather all the patient's belongings and assist with packing.
19. If a patient says she intends to leave without permission you should
    a. do nothing. It is the patient's decision.
    b. report immediately to your supervisor.
    c. start gathering the patient's belongings.
    d. call the doctor.
20. The patient is weighed on admission and you find the weight to be 158 lbs. This is equal to
    a. 60 kilograms.
    b. 64.4 kilograms.
    c. 71.8 kilograms.
    d. 75 kilograms.
21. The patient is measured at 68 inches. This equals
    a. 5 feet 3 inches.
    b. 5 feet 4 inches.
    c. 5 feet 6 inches.
    d. 5 feet 8 inches.
22. The patient is 5 ft 2 inches. This may be expressed as
    a. 120 centimeters.
    b. 130 centimeters.
    c. 145 centimeters.
    d. 155 centimeters.
23. On admission the patient should have his
    a. temperature taken.
    b. pulse determined.
    c. weight determined.
    d. All of the above.
24. Identify the patient by asking his name and
    a. checking his chart.
    b. asking a visitor.
    c. asking the charge nurse.
    d. checking the identification bracelet.
25. Valuables brought with the patient to the hospital should be listed and left
    a. in the patient's locker.
    b. at the bedside.
    c. in the hospital safe.
    d. on the patient.

Unit 17 Patient Bathing

OBJECTIVES

As a result of this unit, you will be able to:

- Assist the patient with a tub bath or shower.
- Give a bed bath.
- Give a partial bath.
- Assist with the other aspects of patient bathing: giving female perineal care, giving routine hand and fingernail care, and giving routine foot and nail care.
- Give a bed shampoo.

A daily bath is as important for the patient as it is for you. A bath with warm water and mild soap not only removes dirt and perspiration, but it increases circulation, and provides the patient with a mild form of exercise. The patient feels clean, relaxed, and refreshed. You, as the care giver, are able to see first-hand how the patient's strength is improving, decreasing or changing in any way.

PATIENT BATHING

The patient receiving an IV or who has drainage tubes or oxygen requires special attention. Be very careful as you bathe and move the patient that you do not put stress on the tubes. Never lower the IV bottle below the level of the infusion site or raise the drainage tube above the drainage site.

With the doctor's permission, the patient may be allowed to take regular tub baths or showers. Other patients will be bathed in bed. Care of the hair, teeth, and nails usually follow the bath procedure.

Safety Measures

The room should be comfortably warm and free from drafts, and the patient must be guarded against chilling; cotton bath blankets can be used to cover the patient during a bed bath and may be used for added warmth following the tub bath or shower. The temperature of the water, whether shower, tub, or bed bath, should be maintained at about 105 degrees F.

Falls during the tub and shower bath can be avoided when nonskid strips are placed in the tub and floor of the shower and handrails are secured to the walls. Assisting the patient in and out of the tub will also help to prevent falls. Sometimes a chair placed in the shower will enable the patient to bathe more easily.

Since the warm water and exertion of bathing may tire the patient or make him feel faint, be sure (1) that the bathroom door remains unlocked and (2) that you check on the patient every 5 minutes. If a patient should fall or feel faint do not leave him alone. Signal for help, using the emergency call button in the bathroom.

Procedure

ASSISTING WITH THE TUB BATH OR SHOWER

1. Wash hands and assemble the following equipment:
   - Soap
   - Washcloth
   - 2–3 bath towels
   - Bath blanket
   - Bath thermometer
   - Bath powder
   - Chair or stool
   - Patient's gown, robe, and slippers
   - Bathmat
2. Identify patient and explain what you plan to do.
3. Take the supplies to the bathroom and prepare it for the patient, Figure 17-1. Make sure the tub is clean.
4. Fill tub half full with water 95–105°F or adjust shower flow. If a bath thermometer is not available, the health assistant can test the water with an elbow. The water should feel comfortably warm.
5. Assist patient with robe and slippers.
6. Place a towel in the bottom of the tub to prevent patient from slipping.
7. Help the patient to undress. Give the male patient a towel to wrap around his *midriff*.
8. Assist the patient into the tub or shower.
9. Wash the patient's back. Observe the skin for signs of redness or breaks. See Unit 30 for information on caring for pressure sores or other skin lesions. The patient may be left alone to wash the *genitalia*. If the patient

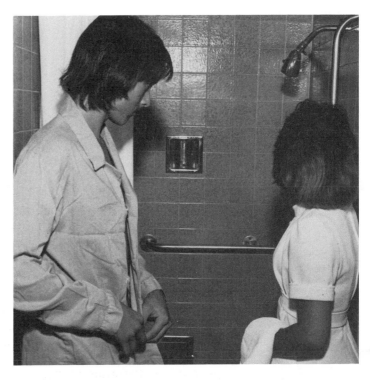

FIGURE 17-1. Preparing for a shower

shows any signs of weakness, remove the plug and let the water drain out, or turn off the shower. Allow the patient to rest until feeling better before making any attempt to assist him out of the tub or shower. Keep the patient covered with a bath towel to avoid chilling.

10. Hold the bath blanket around the patient who is stepping out of the tub. The male patient may choose to remove wet towel under bath blanket.
11. Assist the patient to dry, powder, dress, and return to the unit.
12. Return supplies to the patient's unit.
13. Clean the bathtub. Wash hands.
14. Report completion of task to nurse.
15. Record on chart:
    - Date
    - Time
    - Tub bath/shower
    - Patient's reaction

Procedure
GIVING A BED BATH

1. Wash hands and assemble the following equipment:
   - Bed linen
   - Bath blanket
   - Laundry bag or hamper
   - Bath basin: on filling, the water should be 105°F
   - Bath thermometer
   - Soap and soap dish
   - Washcloth
   - Face towel
   - Bath towel
   - Hospital gown or the patient's night clothes
   - Alcohol or lotion, powder
   - Equipment for oral hygiene
   - Nail brush and emery board
   - Brush and comb
   - Bedpan or urinal and cover
2. Identify patient and explain what you plan to do and how you can be assisted.
3. Make sure windows and door are closed to prevent chilling the patient.
4. Screen the unit.
5. Put towels and linen on chair in order of use. Place laundry hamper conveniently.
6. Offer bedpan or urinal (see Unit 18). Empty and clean before proceeding with bath. Wash hands.
7. Lower the back of the bed and the siderails if permitted.
8. Loosen top bedclothes. Remove and fold blanket and spread. Place bath blanket over top sheet and remove by sliding it out from under the bath blanket.
9. Leave one pillow under patient's head. Place other pillow on chair.
10. Remove patient's night wear and place in laundry hamper.
    a. Loosen gown from neck.
    b. Slip gown from free arm.
    c. Make sure patient is covered by bath blanket.
    d. Slip gown away from body toward arm with IV line in place.
    e. Gather gown at arm and slip downward over arm and line, being careful not to disturb line.
    f. Gather material of gown in one hand so there is no pull or pressure on line and slowly draw gown over tip of fingers.

g. With free hand, lift IV free of standard and slip gown over bottle. Be sure at no time to lower the bottle; raise the gown.

11. Fill bath basin two-thirds full with water 105°F.

12. Assist patient to move to the side of the bed nearest you.

13. Fold face towel over upper edge of bath blanket to keep it dry.

14. Form a *mitten* by folding washcloth around hand, Figure 17-2. Wet washcloth; wash eyes, using separate corners of cloth. Do not use soap near eyes.

15. Rinse washcloth and apply soap if patient desires. Squeeze out excess water.

16. Wash and rinse patient's face, ears, and neck well. Use towel to dry.

17. Expose patient's far arm. Protect bed with bath towel placed underneath arm. Wash, rinse and dry arm and hand. Repeat for other arm. Be sure *axillae* (armpits) are clean and dry. Apply deodorant and powder if patient requests them or needs them.

18. Care for hands and nails as necessary.
   a. Wash each hand carefully. Rinse and dry. Push *cuticle* (base of fingernails) back gently with towel while wiping the fingers.

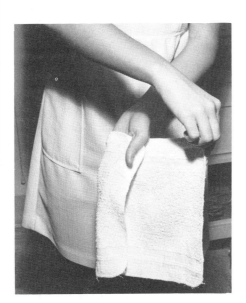
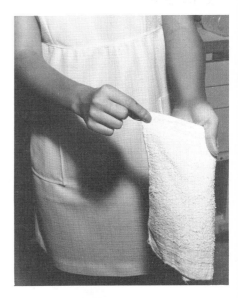
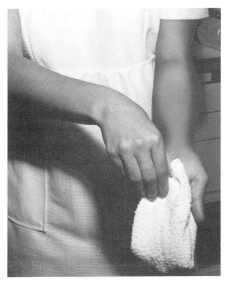

FIGURE 17-2. Making a washcloth "mitten"

   b. Clean under nails and shape with emery board. Be careful not to file nails too close. Do not cut nails if patient is diabetic. Inform the nurse if attention is needed.
19. Repeat procedure with near arm.
20. Put bath towel over patient's chest. Then fold blanket to waist. Under towel, wash, rinse, and dry chest. Rinse and dry folds under breasts of female patient carefully to avoid irritating the skin. Powder lightly if necessary. Do not allow powder to cake.
21. Fold bath blanket down to *pubic* area. Wash, rinse, and dry abdomen. Fold bath blanket up to cover abdomen and chest. Slide towel out from under bath blanket.
22. Ask patient to flex knee if possible. Fold bath blanket up to expose thigh, leg and foot. Protect bed with bath towel. Put bath basin on towel. Place patient's foot in basin. Wash and rinse leg and foot. When moving leg, support leg properly, Figure 17-3.
23. Lift leg and move basin to the other side of the bed. Dry leg and foot. Dry well between toes.
24. Repeat for other leg and foot. Take basin from bed before drying leg and foot.
25. Care for nails as necessary. Apply lotion to feet of patient with dry skin. File nails straight across. Do not round edges. Do not push back the cuticle because it is easily injured and infected.
26. Change water and check for correct temperature with bath thermometer. It may be necessary to change water before this point in the patient's bath if it becomes cold.
27. Help patient to turn on side away from you. Help him to move toward the center of the bed. Place bath towel lengthwise next to patient's back. Wash, rinse, and dry neck, back, and buttocks. Use long, firm strokes when washing back.
28. A back rub is usually give at this time (see Unit 18).
29. Help patient to turn on back.
30. Place a towel under the buttocks and upper legs. Place washcloth, soap, basin, and bath towel within convenient reach of the patient. Have pa-

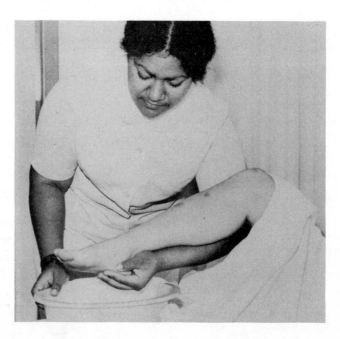

FIGURE 17-3.   Supporting the patient's leg

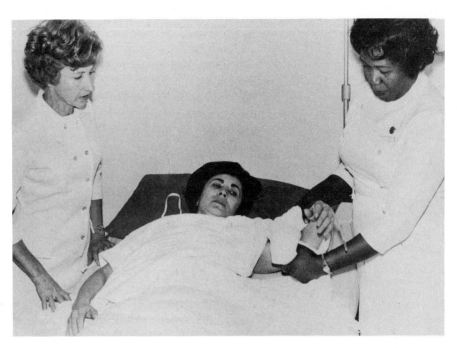

FIGURE 17-4. Note how the gown is gathered and guided toward the IV line.

tient complete bath by washing genitalia. Assist the patient if necessary. The health assistant must assume the responsibility for the procedure if the patient has difficulty. Many times patients are reluctant to acknowledge the need for help. If assisting a female patient, always wash from front to back, drying carefully. If assisting a male patient, be sure to carefully wash and dry penis, scrotum, and groin area.

31. Carry out range of motion exercises as ordered. (See Unit 33 for proper procedure.)
32. Cover pillow with towel and comb or brush hair. Oral hygiene is usually given at this time (see Unit 18).
33. Discard towels and washcloth in laundry hamper.
34. Provide clean gown.
    a. If the patient has an IV, gather the sleeve on the IV side in one hand.
    b. Lift the bottle free of the standard, maintaining height.
    c. Slip the IV bottle through the sleeve from the inside and rehang.
    d. Guide the gown alone the IV tubing to bed, Figure 17-4.
    e. Slip gown over hand. Do this very carefully so as not to disturb the infusion site.
    f. Position gown on infusion arm, then insert opposite arm. Remove gown by reversing procedure.
35. Clean and replace equipment according to hospital policy.
36. Put clean washcloth and towels in bedside stand or hang according to hospital policy.
37. Change the linen following occupied bed procedure. Replace and discard soiled linen in laundry hamper.
38. Leave patient in comfortable position. Place signal cord within reach of patient. Replace furniture. Leave unit in order. Wash hands. Turn out ceiling light, if used.
39. Report completion of the tasks and any important observations to the nurse.

Procedure

GIVING A PARTIAL BATH

Note: A partial bath assures cleaning of the hands, face, axillae, buttocks, and genitals. It is very refreshing and many patients will be able to help with the bath process and, whenever possible, should be encouraged to do so.

1. Wash hands and assemble the following equipment:
   - Bed linen
   - Bath blanket
   - Bath thermometer
   - Soap and soap dish
   - Washcloth
   - Face towel
   - Bath towel
   - Gown
   - Laundry bag or hamper
   - Bath basin—water 105°F
   - Alcohol or lotion, powder
   - Equipment for oral hygiene
   - Nail brush and emery board
   - Brush, comb, and deodorant
   - Bedpan or urinal and cover
   - Paper towels or protector
2. Identify patient and explain what you plan to do.
3. Make sure windows and door are closed to prevent chilling the patient.
4. Screen the unit.
5. Put towels and linen on chair in order of use. Place laundry hamper conveniently.
6. Offer bedpan or urinal (see Unit 18). Empty and clean before proceeding with bath. Wash hands.
7. Elevate head rest, if permitted, to comfortable position.
8. Loosen top bedclothes. Remove and fold blanket and spread. Place bath blanket over top sheet and remove by sliding it out from under the bath blanket.
9. Leave one pillow under patient's head. Place other pillow on chair.
10. Assist patient to remove gown and place in laundry hamper.
11. Place paper towels or bed protector on overbed table.
12. Fill bath basin two-thirds full with water 105°F and place on overbed table.
13. Push overbed table comfortably close to patient.
14. Place towels, washcloth, and soap on overbed table with easy reach.
15. Instruct patient to wash as much as he is able and that you will return to complete the bath.
16. Place call bell within easy reach. Ask patient to signal when ready.
17. Wash hands and leave unit.
18. Wash hands and return to unit when patient signals.
19. Change the bath water. Complete bathing those areas the patient couldn't reach. Make sure the face, hands, axillae, buttocks, back, and genitals are washed and dried.
20. Give a back rub with lotion or alcohol and powder.
21. Assist the patient in applying deodorant and/or powder and a fresh gown.
22. Cover pillow with towel and comb or brush hair. Assist with oral hygiene if needed (see Unit 18).
23. Clean and replace equipment according to hospital policy.
24. Put clean washcloth and towels in stand or hang according to hospital policy.
25. Change the linen following occupied bed procedure. Replace and discard soiled linen in laundry hamper.
26. Leave patient in comfortable position with siderails up and bed in lowest horizontal position. Place signal cord within reach of patient.
27. Replace furniture. Leave unit in order. Turn out ceiling light, if used.
28. Wash hands.
29. Report completion of the tasks and any important observations to the nurse.

Procedure

GIVING FEMALE PERINEAL CARE

1. Wash hands and assemble the following equipment:
   - Bath blanket
   - Bedpan and cover
   - Graduate pitcher
   - Cotton balls
   - Disposable gloves
   - Bed protector or bath towel
   - Ordered solution (if other than water)
   - Plastic bag to dispose of used cotton balls
   - Perineal pad and belt, if needed
2. Identify patient and explain what you plan to do.
3. Fill pitcher with warm water (or ordered solution) approximately 100°F and take to bedside.
4. Screen unit.
5. Lower siderail and position bed protector (or towel) under patient's buttocks.
6. Fanfold spread to foot of bed.
7. Cover patient with bath blanket and fanfold sheet to foot of bed.
8. Position patient on bedpan.
9. Put on disposable gloves.
10. Have patient flex and separate knees.
11. Draw bath blanket upward to expose perineal area only.
12. Unfasten perineal pad if in use. Touch only the outside. Note amount and color of discharge. Fold with the insides together and place in plastic bag.
13. Holding pitcher of water approximately 5 inches above the pubis, allow all the water to flow downward over vulva and into the bedpan.
14. Dry vulva using cotton balls in the following manner:
    a. Use each cotton ball once only and dispose of into plastic bag.
    b. Bring one or more cotton balls down one side of vulva from pubis to perineum until dry.
    c. Repeat on opposite side of vulva. Remember, use each cotton ball only once and discard.
    d. Dry area over center of vulva.
14. Remove and dispose of disposable gloves.
15. Ask patient to raise hips and carefully remove bedpan. Cover and place on chair.
16. Apply perineal pad if needed and secure to belt. Never touch fingers to inside of pad. Apply from front to back, then fasten belt.
17. Remove bath towel or disposable pad and dispose of according to hospital policy.
18. Draw sheet and spread up over patient and remove bath blanket.
19. Fold bath blanket and store in bedside stand.
20. Make patient comfortable and leave unit tidy.
21. Clean equipment and discard disposables according to hospital policy.
22. Wash hands.
23. Report completion of task and observations to the nurse.

Procedure

GIVING HAND AND FINGERNAIL CARE

Note: This procedure can be carried out independently or can be modified and incorporated with the bath procedure.
1. Wash your hands and assemble the following equipment:

• Basin	• Plastic protector
• Soap	• Nail clippers
• Bath towel	• Nail file
• Lotion	• Orangewood stick

2. Identify patient and explain what you plan to do.
3. Screen unit.
4. Elevate head of bed, if permitted, and adjust overbed table in front of patient. If patient is allowed out of bed, assist to transfer to a chair and position overbed table waist high across lap.
5. Place plastic protector over the bedside table.
6. Fill basin with warm water approximately 105°F and place on overbed table.
7. Instruct patient to put hands in basin and soak for approximately 20 minutes. Place towel over basin to help retain heat. Add warm water if necessary.
8. Wash hands. Push cuticles back gently with wash cloth.
9. Lift hands out of basin and dry with towel.
10. Use nail clippers to cut fingernails straight across. Do not cut below tips of fingers. Keep nail cuts on protector to be discarded.
11. Shape and smooth fingernails with nail file.
12. Pour small amount of lotion in your palms and gently smooth on patient's hands.
13. Empty basin of water. Gather equipment. Clean and store according to hospital policy.
14. Return overbed table to foot of bed. If patient has been sitting up for the procedure, assist into bed.
15. Lower head of bed and make patient comfortable. Leave call bell within easy reach. Make sure bed is in lowest position and siderails are up.
16. Leave unit tidy.
17. Wash hands.
18. Report completion of your task and any observations to the nurse.

Procedure
GIVING FOOT AND TOENAIL CARE

1. Wash hands and assemble the following equipment:
   - Wash basin
   - Soap
   - Bath mat
   - Lotion
   - Disposable bed protector
   - Bath towel/washcloth
   - Orangewood stick
2. Identify patient and explain what you plan to do.
3. If permitted, assist patient out of bed and into chair.
4. Place bath mat on floor in front of patient.
5. Fill basin with warm water (105°F). Put basin on bathmat.
6. Remove slippers and allow patient to place feet in water. Cover with bath towel to help retain heat.
7. Soak feet approximately 20 minutes. Add warm water as necessary. Lift feet from water while warm water is being added.
8. At end of soak period, wash feet with soap. Use wash cloth to scrub roughened areas. Rinse and dry. Note any abnormalities like corns or callouses.
9. Remove basin, covering feet with towel.
10. Use the orangewood stick to gently clean toenails. If nails are long and need to be cut, report this fact to the nurse. *Do not* undertake this task yourself.
11. Dry feet.
12. Pour lotion into palms of hands. Hold hands together to warm lotion and apply to feet.
13. Assist patient with slippers and to return to bed unless ambulatory.
14. Make patient comfortable.

15. Gather equipment, clean and store according to hospital policy. Leave unit tidy.
16. Wash hands.
17. Report completion of task and your observations to the nurse.

Procedure
GIVING A BED SHAMPOO

1. Wash hands and assemble the following equipment and supplies:
   • Shampoo tray—plastic sheeting which has the top and 2 sides rolled forming a drain may be used if regular tray is not available, Figure 17-5A.
   • Shampoo
   • Wash cloths

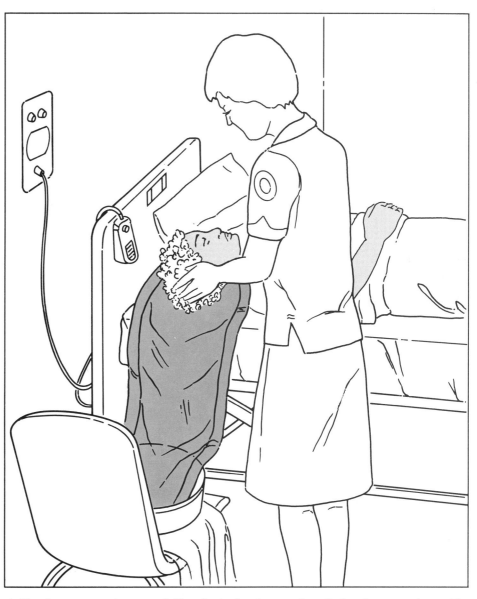

A. If a shampoo tray is not available, plastic sheeting may be rolled at the top and two sides to form a trough for the water.

FIGURE 17-5.

- 3 bath towels
- Bath blanket
- Basin of water (105°F)
- Safety pin
- 2 bed protectors
- Waterproof covering for pillow
- Large basin to collect used water
- Hair dryer if available (portable)
- Hairbrush and comb
- Small empty pitcher or cup
- Large pitcher of water (115°F)—use if additional water is needed

2. Screen unit.
3. Identify patient and explain what you plan to do.
4. Place chair beside head of bed. Cover seat with bed protector. Place large, empty basin on chair.
5. Arrange on bedside stand within easy reach:

   - Basin of water (105°)   • 2 bath towels
   - Pitcher of water (115°)   • Shampoo
   - Wash cloth   • Empty pitcher

6. Replace top bedding with bath blanket.
7. Ask patient to move to side of bed nearest you.
8. Replace pillow case with waterproof covering.
9. Cover head of bed with bed protector. Be sure it goes well under the shoulders.
10. Loosen neck ties of gown.
11. Place towel under patient's head and shoulders. Brush hair free of tangles, working snarls out carefully.
12. Bring towel down around patient's neck and shoulders and pin. Position pillow under shoulders so that head is tilted slightly backward.

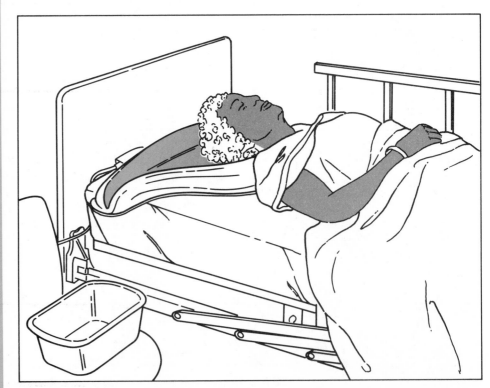

B. A shampoo tray or trough is placed under the patient's head when shampooing the patient's hair. The tray allows water to drain into the collecting basin.

FIGURE 17-5. Continued

13. Raise bed to high horizontal position.
14. Raise patient's head and position shampoo tray so that drain is over the edge of bed directly above basin in chair, Figure 17-5B.
15. Give patient wash cloth to cover eyes.
16. Recheck temperature of water in the basin. Using the small pitcher, pour a small amount of water over hair until thoroughly wet. Use one hand to help direct the flow away from the face and ears.
17. Apply a small amount of shampoo, working up a lather. Work from scalp to hair ends.
18. Massage scalp with tips of fingers. Do not use fingernails.
19. Rinse thoroughly, pouring from hairline to hair tips directing flow into drain. Use water from pitcher if needed but be sure to check temperature of water before use.
20. Repeat procedure a second time.
21. Lift patient's head. Remove tray and bed protector. Adjust pillow and slip a dry bath towel underneath head.
22. Place tray on basin and wrap hair in towel. Be sure to dry face, neck and ears as needed.
23. Dry hair with towel. If available and not otherwise counterindicated, a portable hair dryer may be used to complete the drying process. Brushing the hair as you blow dry facilitates drying. Be sure to keep the dryer moving and not too close to the hair.
24. Comb hair appropriately and remove protective pillow cover. Replace with cloth cover.
25. Lower height of bed to comfortable working position.
26. Replace bedding and remove bath blanket. Help patient assume a comfortable position and lower bed to lowest horizontal position. Allow patient to rest undisturbed. Length of procedure may tire patient.
27. Empty water from collection basin.
28. Clean equipment per hospital policy and return to proper area.
29. Be sure unit is left in proper order. Wash your hands.
30. Report and record procedure:
    - Bed shampoo
    - Patient's reaction

Summary

The bath is an important part of daily patient care and patients should be allowed to help as much as possible. The bath refreshes the patient. Range of motion exercises are usually performed following the bath procedure according to the patient's needs and orders. The health assistant is responsible for seeing that the bath is properly completed. The method of bathing will vary according to the condition of the patient. An order is required before a shampoo is given. However, it can contribute greatly to the cleanliness and comfort of the patient.

SUGGESTED ACTIVITY

1. Practice giving the bed bath and assisting with tub bath and shower.

VOCABULARY

Learn the meaning and correct spelling of the following words.

axillae	genitalia	pubic
cuticle	midriff	shampoo tray

UNIT REVIEW

A. Brief Answer. Answer the following questions.

1. Why should the cleansing bath be given daily to the bed patient if his condition permits?

2. Why should the patient help you with the bed bath as much as his condition permits?

3. How should the toenails be cut?

4. What is the assistant's responsibility when the patient is unable to complete his bath?

5. What other procedures may be carried out in conjunction with the bath procedure?

B. Clinical Situations. Briefly describe how a health care assistant should react to the following situations.

1. Your patient feels weak or faint during a tub bath.

2. You have not yet finished bathing the legs of a bed patient and the water feels cool.

3. Your patient is a diabetic and his toenails need cutting.

Unit 18 General Comfort Measures

OBJECTIVES

As a result of this unit, you will be able to:

- Assist the patient with personal hygiene.
- Give a back rub.
- Explain the use of comfort devices.
- Assist the patient with use of the bedpan, urinal, or commode.

There is much that you can do for your patients which will add to their general comfort and feeling of well-being. These include caring for *oral hygiene*, giving back rubs, brushing hair, and shaving male patients. Pillows and special equipment may also be used to make the patient more comfortable.

ORAL HYGIENE

Oral hygiene, or care of the mouth and teeth, should be performed at least three times a day. The patient should be allowed to do as much as possible for himself. Special oral hygiene is the cleansing of the mouth of the helpless patient, Figure 18-1, and is presented in this unit. Commercially prepared lemon and glycerine swabs are available for this purpose. A patient who is unconscious, has a high temperature, or breathes with his mouth open may require more frequent mouth care. Proper cleansing of the teeth and mouth will help prevent tooth decay (*caries*) and bad breath (*halitosis*).

Procedure

ASSISTING WITH ROUTINE ORAL HYGIENE

1. Wash hands and assemble the following equipment:
   - Toothbrush
   - Toothpaste or powder
   - Mouthwash solution in cup
   - Emesis basin
   - Paper bag
   - Bath towel
   - Drinking tube
   - Tissues
   - Cup of fresh water
2. Identify and tell patient what you plan to do.
3. Screen the unit.
4. Raise back of bed so that the patient may sit up if his condition permits.
5. Place bath towel over patient's gown and bedcovers.
6. Pour water over toothbrush and put toothpaste on brush. Brush patient's teeth carefully and thoroughly. Insert toothbrush into the patient's mouth with the bristles in a downward position. Turn toothbrush with bristles toward teeth and brush all tooth surfaces with an up-and-down motion.
7. Give patient water in cup to rinse his mouth. Use straw if necessary.

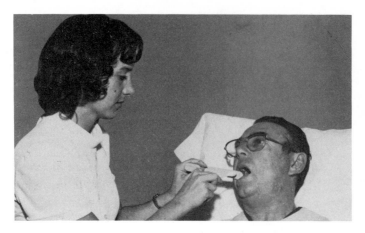

FIGURE 18-1.   Oral hygiene means care of the mouth and teeth.

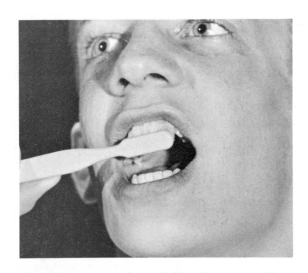

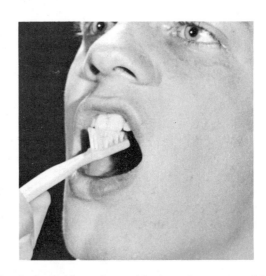

A. Brush the outer surfaces of all teeth, upper and lower.

B. Brush the inside surfaces of back teeth, upper and lower.

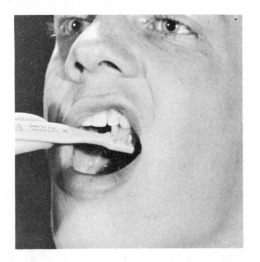

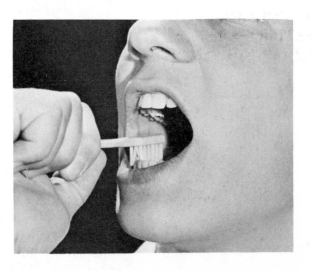

C. Brush the inside surfaces of front teeth, upper and lower.

D. Brush the chewing surfaces of upper and lower teeth.

FIGURE 18-2.   Brush the teeth as they grow and across the chewing surfaces. *(Photos courtesy of the American Dental Association.)*

Turn the patient's head to one side with emesis basin near chin for return of fluid.
8. Repeat steps 6 and 7 as necessary. Offer mouthwash.
9. Remove basin. Wipe mouth and chin with tissue. Discard in paper bag.
10. Remove towel.
11. Rinse toothbrush with water.
12. Clean and replace equipment according to hospital policy. Wash hands.

Procedure

ASSISTING WITH SPECIAL ORAL HYGIENE

1. Wash hands and assemble the following equipment:
   • Mouthwash or solution in cup or
   • Mixture of glycerine in lemon juice
   • Emesis basin
   • Bath towel
   • Paper bag
   • Applicators
   • Tissues
   • Tongue depressor
   • *Lubricant* for lips
2. Identify patient and explain what you plan to do.
3. Cover pillow with towel and turn patient's head to one side. Place emesis basin under patient's chin.
4. Open mouth gently with tongue depressor.
5. Dip applicators into mouthwash solution or glycerine mixture. (In some cases, a physician may order hydrogen peroxide solution.)
6. Using moistened applicators, wipe gums, teeth, tongue, and inside of mouth.
7. Discard used applicators in paper bag.
8. Lubricate lips with cold cream or petroleum jelly.
9. Clean and replace equipment. Wash hands.

Procedure

ASSISTING PATIENT TO BRUSH HIS TEETH

1. Wash hands and assemble the following equipment:
   • Emesis basin   • Mouth wash (if permitted)
   • Toothbrush   • Hand towel
   • Toothpaste   • Bed protector
   • Glass of cool water
2. Identify patient and explain what you plan to do to help. Screen unit.
3. Elevate the head of bed. Help patient into a comfortable position.
4. Lower siderails and position overbed table across patient's lap.
5. Cover table with plastic protector.
6. Place emesis basin and glass of water on overbed table.
7. Place towel across patient's chest.
8. Be prepared to help as patient brushes teeth.
9. After patient has brushed his teeth, push overbed table to the foot of the bed. Remove towel, fold and place on table. Help patient to assume a comfortable position and adjust bedding to leave the unit tidy.
10. Raise siderails.
11. Gather equipment. Clean and store according to hospital policy. Discard soiled linen in proper receptacle.
12. Wash hands.
13. Report completion of task and your observations to the nurse.

DENTURES AND EYEGLASSES

When a patient wears dentures, it is the assistant's responsibility to see that they are kept clean and do not become lost or broken. Extreme care must be used when handling dentures.

When the patient is not wearing them, dentures should be kept in the bedside table in a container labeled with the patient's name. Vulcanite dentures should be covered with mild antiseptic solution. Plastic dentures may be kept dry.

Dentures are cleaned in much the same way as natural teeth, with a toothbrush and denture toothpaste or powder. The container for the dentures should also be cleaned and filled with fresh antiseptic solution, if necessary, when the dentures are cleaned. The patient may feel embarrassed about wearing dentures. Therefore, the assistant should provide privacy when they are removed and cleaned. Allow the patient to rinse his mouth out with a gentle mouthwash before returning dentures.

Eyeglasses need special care and attention. They should be kept clean with special lens paper or soft, nonabrasive tissue. When not in use, they should be stored in their case in the bedside stand, within easy reach of the patient.

Procedure

CARING FOR DENTURES

1. Wash hands and assemble the following equipment:
   - Tissues
   - Emesis basin
   - Toothbrush or denture brush
   - Toothpaste or powder
   - Gauze squares
   - Denture cup
2. Tell the patient what you plan to do.
3. Screen the unit.
4. Allow the patient to clean dentures if able to do so. If the patient cannot, give tissue to patient and ask him to remove dentures. Assist if necessary.
5. Place dentures in denture cup padded with gauze squares. Take to bathroom or utility room.
6. Put toothpaste or tooth powder on toothbrush. Place dentures in palm of hand and hold them under a gentle stream of warm water. Brush

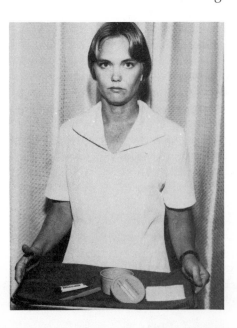

FIGURE 18-3. The emesis basin and box of tissues may be added from the bedside equipment in setting up the denture care tray.

until all surfaces are clean. Note: Dentures may be soaked in a solution with a cleansing tablet before brushing, if necessary.

7. Rinse dentures thoroughly under cold running water. Rinse denture cup.
8. Place fresh gauze squares in denture cup. Place dentures in cup and take them to bedside.
9. Assist patient to rinse mouth with mouthwash.
10. Use tissue or gauze to hand the wet dentures to patient. Insert if necessary.
11. Clean and replace equipment according to hospital policy. Wash hands.
12. Store dentures in a denture cup inside the bedside stand when not in use. Some patients prefer storing their dentures dry while others prefer to store their dentures in a special solution.

BACK RUBS

Unless contraindicated, the back rub is given routinely as part of the cleansing bed bath or partial bath. It may also be given following use of the bedpan or when changing the position of the helpless patient.

The assistant's nails should be kept short to prevent injuring the patient during the back rub. A good back rub takes from 3 to 5 minutes. When performed properly with long, smooth strokes, it stimulates the patient's circulation and aids in preventing decubiti. It is also soothing and refreshing.

Procedure
GIVING A BACK RUB

1. Wash hands and assemble the following equipment:
   • Basin of water (105°F)
   • Bath towel
   • Soap, alcohol, or lotion
   • Body powder
2. Tell the patient what you plan to do.
3. Screen the unit.
4. Place alcohol or lotion in basin of water to warm.
5. Turn the patient on his side with his back toward you.
6. Expose and wash the back.
7. Pour a small amount of lotion into one hand. Apply to the skin and rub with a gentle but firm stroke. Give special attention to all bony prominences. Rubbing alcohol may also be used in some cases, if ordered by a physician.
8. Begin at the base of the spine and with long, soothing strokes rub up the center, around the shoulders and down the sides of the back and buttocks, Figure 18-4. This procedure stimulates circulation over the bony prominences.
   a. Repeat this step four times, using the long, soothing upward stroke and a circular motion on the downstroke, Figure 18-5.
   b. Repeat, but on the downward stroke, rub in a small circular motion with the palm of the hand, Figure 18-6. Be sure to include area over coccyx.
   c. Repeat the long, soothing strokes to muscles for 3–5 minutes, Figure 18-7.
   d. Dry and apply powder.
   e. If pressure areas are noted, be sure to report to the nurse. (See Unit 30 for information on care and treatment of pressure sores.)
9. Straighten drawsheet.

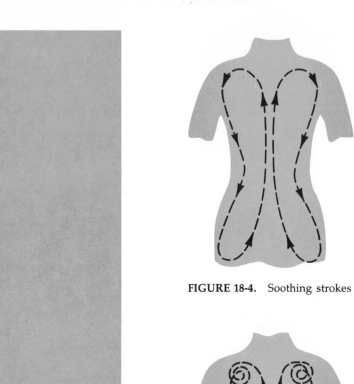

FIGURE 18-4.   Soothing strokes   **FIGURE 18-5.**   Circular movement

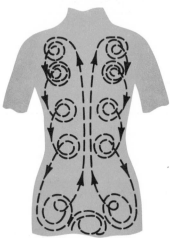

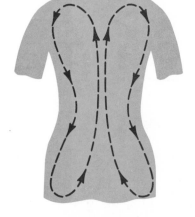

FIGURE 18-6.   Passive movement   **FIGURE 18-7.**   Soothing strokes

10. Change the patient's gown if needed.
11. Replace equipment. Wash hands.

DAILY SHAVING

Daily shaving is part of the routine self-care of most men and should not be neglected in the hospital. When patients are unable to shave themselves and a barber is not available, it is the assistant's responsibility, Figure 18-8. Use the patient's own shaving equipment if possible.

If the patient is receiving anticoagulants, an electric razor provides greatest safety. If oxygen is being given, it should be discontinued during this procedure, if possible; otherwise a safety razor should be used.

Procedure
SHAVING A PATIENT

1. Wash hands and assemble the following equipment:
   • Electric shaver or safety razor
   • Shaving lather or an electric preshave lotion
   • Basin of water (115°F)

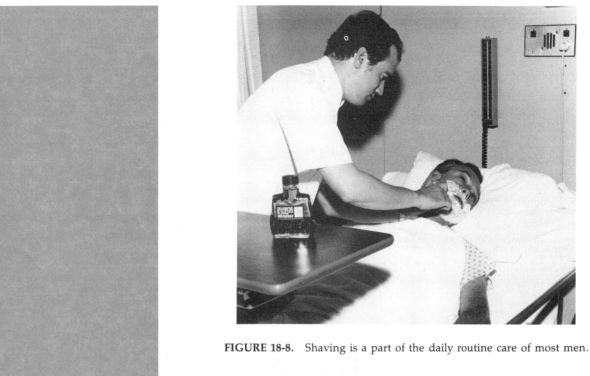

FIGURE 18-8. Shaving is a part of the daily routine care of most men.

- Face towel
- Mirror
- Aftershave lotion or powder
2. Identify the patient and explain what you plan to do. Let him help as much as possible.
3. Screen unit.
4. Raise the head of the bed. Place equipment on overbed table.
5. Place face towel across patient's chest.
6. Moisten face and apply lather.
7. Starting in front of the ear, hold skin taut and bring razor down over cheek toward chin. Repeat until lather on cheek is removed and area has been shaved. Repeat on other cheek. Use firm short strokes, rinsing razor frequently.
8. Lather neck area and stroke up toward the chin in a similar manner.
9. Wash face and neck and dry thoroughly.
10. Apply aftershave lotion or powder if desired.
11. If the skin is nicked, apply pressure directly over the area and then an antiseptic. Report incident to nurse.
12. Clean and replace equipment. Wash hands.

DAILY HAIR CARE

Daily care of the hair, for both male and female patients, is usually performed after the patient's bed bath. It involves brushing the hair which stimulates circulation of the scalp, refreshing the patient. It also removes dust and lint and helps to keep the hair shiny and attractive.

If additional care is needed, a fluid dry cleaner to shampoo the hair is available. It leaves the hair soft and manageable and the hair set intact. This procedure is so simple that it is often used instead of the regular shampoo for bed patients.

Sometimes, however, a shampoo may be advisable for the patient in bed. Approval for the procedure must be obtained from the doctor. Bed shampoos should be given every two weeks when the patient is bed bound for a protracted period.

The following procedure assumes that the patient is a female. Hair care for a male is very similar, however, so the procedure can easily be adapted.

Procedure
GIVING DAILY CARE OF THE HAIR

1. Wash hands and assemble the following equipment:
   - Towel
   - Comb and brush
   - Alcohol or petroleum jelly
2. Identify patient and ask her to move to the side of the bed nearest you or let the patient sit in a chair if permitted.
3. Screen the unit.
4. Cover the pillow with a towel.
5. Part or section hair and comb with one hand between scalp and end of hair.
6. Brush carefully and thoroughly.
7. Have patient turn so hair on the back of the head may be combed and brushed. If hair is snarled, working section by section, apply alcohol to oily hair or petroleum jelly to dry hair as needed. Unsnarl the hair, beginning near the ends and working toward the scalp. Gum may be removed with ice.
8. Complete brushing and arrange attractively. Braid long hair to prevent repeated snarling.
9. Clean and replace equipment according to hospital policy. Wash hands.

COMFORT DEVICES

Bed Cradle

The bed cradle, Figure 18-9, prevents the weight of the bedclothes from falling on some part of the body. It is used over fractured limbs, burns, and skin lesions. Coverings which maintain some degree of warmth within the cradle may also be needed to keep the patient comfortable. Lights may be suspended from a cradle to provide extra external head to promote healing. An order is required for this procedure.

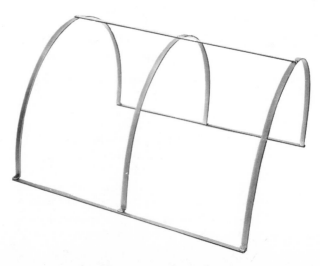

FIGURE 18-9.   The bed cradle

Footboard or Footrest

The footboard or footrest is a device placed between the mattress and bed to maintain the foot at right angles to the legs (natural standing position). It is used to prevent footdrop, a hazard when the patient must remain in bed over a long period of time. In footdrop, the muscle in the calf of the leg tends to tighten, causing the toes to point downward. Even a period of three weeks in bed is sufficient to cause a degree of footdrop which makes walking difficult when the patient does get out of bed.

Pillows

Pillows can be used as comfort devices when properly arranged. Figures 18-10 through 18-14 show different arrangements. Pillows are also used to relieve pressure. This technique is called *bridging*, Figure 18-15.

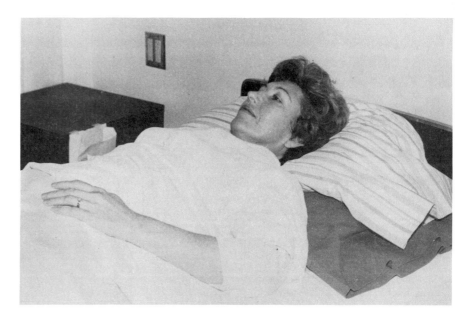

FIGURE 18-10. One pillow is placed crosswise under the patient's shoulders, and the other under her head.

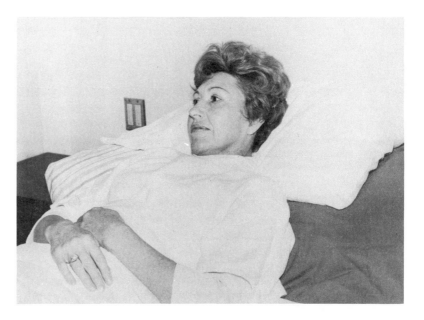

FIGURE 18-11. One pillow is placed lengthwise under each shoulder, and the third supports the patient's head.

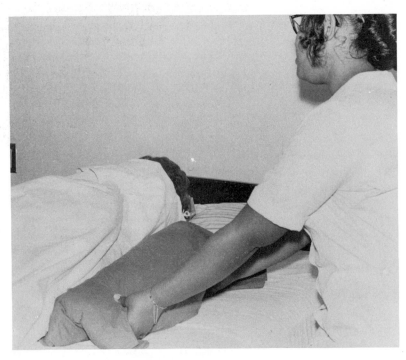

FIGURE 18-12. The patient is lying on her side, and a pillow is doubled over and placed lengthwise to support her back.

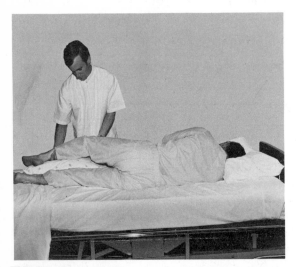

FIGURE 18-13. A pillow is placed under the uppermost leg to keep the pelvis in good position.

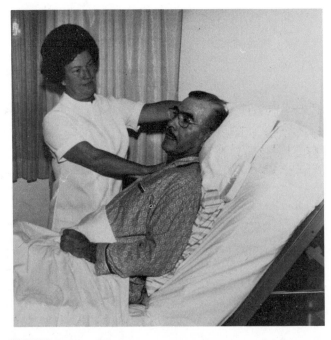

FIGURE 18-14. Pillows are used under the lower back and head for support.

ELIMINATION NEEDS

Regular, periodic elimination of body wastes is essential for maintaining health. Patients who are confined to bed must rely on the health care assistant to help them with this physical task. You will learn more about the *urinary system* and the *bowel* in Units 36 and 37. For now, you should know that the patient must regularly empty the bladder by *urinating*

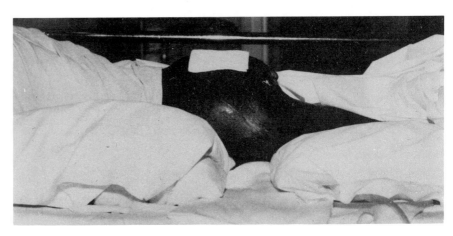

FIGURE 18-15. This patient is positioned on his abdomen and pillows are used to form a bridge, preventing pressure on his genitals.

or *voiding*. A urinal is used by male patients when they need to urinate, whereas a bedpan is used by female patients who are confined to bed.

A regular *bowel movement* (which is the discharge of solid waste from the body) is also important to a patient's health. You will be assisting your patients in this important physical process, too. The solid waste produced by the patient is called *feces* or *stool*.

Many patients are somewhat sensitive about using a bedpan or urinal. The health care assistant must provide privacy for the patient, and should try to make the patient as comfortable as possible during this procedure.

Personal hygiene is exceedingly important in carrying out these procedures properly. *Health care assistants mush wash their hands immediately before and after the procedure in order to prevent transmission of any disease to others.*

Procedure
GIVING AND RECEIVING THE BEDPAN

1. Wash hands; assemble the following equipment:
   - Bedpan and cover
   - Toilet tissue
   - Basin of warm water
   - Soap
   - Washcloth
   - Towel
2. Identify the patient and explain what you plan to do.
3. Screen the unit.
4. Lower the head of the bed.
5. Take the bedpan and tissue from the bedside stand and place the bedpan, Figure 18-16, on the bedside chair. Never place it on the side stand or overbed table. Put tissue on the bedside stand within easy reach of the patient. Put the remainder of the articles on the bedside table.
6. Place bedpan cover at the foot of the bed between the mattress and springs. The bedpan may be warmed by running hot water into it and emptying it. In hot weather, talcum powder may be used on the bedpan to prevent the patient's skin from sticking to it. Plastic bedpans may be comfortable without warming.
7. Fold top bedcovers back at a right angle and raise the patient's gown. Pad the bedpan with a folded towel if the patient is thin or has a pressure sore.
8. Ask patient to flex knees and rest weight on heels if able.
9. Help the patient to raise buttocks by putting one hand under the small of the patient's back and lifting gently and slowly with one hand. With the other hand, place the bedpan under the patient's hips. If the patient is unable to raise the buttocks, two assistants may be needed to lift, or the pan may be placed by rolling the patient to one side, positioning

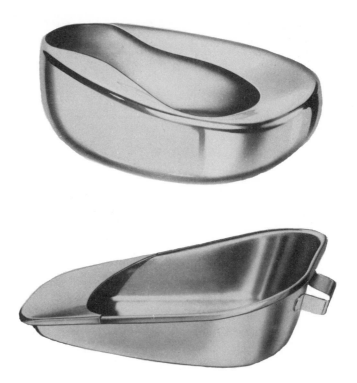

FIGURE 18-16.   Regular adult bedpan (top) and orthopedic bedpan (bottom).

the bedpan against the buttocks, and rolling the patient back on it, Figure 18-17. Alternatively, if a trapeze is in place over the bed, the assistant places the bedpan under the patient as the patient lifts herself using the trapeze, Figure 18-18. The patient's buttocks should rest on the rounded shelf of the bedpan. The narrow end should face foot of bed.

10. Replace top bedcovers. Raise the head of the bed to a comfortable height.
11. Make sure the signal cord is within easy reach of the patient. Leave the patient alone unless contraindicated.

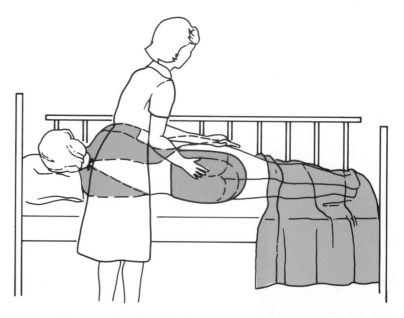

FIGURE 18-17.   The assistant rolls the patient away from her. She supports the patient with one hand on her hip and arm and places the bedpan with her other hand. Then she rolls the patient toward her and onto the bedpan.

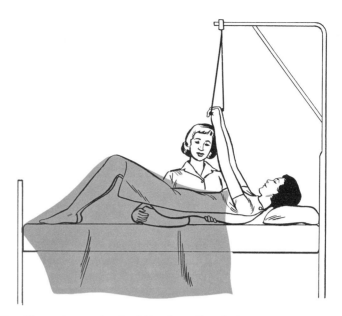

FIGURE 18-18. The patient assists by lifting herself with the trapeze as the assistant places the bedpan under her. Note that the assistant supports the patient's back with her hand.

12. Answer the patient's call signal immediately. Fill the basin with warm water and get soap, washcloth, and towel. Lower the head of the bed.
13. a. Ask the patient to flex knees and rest weight on heels. Place one hand under the small of the back and lift gently to help raise the buttocks off bedpan. Take the bedpan with the other hand. Cover it and place it on the chair.
    b. If the patient is unable to raise the buttocks, two assistants may be needed to lift. Otherwise, roll the patient off the pan to the side and remove the pan. Lift and move carefully. Hold the pan firmly with one hand.
    c. Many patients have difficulty cleaning adequately after using the bedpan. You may need to clean and dry the patient yourself.
14. Assist the patient to a clean area of the bed, if necessary. Discard tissue in bedpan unless specimen is to be collected. Cover the bedpan again and place on chair. Cleanse patient with warm water and soap, if necessary.
15. Replace bedclothes. Encourage the patient to wash hands and freshen up after the procedure. Change the linen or protective pads as necessary.
16. Take the bedpan to the bathroom or utility room and observe contents. Measure, if required.
17. Empty bedpan. Rinse with cold water and disinfectant; rinse, dry and cover the bedpan.
18. Put bedpan inside patient's bedside table. Clean and replace other articles.
19. Wash hands. Leave unit in order.
20. Report any unusual observations to your supervisor, and chart according to hospital policy.

Procedure

GIVING AND RECEIVING THE URINAL

1. Wash hands and assemble the following equipment:
   - Urinal and cover
   - Basin of warm water
   - Soap
   - Washcloth
   - Towel
2. Identify the patient and explain what you plan to do.

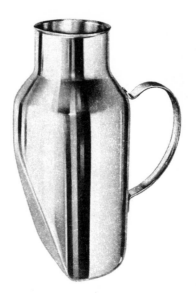

FIGURE 18-19.   Male urinal

3. Screen the unit.
4. Lift the top bedcovers and place the urinal under the covers so the patient may grasp the handle.
5. Make sure the signal cord is within easy reach of the patient. Leave the patient alone if possible.
6. Answer the patient's signal immediately. Fill a basin with warm water, and lay out the soap, washcloth and towel, so patient can wash and dry hands.
7. Ask the patient to hand the urinal to you. Cover it, and rearrange bedclothes if it is necessary.
8. Take the urinal to the bathroom or utility room and observe the contents. Measure, if required. Do not empty urinal if anything unusual (such as blood) is observed. Rather, save the contents of the urinal for your supervisor's inspection.
9. Empty the urinal. Rinse with cold water, and clean with warm soapy water. Rinse, dry, and cover urinal.
10. Place urinal inside patient's bedside table. Clean and replace other articles. Leave patient comfortable and unit tidy.
11. Wash your hands.
12. Report any unusual observations to supervisor, and chart according to hospital policy.

Procedure

ASSISTING WITH THE USE OF THE BEDSIDE COMMODE

1. Wash hands and assemble the following equipment:
   - Portable commode
   - Toilet tissue
   - Basin of warm water
   - Wash cloth and soap
   - Towel
2. Identify patient and explain what you plan to do.
3. Draw curtains for privacy.
4. Place tissue on bedside table within reach of patient.
5. Position commode beside bed—facing head. Lock wheels and remove cover. Be sure receptacle is in place under seat.
6. Lower siderails and bed to lowest horizontal position.
7. Assist patient to sitting position. Swing legs over edge of bed.
8. Put slippers on and assist patient to stand.
9. Have patient place his or her hands on your shoulders.

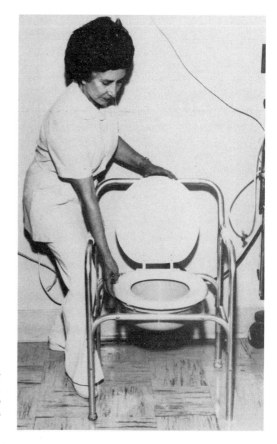

FIGURE 18-20. The bedside commode is convenient for patients who can sit up, but who cannot ambulate. Be sure to clean the receptacle promptly and keep the cover in place when not in use.

10. Support under the arms and pivot patient to the right and lower to commode.
11. Leave call bell and tissue within reach.
12. When patient signals, return promptly. Draw warm water in basin and bring to bedside along with soap, towel, and wash cloth.
13. Assist patient to stand.
14. Cleanse anus or perineum if patient is unable to help self.
15. Allow patient to wash and dry hands.
16. Assist patient to return to bed. Adjust bedding and pillows for comfort.
17. Put cover on commode.
18. Remove receptacle. Cover with bedpan cover.
19. Take to bathroom. Note contents and measure if required.
20. Empty and clean per hospital policy. Return to commode. Clean remainder of articles and return to their place.
21. Put commode in proper place (it will probably be kept in the corner of the room).
22. Wash hands.
23. Report completion of task. Indicate:
    • Any unusual observations
    • Record on appropriate record form.

Summary

There are several measures that the health assistant can take which will greatly add to the general comfort of the patient. These measures include care of the teeth and hair, shaving, and the use of specific devices.

Patients find that back rubs can be both soothing and stimulating when properly administered. Elimination needs must be promptly met, and the patient's need for privacy considered carefully.

SUGGESTED ACTIVITIES

1. Practice giving oral hygiene to a fellow student who is role playing being unconscious.

2. Practice brushing the teeth of other students to acquire skill.

3. Practice giving back rubs.

4. Practice cleaning dentures.

5. Practice procedure for shaving a male patient, using the Chase mannequin or a male classmate.

6. Set up for and give hair care to fellow students.

VOCABULARY   Learn the meaning and correct spelling of the following words.

bridging	dentures	lubricant
caries	halitosis	oral hygiene

UNIT REVIEW   **A. Brief Answer.** Answer the following questions.

1. Why is oral hygiene important?

2. How are dentures kept when the patient is not wearing them?

3. Why are frequent back rubs given to the patient who is not permitted out of bed?

4. Why should assistants keep their fingernails short?

5. Why should the skin be held taut while using the razor?

6. What should you do if you accidentally nick a patient during the shaving procedure?

7. What solution is used when there are snarls in oily hair?

8. Why should most patients be left alone when using a bedpan, urinal, or commode?

B. **Clinical Situations.** Briefly describe how a health care assistant should react to the following situations.

1. You note a pressure area on your patient's hip while giving a backrub.

2. Your patient needs a shave, but he is receiving oxygen, and the orders require that the oxygen be administered without interruption.

3. Your patient needs to use the bedpan, but cannot lift her buttocks off the bed.

Unit 19 Early Morning and Bedtime Care

OBJECTIVES

As a result of this unit, you will be able to:

• Demonstrate the procedures for early morning care.
• Demonstrate the procedures for bedtime care.
• Discuss the reasons for early morning and bedtime care.

WHEN CARE IS GIVEN

The patient is awakened before breakfast and given an opportunity to freshen up and go to the bathroom. This initial care is called early morning or AM care and helps to set the tone for the entire day. If the patient is refreshed and comfortable before eating breakfast, the day is off to a good start.

Patients should be awakened gently. Place your hand on the patient's arm and say his name. Never awaken a patient abruptly. Patients going to surgery or having tests that prohibit eating are not usually awakened early.

The care given to the patient just before bedtime is very similar to that given in the early morning. Bedtime care is also called PM care. A quiet, unrushed approach will help the patient settle down more easily for sleep. PM care should be completed before medication for sleep is given by the nurse.

Procedure
PROVIDING AM CARE

1. Wash hands. Awaken patient gently by placing your hand on the patient's arm and saying his name.
2. Tell the patient what you plan to do.
3. Screen the unit and elevate the bed if permitted.
4. Offer the bedpan or urinal. Save specimens if ordered (see Unit 39).
5. Routine vital signs (temperature, pulse, and respiration) may be taken at this time. See Section 8.
6. Provide wash water and toilet articles, Figure 19-1. Assist the patient if necessary.
7. Provide for care of mouth and hair (see Unit 18). Assist the patient as necessary.
8. Give back rub. Give special attention to pressure areas (see Unit 18).
9. Tighten the lower sheet and straighten the top linen.
10. Change the patient's gown if soiled.
11. Clear the overbed table and adjust the height of the bed if permitted so that breakfast may be served to the patient.
12. Leave fresh water and signal cord within reach of patient.
13. Wash hands.

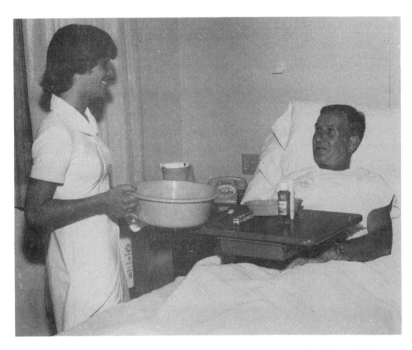

FIGURE 19-1.   Provide patients with wash water and toilet articles.

Procedure
PROVIDING PM CARE

1. Wash hands, identify patient, and explain what you plan to do.
2. If permitted, offer nourishment, Figure 19-2.
3. Screen the unit.
4. Offer bedpan or urinal.
5. Provide wash water and toilet articles. Assist with hair and mouth care as necessary (Unit 18).
6. Give back rub. Give special attention to pressure areas (see Units 18 and 30).
7. Tighten lower sheet. Then straighten the top linen.
8. Change patient's gown if soiled.
9. Push overbed table to foot of bed or place it parallel to the bed with water within reach. Put bed in lowest horizontal position and siderails up, Figure 19-3.

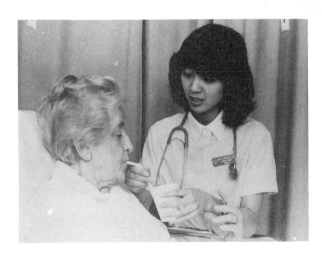

FIGURE 19-2.   Patients may be assisted in taking liquids during PM.

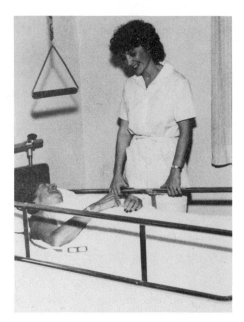

FIGURE 19-3. Siderails must be in position. Check to be sure they are secure.

10. Remove flowers and any unnecessary equipment from room according to hospital policy.
11. Leave fresh water and signal cord within reach of patient.
12. Wash hands.

Summary

Early morning care refreshes the patient before breakfast and prepares him for the day. A similar procedure is followed in the evening to help him relax and prepare him for sleep.

SUGGESTED ACTIVITY

1. Practice carrying out the procedures for AM and PM care.

UNIT REVIEW

A. Brief Answer.

1. The procedures for AM and PM care have much in common. How do they differ?

	AM	PM
Position of head of bed Siderails Overbed table		

2. Why is mouth care given before the patient has breakfast?

3. Why is a back rub given to the patient at bedtime?

4. How do you wake the patient?

B. Clinical Situations. Briefly describe how a health care assistant should react to the following situations.

1. You were giving PM care and the patient had flowers.

2. Your patient was scheduled for 9 AM surgery and you were assigned to give AM care to the patient in that room.

Section Seven
Self-evaluation

A. Choose the phrase which best completes each of the following sentences by encircling the proper letter.
  1. The proper temperature of bath water is
     a. 80°–90° F.
     b. 95°–105° F.
     c. 105°–115° F.
     d. 115°–120° F.
  2. Health care assistants are responsible for seeing to the completion of the patient's bathing
     a. if they feel like it.
     b. if the supervisor tells them.
     c. if the patient cannot.
     d. if the patient asks.
  3. When giving a bed bath, expose
     a. the entire body at one time.
     b. the part to be washed.
     c. both legs at one time.
     d. one whole side of the body.
  4. A female health assistant may refuse to wash the genitals of a helpless male patient
     a. because she doesn't want to be embarrased.
     b. because someone else will do it.
     c. because no one will know.
     d. No answer applies.
  5. If the patient is receiving an IV and his gown needs to be changed, the assistant will
     a. discontinue the IV.
     b. call the team leader to disconnect the IV.
     c. remove the patient's gown using the proper technique, keeping the IV flowing.
     d. cut the patient's gown off.
  6. Patients should be encouraged to help as much as possible during morning care because
     a. the assistant has many patients and the work will be done faster.
     b. it stimulates the patients general physiology.
     c. you don't want the patient to get too tired.
     d. No answer applies.
  7. A good back rub should take about
     a. 1 minute.
     b. 3–5 minutes.
     c. 10 minutes.
     d. 20 minutes.
  8. When not in the patient's mouth, dentures should be
     a. left on the bed.
     b. placed on the bedside table.
     c. placed in a container on bedside table.
     d. left on the bathroom shelf.
  9. When giving a bedpan or urinal always
     a. pad the receptacle.
     b. provide privacy.
     c. allow visitors to remain.
     d. disconnect the call bell.
  10. To waken a patient
     a. rap loudly on the door.
     b. call the patient's name loudly.
     c. gently place your hand on their arm.
     d. shake the patient vigerously.
  11. Bedtime care includes
     a. offering the bedpan.
     b. washing hands and face.
     c. giving a backrub.
     d. All of the above.

12. At bedtime flowers are sometimes removed from the room because
    a. they may be knocked over in the dark.
    b. its cooler in the hallways.
    c. it allows others to see them.
    d. they use up the oxygen in the room.
13. At bedtime the overbed table should be
    a. moved from the room.
    b. left in the bathroom.
    c. pushed to the foot of the bed.
    d. pushed close to the head of the bed.
14. Before the bath procedure
    a. tighten the bottom bedding.
    b. loosen the top bedding.
    c. place two pillows under the patient's head.
    d. remove the laundry hamper from the room.
15. When preparing to give a bed bath include in your supplies
    a. bed linen and gown.   c. lotion or powder.
    b. bath basin.   d. All of the above.

B. Match Column I with Column II.
   Column I   Column II
16. caries   a. artificial teeth
17. halitosis   b. toes involuntarily point down
18. dentures   c. dental cavities
19. foot drop   d. care given before breakfast
20. early (AM) care   e. care given before bedtime
                                       f. unpleasant breath

C. Answer the following questions true or false.
   21. Nail care is not part of the routine morning care.
   22. If a patient feels faint while taking a shower stay and signal for help.
   23. The bathtub need only be rinsed between patients.
   24. Bed shampoos may be given without a physician's order.
   25. A patient going to surgery at 8 AM should be wakened for breakfast.

Unit 20 Body Temperature

OBJECTIVES

As a result of this unit, you will be able to:

- Name and identify the three types of clinical thermometers and tell their uses.
- Read a thermometer.
- Demonstrate the procedure for using each type of clinical thermometer.
- Convert thermometer readings between Fahrenheit and Centigrade (Celsius).

The temperature, pulse, respiratory rate: known as TPR, and blood pressure readings are referred to as the patient's *vital signs*. Specific equipment is used to determine or measure these vital signs. They must be accurately taken because they tell us a great deal about the patient's condition. Never tell the patient the results: this is the physician's function. Each vital sign will be discussed in separate units, although they are usually determined as a combined procedure.

DEFINITION OF TEMPERATURE

Temperature is the measurement of body heat. It is the balance between the heat produced by the body and the heat that is lost. Normal body temperature is 98.6 degrees Fahrenheit or 37 degrees Celsius (or Centigrade).

Clinical Thermometers

A patient's temperature is determined by using a thermometer. Three types of glass clinical thermometers are in general use, Figure 20-2. They are the oral, security, and rectal thermometers. They differ mainly in the size and shape of the bulb, which is the end that is inserted into the patient. When only the security or stubby type is in use, the rectal thermometers are marked with a red dot at the end of the stem.

The electronic thermometer, Figure 20-3, is currently being used in some hospitals. It is battery-operated and registers the temperature on the viewer in a few seconds. The portion called the probe is inserted into the patient. The probes are colored red for rectal use and blue for oral use.

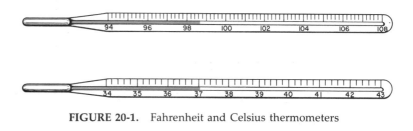

FIGURE 20-1. Fahrenheit and Celsius thermometers

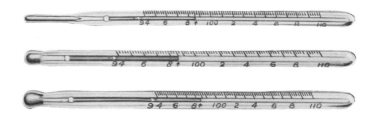

FIGURE 20-2. Clinical thermometers. From top to bottom: oral, security, and rectal.

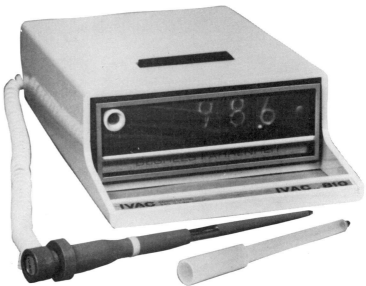

FIGURE 20-3. An electronic thermometer. The temperature is registered in large, easy-to-read numerals. The disposable, protective sheath is placed over thermometer tip. The tip is then inserted into patient's mouth in the usual manner. *(Photo courtesy of Ivac Corporation)*

The probe is covered by a plastic sheath before use which stays on during use and is discarded after use.

Plastic thermometers are used in some facilities. One unit can serve many patients by simply changing the disposable tips. The plastic thermometer has dots which are treated to change color from brown to blue according to the patient's temperature, Figure 20-4.

Reading the Thermometer

Mercury (the solid color line shown in Figure 20-5) in the bulb of the thermometer rises in the hollow center of the stem. To read the thermometer, hold it at eye level. Find the solid column of mercury. Look along the sharper edge between the numbers and lines. Starting with 94 degrees Fahrenheit (34 degrees Celsius or Centigrade), each long line indicates a 1-degree elevation in temperature. Only every other degree is marked with a number. In between each long line are four shorter lines. Each shorter

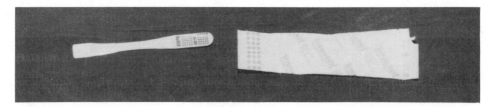

FIGURE 20-4. Look for changes in the color of the dots, indicating the temperature reading on plastic thermometers. The whole numbers represent whole degrees Fahrenheit. Each dot beside the whole number represents 0.2 of one degree. Read the whole number and add each dot which has turned from brown to blue as 0.2. For example, if four dots beside 99° have turned blue, the temperature would be 99.8°F.

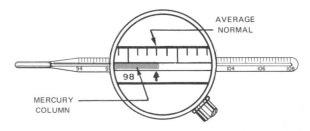

FIGURE 20-5. Reading a thermometer. This thermometer reads 98.6°F.

line equals two-tenths (2/10 or .2) of 1 degree. The thermometer is read at the point at which the mercury ends. If it falls between two lines, read it to the closest line.

Methods of Converting Temperatures

A formula can be used to convert temperatures from Celsius to Fahrenheit and from Fahrenheit to Celsius. See Figure 20-6 for some important equivalents and formulas for conversion.

METHODS OF TAKING TEMPERATURE

There are three methods of taking the temperature. They are:

- *Oral*—most common
- *Rectal*—most accurate (Rectal temperature registers 1 degree higher than oral.)

	CELSIUS (C)	FAHRENHEIT (F)
Freezing	0°	32°
Body Temp.	37°	98.6°
Pasteurization	63°	145°
Boiling	100°	212°
Sterilizing (Autoclave)	121°	250°

CONVERSION FORMULAS
F → C   C = 5/9 (F − 32)
C → F   F = 9/5 (C + 32)

For example: To convert a Celsius temperature of 100 to Fahrenheit, follow the procedure:

$$F = 9/5 \times 100 = \frac{900}{5} = 180 + 32 = 212°$$

For example: To convert a Fahrenheit temperature of 212 to Celsius, follow the procedure:

$$C = 5/9 (212 − 32) \quad 212 − 32 = 180 \times \frac{5}{9} = 100°$$

FIGURE 20-6. Formulas for converting Fahrenheit and Celsius temperature readings

• *Axillary* or *groin*—less accurate (This method is used only when the patient's condition does not permit the use of oral or rectal thermometers. Axillary temperatures register 1 degree Fahrenheit (or 0.6 degree Celsius) below oral temperature.)

The oral method to determine temperature is—as just said—the most common technique used. Special circumstances may make oral temperature taking inadvisable, however. If the patient is a child or irrational, a glass thermometer in the mouth could result in injury. Patients with respiratory problems, mouth breathers, or those who are very weak or unconscious may not be able to maintain the oral thermometer in their mouths for a period long enough to assure an accurate recording. In these situations a rectal thermometer inserted in the anus for the proper time is the best choice for temperature determination. Be sure to continuously hold the rectal thermometer.

When the mouth and anus are both unavailable for thermometer insertion, the axillary or groin area may have to be used.

Procedure

TAKING AN ORAL TEMPERATURE (GLASS THERMOMETER)

Note: To take oral temperatures accurately, wait 15 minutes for patients who have been smoking or drinking hot or cold liquids.
1. Wash hands and assemble the following equipment on a tray:
   • Container with clean thermometers
   • Container for used thermometers
   • Container for soiled tissues
   • Container with tissues
   • Pad and pencil
   • Watch with second hand
2. Identify patient and explain what you plan to do.
3. Have patient rest in a comfortable position in bed or chair.
4. Remove thermometer from container by holding stem end. Wipe with tissue and check to be sure the thermometer is intact. Read mercury column. It should register below 96 degrees F. If necessary, shake down. (To shake down, move away from table or other hard objects. Grasp stem tightly between thumb and fingers. Shake down with downward motion.)
5. Insert bulb end of thermometer under patient's tongue, toward side of mouth, Figure 20-7. Tell patient to hold thermometer gently with lips closed for 3 minutes.
6. Remove thermometer, holding by stem. Wipe from stem end toward bulb end.
7. Discard tissue in proper container.
8. Read thermometer and record on pad.

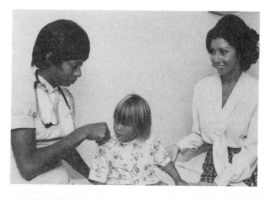

FIGURE 20-7.   The bulb end of the thermometer is inserted under the patient's tongue.

9. Place thermometer in container for used thermometers. If thermometer is to be reused for this patient, be sure to wash it in cold water and soap and dry it. Return it to the individual disinfectant-filled holder.
10. Clean and replace equipment according to hospital policy. Wash hands.
11. A record of the temperature is made on the patient's chart. Record on patient's chart as soon as possible for physician's information. Report any unusual variation in reading immediately to supervising nurse.

Procedure

TAKING AN ORAL TEMPERATURE (PLASTIC THERMOMETER)

Note: Latest findings indicate that temperature readings taken with this type of thermometer may not be entirely accurate.
1. Wash hands and obtain an unused packaged plastic thermometer.
2. Identify patient and explain what you plan to do.
3. Open package by grasping separated end (indicated by the words "open here").
4. Expose end of thermometer to be handled.
5. Remove thermometer from package but do not touch end to go in patient's mouth.
6. Place tip in patient's mouth under tongue in the usual manner.
7. Leave thermometer in place one minute.
8. Remove thermometer and read at once.
9. Dispose of thermometer per hospital policy. Wash hands.
10. Record temperature reading.

Procedure

TAKING AN ORAL TEMPERATURE (ELECTRONIC THERMOMETER)

1. Wash hands and assemble the following equipment:
   • Electronic thermometer
   • Sheaths
2. Identify patient and explain what you plan to do.
3. Cover probe (blue) with protective sheath.
4. Insert covered probe under patients tongue toward side of mouth.
5. Hold probe in position.
6. When buzzer signals temperature has been determined, take reading and record on pad.
7. Discard sheath in wastepaper basket. Do not touch sheath.
8. Return probe to proper position and entire unit to charging stand. Wash hands.
9. Record the temperature on the patient's chart and note the time it was taken. Report any unusual variations in reading to the supervising nurse.

Procedure

TAKING A RECTAL TEMPERATURE (GLASS THERMOMETER)

1. Wash hands and assemble equipment as for oral temperature, except use a rectal thermometer with rounded bulb end. Add lubricant.
2. Identify patient and explain what you plan to do.
3. Screen the unit.
4. Lower backrest of bed. Ask patient to turn on his side. Assist if necessary.
5. Place small amount of lubricant on tissue.
6. Remove thermometer from container by holding stem end and read mercury column. Be sure it registers below 96 degrees F. Check condition of thermometer.
7. Apply small amount of lubricant to bulb with tissue.
8. Fold the top bedclothes back to expose anal area.
9. Separate buttocks with one hand. Insert the thermometer gently into

rectum 1 1/2 inches. Hold in place. Replace bedclothes as soon as thermometer is inserted.

10. Thermometer should remain inserted for 2 minutes.

11. Complete procedure as given for oral temperature, steps 6 to 11.

12. Record an *R* beside temperature reading on the graph. Normal rectal temperature is 99.6°.

Procedure

TAKING A RECTAL TEMPERATURE (ELECTRONIC THERMOMETER)

1. Wash hands and assemble the following equipment:
   • Electronic thermometer
   • Red sheaths
2. Identify patient and explain what you plan to do.
3. Screen unit.
4. Lower backrest of bed. Ask patient to turn on his side. Assist, if necessary.
5. Place a small amount of lubricant on the tip of the sheath.
6. Fold the top bedclothes back to expose anal area.
7. Separate buttocks with one hand. Insert sheath-covered probe about one-half inch into rectum. Hold in place. Replace bedclothes as soon as thermometer is inserted.
8. Read temperature when registered on digital display.
9. Remove probe and discard sheath.
10. Assist the patient to a comfortable position.
11. Wash hands and return equipment to proper location.
12. Record the temperature reading on the graph.

Procedure

TAKING AN AXILLARY OR GROIN TEMPERATURE (GLASS THERMOMETER)

1. Wash hands and assemble equipment as for oral temperature. The procedure for taking temperature in the groin or axilla (underarm) is basically the same as taking temperatures in the mouth or rectum.
2. Identify patient and explain what you plan to do.
3. Wipe the area dry and place the thermometer. The patient's arm is kept close to his body if axillary site is used, Figure 20-8. Thermometer must be in the fold against the body if groin site is used. The thermometer is left in place 10 minutes.

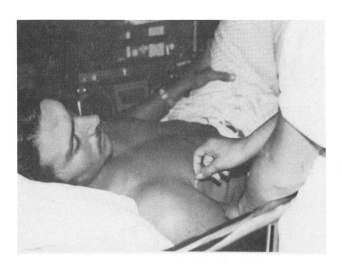

FIGURE 20-8.   Axillary thermometer in position

4. In recording the axillary temperature, place *AX* after the degree, such as 98 degrees *AX*. For a groin temperature use the abbreviation *GR*, as in 98 degrees *GR*. Normal axillary temperature is 97.6°.

Procedure

TAKING AN AXILLARY TEMPERATURE (ELECTRONIC THERMOMETER)

1. Wash hands and assemble equipment as for procedure using oral thermometer but substitute an oral electronic thermometer with an oral probe (blue) and disposable sheaths.
2. Identify the patient and explain what you plan to do.
3. Wipe axillary area dry and place covered probe in place. Keep patient's arm close to the body. Hold probe in place until temperature records on digital display.
4. Remove thermometer probe and dispose of sheath. Return equipment.
5. Wash hands and record axillary temperature, placing *AX* after the reading on the graphic chart.

Summary

Temperature, pulse, respiration, and blood pressure are considered vital signs. Equipment used to take vital signs include the clinical thermometers, stethoscope, blood pressure cuff, and watch with a second hand. Clinical thermometers can be identified by the shape of their bulbs. Electronic thermometers are also available. The procedures for properly taking temperatures and reading thermometers should be carefully followed.

SUGGESTED ACTIVITIES

1. Prepare a rectal thermometer tray for use.
2. Practice shaking down thermometers to below 96 degrees F.
3. Practice taking and reading oral temperatures. A glass of warm water may be used to vary thermometer readings. Students should check each other's readings.
4. Practice insertion of a rectal thermometer on the Chase mannequin.
5. Investigate the different types of thermometers used at your facility.

VOCABULARY   Learn the meaning and correct spelling of the following words.

axillary	Fahrenheit	rectal
blood pressure cuff	groin	stethoscope
Celsius	oral	vital signs

UNIT REVIEW   **A. Brief Answers.** Answer the following questions.

1. What method of taking temperature is the most common?

2. Which method of taking a temperature is the least accurate?

3. How can a rectal thermometer be distinguished from an oral thermometer?

4. How long should you wait to take an oral temperature after a patient has had something hot to drink?

B. Clinical Situations. Briefly describe how a health care assistant should react to the following situations.

1. You wish to take an oral temperature and your patient just drank a glass of water.

2. The rectal thermometer registers 98°F before insertion.

3. Your patient's temperature was 39°C and you need to record it in the chart in Fahrenheit degrees.

C. Identification. Identify the following thermometers.

1.

2.

3.

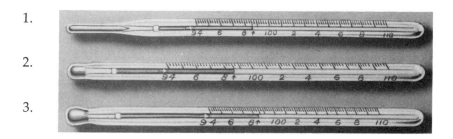

4.

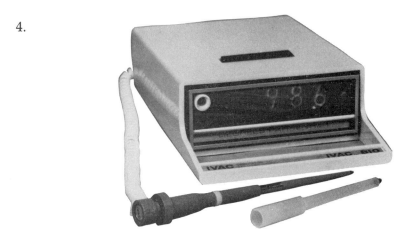

5.

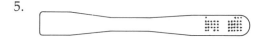

Unit 21 Pulse and Respiration

OBJECTIVES

As a result of this unit, you will be able to:

- Define what a pulse is.
- Locate the pulse areas.
- List the characteristics of the pulse and respiration.
- Take pulse and respiration of a patient.

The pulse and respiration of the patient are usually counted during the same procedure. Because breathing is partly under *voluntary* control, a person is able to stop or alter breathing temporarily for a short period. For example, when a patient realizes that his breathing is watched and being counted, he alters his breathing pattern without meaning to do so. To avoid this, the respirations are counted immediately following the pulse count without appearance of doing so. The patient's hand is kept in the same position, and your fingers remain upon the pulse, ostensibly still taking the pulse.

THE PULSE

Pulse is the pressure of the blood felt against the wall of an artery as the heart alternately beats (contracts) and rests (relaxes). It is more easily felt in arteries which come fairly close to the skin and can be gently squeezed against a bone by the finger. The pulse rate and its character provide a good indication of how the cardiovascular system is able to meet body needs.

Radial Pulse

Figure 21-1 shows the most common body sites for taking the pulse. You will usually take the pulse over the *radial artery*. The age, sex, size, and condition of the patient may influence the pulse *rate* (speed), *rhythm* (regularity), and *volume* (fullness). Rate and *character* (rhythm and volume) should be noted when taking the pulse. See Figure 21-2 for average pulse rates.

An unusually fast heartbeat is called *tachycardia*. An unusually slow heartbeat is called *bradycardia*. Both extremes should be reported immediately. Pulse rates under 60 or over 90 should be reported.

Procedure
TAKING A RADIAL PULSE

1. Wash hands and go to bedside. Identify patient and explain what you plan to do.
2. Place patient in a comfortable position. The palm of his hand should be down and his arm should rest across his chest, Figure 21-3.
3. Locate the pulse on the thumb side of the wrist with the tips of your first three fingers, Figure 21-4. Do not use your thumb since it contains a pulse which may be confused with the patient's pulse.
4. When pulse is felt, exert slight pressure. Use second hand of watch

212

and count for 1 minute. It is the practice in some hospitals to count for one-half minute and multiply by 2 and to record the rate for 1 minute. A 1 minute count is preferred.

5. Wash hands.
6. Record the rate and character of the pulse.

Apical Pulse

The surge of blood along the arteries as the ventricles contract is felt as the pulse, unless the contraction is too weak and the flow too little. This condition is frequently seen in patients with congestive heart failure where the heart contracts more often than a radial pulse can detect accurately. Therefore, an apical pulse is usually the more accurate way to check this type of heart rate. The difference between the approximate apical pulse and the radial pulse is called the *pulse deficit.*

An apical pulse is taken by placing the stethoscope over the tip (apex) of the heart. This may be found on the left side of the front of the chest between the fifth and sixth ribs or just below the left nipple. Listen carefully and two sounds will be heard. The louder sound corresponds to the contraction of the ventricles pushing the blood forward through the arteries

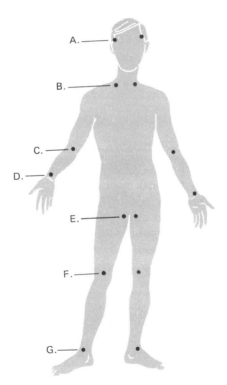

FIGURE 21-1.   Pulse sites in the body. A—temporal (at side of forehead); B—carotid (at the neck); C—brachial (inner aspect of the forearm); D—radial (inner aspect of the wrist, above the thumb); E—femoral (inner aspect of the upper thigh); F—popliteal (behind knee); G—dorsalis pedis (top of foot arch). *(From Simmers,* Diversified Health Occupations, *1983, Delmar Publishers Inc.)*

Adult men:	60–70	beats per minute
Adult women:	65–80	beats per minute
Children over 7 years:	72–90	beats per minute
Children 1 to 7 years:	80–120	beats per minute
Infants:	110–130	beats per minute

FIGURE 21-2.   Average pulse rates

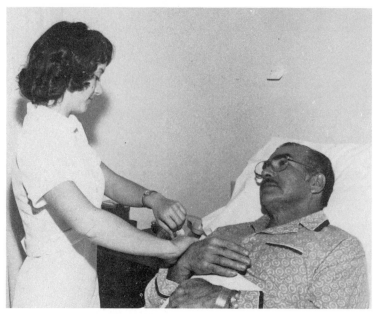

FIGURE 21-3.   Patient's position for taking pulse

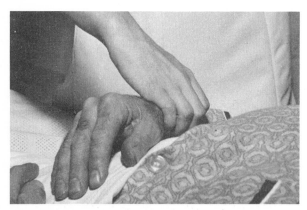 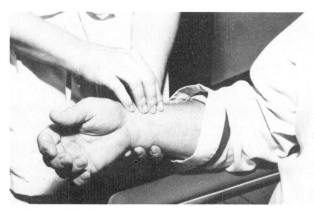

FIGURE 21-4.   The correct position of the hand for taking the pulse. The photo on the right shows how the assistant should place her fingers.

and the closing of the valves to prevent the back flow of blood; this is the sound to be counted. The softer sound corresponds to the relaxation of the ventricles as they fill with blood prior to the next contraction and the closing of the valves to prevent back flow from the arteries.

Apical heart rates are also checked before specific medicines are given which profoundly affect heart rate, and routinely in children whose rapid rates might be difficult to count at the radial artery.

Procedure

TAKING AN APICAL PULSE

1. Wash hands and take stethoscope to bedside. Identify patient and explain what you plan to do.
2. Place the stethoscope earpieces in your ears.
3. Place the stethoscope diaphragm or bell over the apex of the heart. (The apex is the lowest point of the heart and can easily be located near the left nipple or under the left female breast.)
4. Listen carefully for the heartbeat.
5. Count the beats for one minute.
6. Check radial pulse for one minute. Another health assistant may take the radial pulse at the same time the apical pulse is being checked, Figure 21-5.

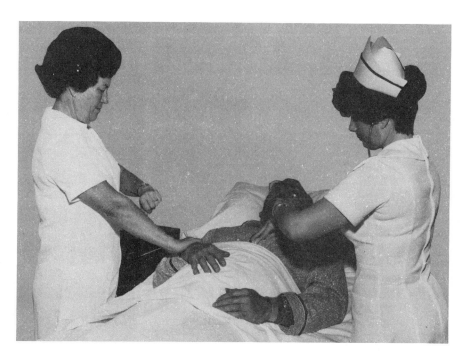

FIGURE 21-5. Checking the apical and radial pulse rates

7. Compare the results. Chart the apical pulse over the radial pulse. For example: $\dfrac{A108}{R82}$. Be sure to indicate character as well as rate differential.

Pulse deficit may also be charted in this way as 26 (108 − 82 = 26).

8. Return stethoscope. Wash hands.

RESPIRATION

The main function of respiration is to supply the cells in the body with *oxygen* and to rid the body of excess *carbon dioxide*. When respirations are inefficient, carbon dioxide accumulates in the bloodstream making the skin "dusky," bluish, or *cyanotic*.

There are two parts to each respiration; one *inspiration* (inhalation) followed by one *expiration* (exhalation). *Dyspnea* describes difficult or labored breathing. A period of no respirations is known as *apnea*. Periods of dyspnea followed by apnea are called *Cheyne-Stokes* respirations. At times fluid *(mucus)* will collect in the air passages, giving rise to characteristic bubbling type of respiration called *rales. Rales* are common in the dying patient.

The character of respirations must be noted as well as rated. Respirations are described as normal, shallow, deep, labored, or difficult. Rate is determined by counting the rise or fall of the chest for 1 minute with a watch equipped with a second hand. The normal rate for adults is 14 to 18 per minute. If the rate is more than 25 per minute, it is said to be accelerated and should be reported.

Procedure
COUNTING RESPIRATIONS

1. When the pulse rate has been counted, you may leave your fingers on the radial pulse and start counting the number of times the chest rises and falls during 1 minute.
2. Note depth and regularity of respirations.
3. Record the time, rate, depth, and regularity of respirations, Figure 21-6.

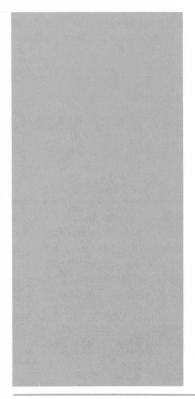

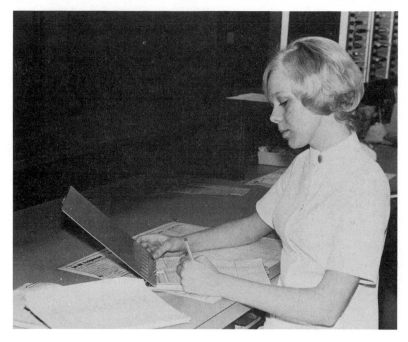

FIGURE 21-6.   TPR may be recorded in a notebook. Information is then transferred to the graphic chart and, sometimes, to the nursing notes.

Summary

The pulse and respiratory rates are usually counted as a continuous procedure. The patient should be unaware that the respiratory rate is being determined. The character of the respirations and pulse as well as the rate should be noted. Determination of vital signs is one of the most common nursing procedures.

SUGGESTED ACTIVITIES

1. Practice taking the pulse in groups of three. One student acts as the patient. A second student takes the pulse at the right radial artery, and a third takes the pulse at the left radial artery simultaneously. Compare the two rates.

2. Practice locating pulses in other areas of the body.

3. Practice counting respirations of fellow students: Two students count the respirations of a third student simultaneously. Compare rates of respiration. Retake respiration after the student has run in place in class. Note the change.

4. Practice counting the apical pulse while another student counts the radial pulse.

VOCABULARY   Learn the meaning and correct spelling of the following words.

accelerated	cyanosis	radial artery
apical pulse	dyspnea	rales
apnea	expiration	rate
bradycardia	inspiration	rhythm
carbon dioxide	mucus	tachycardia
character	oxygen	volume
Cheyne-Stokes respirations	pulse defect	voluntary

UNIT REVIEW   **A. Brief Answer.** Answer the following questions.
1. Over what artery is the pulse usually taken?

2. What are the normal pulse rates of the following?
   a. Adult male _____ beats per minute.
   b. Adult female _____ beats per minute
   c. Child (1–7 years) _____ beats per minute
3. What is an abnormally slow heartbeat called?

4. What is an abnormally fast heartbeat called?

5. What is the normal number of respirations per minute for an adult?

6. Why should the patient be unaware of the procedure when respirations are counted?

B. Clinical Situations. Briefly describe how a health care assistant should react to the following situations.
1. The patient's pulse is 110 and weak.

2. You determined that your patient's pulse seemed irregular and weak and the nurse says she suspects a pulse defect.

C. Completion.
1. The character of the respirations may be described as normal, _____, _____, _____, or _____.
2. The equipment needed to determine an apical pulse is a watch with a second hand and a _____.

Unit 22 Blood Pressure

OBJECTIVES

As a result of this unit, you will be able to:

- Demonstrate the use of the stethoscope.
- Demonstrate the use of the sphygmomanometer.
- Take patient's blood pressure and record.
- Select the proper size blood pressure cuff.
- List precautions associated with use of the sphygmomanometer.

DEFINITION OF BLOOD PRESSURE

Blood pressure is the fourth vital sign. The *systolic* pressure is the greatest force exerted on the walls of the artery by the heartbeat, and the *diastolic* is the least force. Blood pressure is measured by means of a *sphygmomanometer* and a *stethoscope*. Blood pressure is the difference between systolic and diastolic readings.

Blood pressure depends upon the volume (amount) of blood in the circulatory system, the force of the heartbeat, and the condition of the arteries. Arteries which have lost their *elasticity* (stretch) give more resistance, and so the pressure is greater. Blood pressure is also increased by exercise, eating, *stimulants* (substances that speed up body functions) and emotional disturbance. It is decreased by *fasting* (not eating), rest, *depressants* (drugs which slow down body functions) and hemorrhage (loss of blood).

In resting adults, any reading between 100 and 140 mm Hg. systolic and 60 and 90 diastolic is considered normal. Blood pressure rises slightly with age. High blood pressure (greater than 140/90) is called *hypertension*. Low blood pressure (below 100/70) is called *hypotension*. Hypertension can lead to a stroke. Hypotension can lead to shock. In either case, unusual or changed findings must be reported.

EQUIPMENT

The sphygmomanometer consists of a cuff with a bladder (rubber) inside and two tubes, one connected to the pressure control bulb and the other to the pressure gauge. The gauge may be a round dial or a column of mercury, Figures 22-1 and 22-2. Both are marked with numbers. Be sure to use a cuff of the proper size. Cuffs which are too wide or too narrow will give inaccurate readings, Figure 22-3. The width of the cuff should measure approximately two-thirds the diameter of the patient's arm.

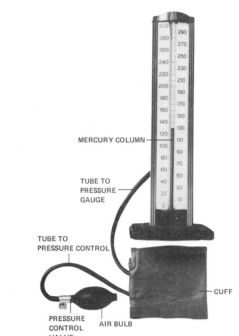

MERCURY COLUMN

TUBE TO
PRESSURE
GAUGE

TUBE TO
PRESSURE CONTROL

CUFF

PRESSURE
CONTROL
VALVE   AIR BULB

FIGURE 22-1.   The mercury gravity sphygmomanometer

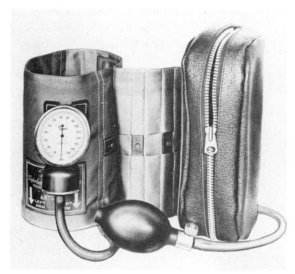

FIGURE 22-2.   The aneroid manometer

HOW TO READ THE GAUGE

The gauges are marked with a series of large lines at 10 mm (milli-meter) intervals. In between the large lines are shorter lines, each of which indicates 2 mm. The first small line above 80 mm is 82 mm. The small line below 80 mm is 78 mm, Figure 22-4. The gauge should be at eye level when reading for accuracy. The mercury column gauge must not be tilted. The reading is taken at the top of the column of mercury, not at the "hump" in the middle of the mercury.

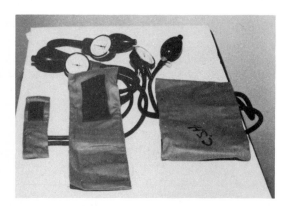

A. Blood pressure cuffs come in various sizes.

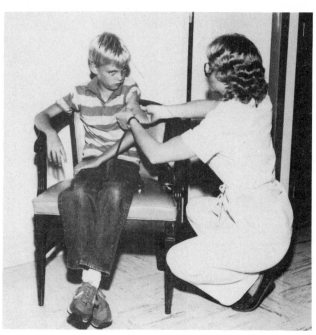

B. The wrong size cuff will cause an inaccurate reading.

FIGURE 22-3.

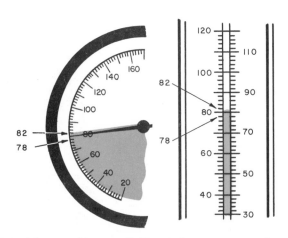

FIGURE 22-4.   The aneroid gauge (left) and the mercury gravity gauge (right)

Procedure

TAKING BLOOD PRESSURE

1. Wash hands and collect the following equipment:
   - Sphygmomanometer
   - Stethoscope (Clean earpieces with antiseptic solution.)
2. Identify patient and explain what you plan to do.
3. Place the patient's arm palm upward and supported on bed or table. The same arm should be used for all readings. Note: Do not attempt to take a blood pressure in the arm that has an IV tube or that is injured.
4. Roll sleeve of gown up about 5 inches above elbow. Be sure it is not tight on the arm.
5. Apply the cuff above the elbow and directly over the *brachial artery*.
6. Wrap the rest of the armband smoothly around the arm. Tuck the ends under a fold, hook to secure, or use the Velcro closure. Be sure cuff is secure but not too tight.

7. Locate the brachial artery with the fingers. The brachial artery is located on the inside of the arm (medial aspect) just inside the elbow (antecubital space), Figure 22-5. Place earpieces in ears. Place stethoscope directly over the artery, Figure 22-6.
8. Close valve attached to hand pump (air bulb) by turning it clockwise. Inflate cuff until indicator registers 20 mm above where pulse ceases to be heard. (Pump and pause to listen.)
9. Open valve of pump and let air escape slowly until the first heart sound is heard.
10. At this first sound, note reading on manometer. This is *systolic pressure*.
11. Continue to release the air pressure slowly until there is an abrupt change of the sound from very loud to soft. The reading at which this change is heard is the diastolic pressure. In some hospitals, the last

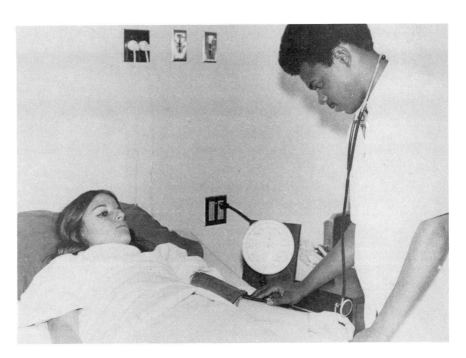

FIGURE 22-5. Using your fingers, locate the brachial artery on the inner aspect of the arm when the palm is turned up.

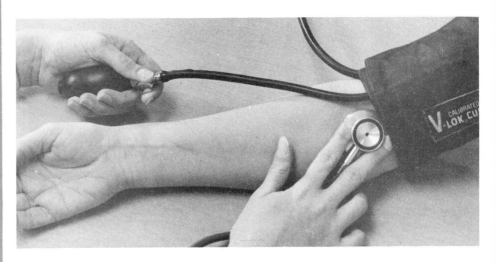

FIGURE 22-6. Place the stethoscope over the brachial artery. (*From Simmers,* Diversified | Health Occupations, *1983, Delmar Publishers Inc.*)

sound heard is taken as *diastolic pressure*. If repeat procedure is necessary, completely deflate cuff, wait one minute and begin again.

12. Remove cuff, expel air from the cuff, and replace apparatus. Clean earpieces of stethoscope with antiseptic solution.

13. Wash hands.

14. Record the time and the blood pressure. The blood pressure is recorded as an inverted or improper fraction. For example, 120/80 means that 120 is the systolic pressure and 80 is the diastolic pressure. Remember, the pulse pressure is the difference between the systolic and diastolic pressures. In this example it is 40.

Summary

Blood pressure, the fourth vital sign, must be determined accurately. The assistant takes the systolic and diastolic pressures at the same time, watching the pressure gauge and listening with a stethoscope.

A recording of the reading is made in inverted fraction form. The systolic reading is placed over the diastolic reading. Unusual readings should be rechecked after one minute and reported.

SUGGESTED ACTIVITIES

1. Practice handling the air release valve until you can manage this operation smoothly.

2. Practice taking blood pressure readings on other students. Compare readings taken while student is: lying down, sitting in a chair, and after running in place.

3. Investigate the procedure and specific type of equipment used for taking blood pressure at your hospital.

VOCABULARY

Learn the meaning and correct spelling of the following words.

brachial artery	fasting	sphygmomanometer
depressant	hypertension	stimulant
diastolic	hypotension	systolic
elasticity	stethoscope	

UNIT REVIEW

A. Clinical Situations. Briefly describe how a health care assistant should react to the following situations.

1. You are not exactly sure you heard the first systolic beat.

2. You determined that the patient's blood pressure was 180/140.

B. Completion. Complete the following sentences.

1. The systolic sound is _____.
2. The diastolic sound is _____.
3. A systolic sound of 140 and a diastolic sound of 80 would be recorded as _____.
4. The difference between systolic and diastolic readings is called the _____.
5. a. Blood pressure is _____ (increased, decreased) by rest.
   b. Blood pressure is _____ (increased, decreased) by stimulants.

6. Blood pressure depends on the volume of _____, the force of _____, and the elasticity of the _____.
7. Another name for the blood pressure apparatus is _____.
8. The brachial artery is located _____.
9. The earpieces of the stethoscope are cleaned with _____ after use.
10. Blood pressure is measured in _____.

Section Eight
Self-evaluation

A. Choose the phrase which best completes each of the following sentences by encircling the proper letter.

1. To read a thermometer properly, you should
   a. hold it straight up and down.
   b. hold it by the bulb.
   c. hold it at eye level.
   d. turn it rapidly.

2. When a patient has just finished a cool drink, it is best to
   a. wait 15 minutes to take the temperature.
   b. take the temperature right away since the mouth will be moist.
   c. omit the temperature until next time temperatures are regularly taken.
   d. take the temperature by the axillary method.

3. In order to take the patient's pulse accurately you will need
   a. a pencil and pad.
   b. a watch with a second hand.
   c. an oral thermometer.
   d. lubricant.

4. When you take a rectal temperature, remember to
   a. hold the thermometer in place.
   b. lubricate the tip.
   c. use a rectal thermometer.
   d. All of the above.

5. When patients have individual thermometer holders by the bedside, remember to
   a. replace the thermometer directly into the solution.
   b. wash the thermometer before putting it back into the solution.
   c. lubricate the thermometer before inserting it into the patient's mouth.
   d. None of the above.

6. To take an axillary temperature accurately, the thermometer must be in place
   a. 2 minutes.
   b. 20 minutes.
   c. 3 minutes.
   d. 10 minutes.

7. The respirations are best counted
   a. without letting the patient know.
   b. while the patient is eating.
   c. while the patient is talking.
   d. after telling the patient what you plan to do.

8. The most common place to take the pulse is at the
   a. temple.
   b. bend in the elbow.
   c. wrist.
   d. knee.

9. The pulse of an adult male patient is 72 beats per minute. You quickly realize this rate is
   a. too fast and must be reported.
   b. too slow and must be reported.
   c. about average for an adult.
   d. about average for a young child.

10. The function of respiration is
    a. to circulate blood.
    b. bring oxygen into the body.
    c. rid the body of carbon dioxide.
    d. Both b and c.

11. When taking blood pressure, it is important that the
    a. mercury column or dial be at eye level.
    b. armband is smooth and tight.
    c. stethoscope is placed over the radial artery.
    d. mercury column or dial be tilted.

B. Read the temperatures on the thermometers.

12. _____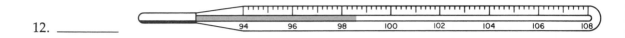

13. _____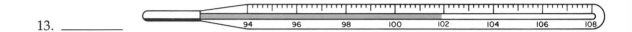

14. _____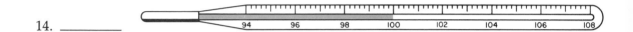

15. _____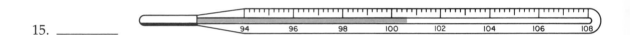

C. Complete the following statements correctly:
16. To indicate on a graphic chart that the temperature has been taken other than orally, you should _____.
17. The following equipment is needed to determine vital signs: _____
_____.
18. Four areas, other than the wrist, where the pulse may be taken are _____
_____.
19. The three types of clinical thermometers in general use are: _____
_____.

D. Match Column I with Column II.

Column I	Column II
20. bubbling respirations	a. bradycardia
21. abnormally slow pulse rate	b. systolic
22. rate of pulse	c. radial
23. very rapid respirations	d. rhythm
24. the highest blood pressure reading	e. volume
25. difficult respirations	f. diastolic
	g. tachycardia
	h. speed
	i. dyspnea
	j. apnea
	k. rales
	l. accelerated

Unit 23 Nutritional Needs and Diet Modifications

OBJECTIVES

As a result of this unit, you will be able to:

- List the four basic hospital diets.
- Name the four basic food groups and list the foods included in each group.
- Feed the helpless patient.
- Use various methods of providing fresh water for the patient.

Nutrition is the entire process by which the body takes in food for growth and repair and uses it to maintain health. The signs of good nutrition include: shiny hair, clear skin and eyes, a well-developed body, an alert expression, a pleasant disposition, and healthy sleep and appetite.

NORMAL NUTRITION

Food is normally taken into the body through the mouth, which is the beginning of the digestive tract. *Digestion* is the process of breaking down foods into simple substances that can be used by the body cells for nourishment.

ALTERNATIVE NUTRITION

When there is disease of the digestive tract or other reasons why food cannot be taken in the normal way, it is necessary to bypass the digestive tract. The essential *nutrients* are given directly to the patient's body through the veins. Remember, this is called an *intravenous infusion* or IV.

The speed at which the IV solution enters the patient's body is called the *flow rate*. The flow rate (rate of flow measured in drops per minute) is ordered by the doctors, Figure 23-1. Know and check the flow rate on patients receiving IVs. Report to the nurse if the drip chamber is full or if the flow rate is slower or faster than ordered or if the drip has stopped. Actual determination of the flow rate is the responsibility of the nurse.

Nutrients may also be provided through a tube leading through the

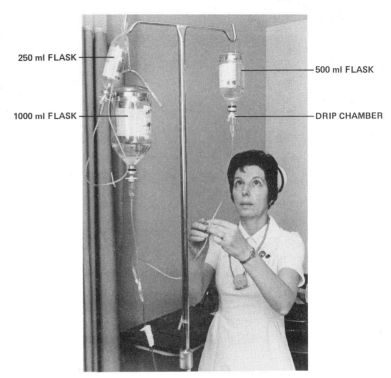

FIGURE 23-1. The nurse establishes the IV flow rate per doctor's orders. Any alteration should be reported. This type of set-up is called a piggy back.

nose and down into the stomach called a *nasogastric tube,* Figure 23-2, or by using a tube leading from the outside directly into the stomach: called a *gastrostomy tube.* Foods are blended into a liquid form and then introduced into the body through the tube. Tube feeding—which is known as gavage—requires special skill to be sure of the correct location of the tube so the nurse will carry out this procedure.

Nurses will also start and monitor intravenous infusions and change bottles or bags when necessary. Be alert to bottles or bags that are nearly empty and call this to the attention of the nurse before the fluid runs out.

ESSENTIAL NUTRIENTS

To be well nourished, we must eat foods which (1) supply heat and energy, (2) build and repair body tissue, and (3) regulate body functions. These foods are called nutrients. The six nutrients essential to maintain health are: *proteins, carbohydrates, fats, minerals, vitamins,* and *water.*

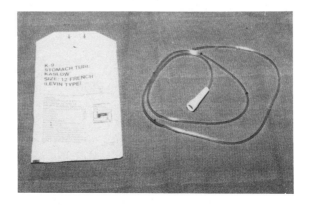

FIGURE 23-2. The nasogastric tube is introduced through the nose and into the stomach.

Protein

Protein is an essential nutrient because it is the basic material of every body cell and it is the only nutrient that can make new cells and rebuild tissue. The foods which contain the greatest amount of protein come from animals. They include meat, fish, poultry, eggs, milk, and cheese.

Carbohydrates and Fats

Carbohydrates and fats are called energy foods because the body uses them to produce heat and energy. When a person eats more energy foods than the body needs, the remainder is stored as fat. Foods which contain the greatest amount of carbohydrates come from plants. They include fruits and vegetables and foods which are made from fruits and vegetables, such as bread, cereals, and macaroni products. Carbohydrate foods also supply the body with roughage (cellulose) which is important in maintaining bowel regularity. Fats come from both plants and animals. Examples of foods rich in fat include butter, pork, nuts and egg yolk.

Vitamins and Minerals

Vitamins are substances that regulate body processes. You probably know them by their letter names: A, B-complex, C, D, E, and K. Vitamins help to build strong teeth and bones, promote growth, aid normal body functioning, and strengthen resistance to disease.

Minerals help to build body tissues, especially bones and teeth. They also regulate body fluids such as blood and digestive juices. The minerals we need in our daily diet include calcium, phosphorus, iodine, iron, and copper. Vitamins and minerals are present in a wide variety of foods.

THE BASIC FOUR FOOD GROUPS

A balanced diet includes the proper amounts of the essential nutrients. The Basic Four Food Groups serve as a guide for selecting balanced meals, Figure 23-3. Although individual food habits usually originate from national or religious customs, the foods used fall into the Basic Four Food Groups.

Vegetables and Fruits

Select four or more servings. Include dark green or yellow vegetables and citrus fruit or tomatoes.

LEAFY, GREEN, AND YELLOW VEGETABLES. Use vegetables raw, cooked, frozen, or canned. This group provides vitamin A, calcium and iron. Leafy green vegetables furnish riboflavin and niacin, which are both B vitamins.

One or More Servings Daily

asparagus: green	mustard greens
beans: snap, green, lima	okra
broccoli	parsley
brussels sprouts	peas: green
cabbage: green	peppers: green and red
carrots	pumpkin
chard	spinach
collards	squash: winter
endive: green	sweet potatoes
escarole	turnip greens
kale	wild greens
lettuce: leaf	other greens including salad greens

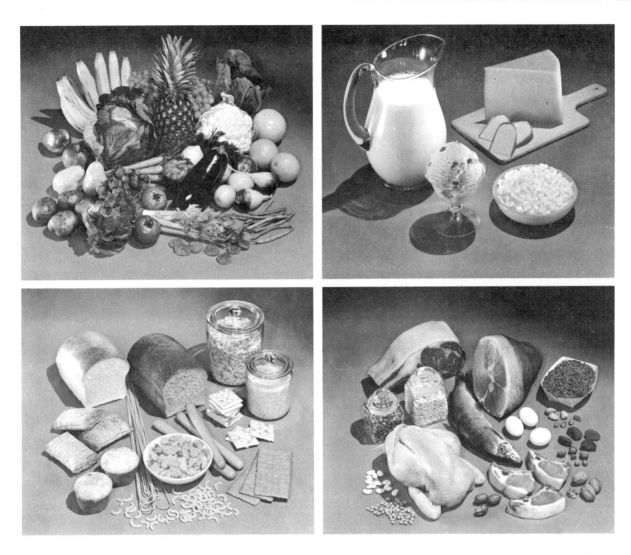

FIGURE 23-3. The basic four food groups: vegetables and fruits, dairy foods, breads and cereals, and meat *(Photos courtesy of the National Dairy Council).*

CITRUS FRUIT, TOMATOES, AND RAW CABBAGE. This group consists of foods high in vitamin C. It also provides vitamin A and the B-complex vitamins. The leafy green vegetables listed provide some iron and calcium.

One or More Servings Daily

broccoli	limes
cabbage: raw	peppers: green, raw
cantaloupe (muskmelon)	oranges
grapefruit	strawberries: raw
grapefruit juice	pineapple: raw
greens: salad	tangerines
kumquats	tomatoes and juice
lemons	turnips: raw

POTATOES AND OTHER VEGETABLES AND FRUITS. Use foods in this group raw, cooked, frozen, canned or dried. When eaten in fairly large amounts, foods in this group provide thiamine, vitamins A and C, calcium and phosphorus.

Two or More Servings Daily

apples	currants	pineapple juice: canned
apricots	dates	plums
artichokes	eggplant	potatoes
avocados	figs	prunes
bananas	grapes	radishes
beets	leeks	raisins
berries	lettuce: head	rhubarb
cabbage: white	mushrooms	rutabaga
cauliflower	onions	salsify (oysterplant)
celery	parsnips	sauerkraut
cherries	peaches	squash: summer
corn: sweet	pears	sweet potatoes
cranberries	persimmons	turnips
cucumbers	pineapple: canned	

Dairy Foods

Children should have three or four glasses of milk daily; teenagers need four or more glasses. Adults should drink two or more glasses. Cheese, ice cream and other milk-made foods can be substituted for part of milk requirement.

This group provides calcium, phosphorus, riboflavin, protein, vitamin A, and fat. Pregnant women should drink at least one quart of milk, or the nutritional equivalent, daily. Nursing mothers should increase the amount of milk in their diet to 1-1/2 quarts daily.

The following dairy foods contain calcium equal to that in one cup of milk and may be substituted for milk:

Milk Substitutes

1 ounce cheddar-type cheese	12 ounces cottage cheese
4 ounces cream cheese	2 to 3 scoops of ice cream

Milk is available in the following forms:

whole milk	evaporated milk	buttermilk
skim milk	condensed milk	dried milk

Breads and Cereals

Select four or more servings. Enriched or whole grain foods with added milk improves nutritional values.

This group provides carbohydrates, thiamine, niacin, iron, and roughage.

Four or More Servings Daily

breads: whole wheat, dark rye, enriched cornmeal, whole grain enriched, or oatmeal

rolls or biscuits made with whole wheat or enriched flour

flour: enriched, whole wheat, other whole grain

grits, enriched cereals: whole wheat, rolled oats, brown rice, converted rice, other cereals, if whole grain or restored

noodles, spaghetti, macaroni

Meat Group

Select two or more servings daily. Alternate dried beans, peas or nuts. These are an incomplete protein.

This group provides protein, some fat, iron, phosphorus, and B-complex vitamins.

One Serving Daily (meat, poultry, fish)

beef	mutton	veal
lamb	game	

pork (except bacon and fatback)
variety meats: liver, heart, kidney, brains, tongue, sweetbreads, tripe
poultry: chicken, duck, goose, turkey
fish, shellfish
lunch meats, such as bologna

Two or More Servings Weekly

dried beans	nuts	soybeans
dried peas	peanuts	soya flour and grits
lentils	peanut butter	

Four or More Servings Weekly (eggs)

BASIC HOSPITAL DIETS

The food you will serve in the hospital will be prepared by the dietary department and will include the essential nutrients. The way in which it is prepared and its consistency will depend on the individual patient's condition and needs. Sometimes very strict dietary control is needed. Special *therapeutic* or treatment diets will be discussed later.

Hospitals usually have four standard diets. They are regular, or house, liquid, soft, and light. The trays will have labels indicating the type of diet, but you should learn to recognize the types of food allowed in these diets to avoid any mistakes. Always double-check the tray before you serve it.

Regular Diet

The regular-select, or house diet is a normal diet, based on the Basic Four Food Groups. It includes a great variety of foods and excludes only the very rich: pastries, heavy cakes, fried foods, and highly seasoned foods, which might be difficult for inactive people to digest. Because an inactive person does not require as many calories as the active person, the calorie count may be somewhat lower than in the normal diet. In many hospitals,

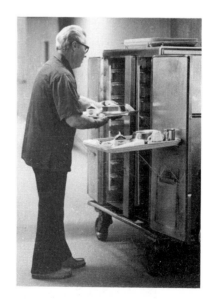

FIGURE 23-4. The food service department prepares and delivers food to the patient care units.

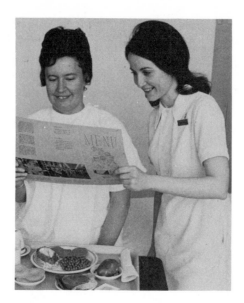

FIGURE 23-5. The select menu allows patients on a regular diet to make individual choices.

patients are given a daily menu from which they may select the foods they desire, Figure 23-5.

Liquid Diets

CLEAR LIQUID DIET. The clear liquid diet consists of liquids that do not irritate, cause gas formation, or encourage bowel movements *(defecation)*. It replaces fluids which may have been lost by vomiting or diarrhea. It is temporary because it is an inadequate diet composed mainly of water and carbohydrates for energy. Feedings are given every 2, 3, or 4 hours as prescribed by the physician. The foods allowed are:

tea, coffee with sugar but without cream
strained fruit or vegetable juice with gelatin (occasionally)
fat-free meat broths
ginger ale (usually) or 7-Up

FULL LIQUID DIET. The full liquid diet does supply nourishment and may be used for longer periods of time than the clear liquid diet. It is given during acute infections, to patients who have difficulty chewing, and to those who have conditions which involve the digestive tract. It includes all of the foods allowed on the clear liquid diet in addition to the following:

strained cereal (gruel)	malted milk
strained soups	milk and cream
sherbet	plain ice cream
gelatin	strained vegetables and fruit juices
eggnog	junket

Six to eight ounces are usually given every two to three hours.

Soft Diet

The soft diet usually follows the full liquid diet. It includes liquids and semi-solid foods that have a soft texture and are easily digested. It is given to patients with infections and fevers, those who have difficulty chewing, and those with conditions which involve the digestive tract. The foods allowed on the soft diet are low-residue, which are almost completely used by the body. The foods are also mildly flavored, slightly seasoned or unseasoned and prepared in a form that is easily digested. Although this diet nourishes the body, between-meal feedings are sometimes given to increase the calorie count. The following foods are usually allowed on the soft diet:

soups
cream cheese and cottage cheese
crackers, toast
fish
white meat of chicken or turkey (boiled or stewed)
fruit juices
cooked fruit (sieved)
tea, coffee
milk, cream, butter
cooked cereals
eggs (not fried)
beef and lamb (scraped or finely ground)
cooked vegetables (mashed or sieved)
angel or sponge cake
small amounts of sugar
gelatin, custard
pudding
plain ice cream

Foods to be avoided are:
coarse cereals
spices
gas-forming foods (onions, cabbage, beans)
rich pastries and desserts
foods high in roughage
fried foods
raw fruits and vegetables
corn

Light Diet

The light or convalescent diet is an intermediate stage between the soft and the regular diets. It is used for convalescent patients, for those with minor illnesses, and sometimes for preoperative or postoperative patients. It differs from the regular diet only in the method of preparing the food. Because digestibility of food is of prime importance, foods should be baked, boiled, or broiled rather than fried. Rich, spicy, and coarse foods should be avoided. The following foods are allowed on the light diet:

soft diet foods
broiled or baked lean meat
fruits, except those high in cellulose
vegetables, except those high in cellulose
refined cereals
any bread except bran
desserts, except the rich pastries
butter, cream, bacon
small amounts of sweets
tea, coffee

Foods to be avoided are:
rich pastries
heavy salad dressings

fried foods
coarse cereals
pork (except bacon)
vegetables and fruits high in cellulose

SPECIAL DIETS

Standard diets are modified to conform with special dietary requirements. For example, an order might be written for a low sodium soft diet when a patient has poor dentures and heart disease.

Three commonly prescribed special diets are the diabetic diet, the sodium-restricted diet and the calorie-restricted diet. Figure 23-6 gives a partial listing of some special diets that are ordered.

The Diabetic Diet

Diet is an integral part of the therapy of the patient with diabetes mellitus. Some physicians prescribe a very carefully balanced diet and insulin which maintains the level of blood sugar (glucose) within normal limits. The diet requires the weighing of all foods and repeated injections of insulin. Other physicians are much more liberal in their approach, permitting an unmeasured diet, limiting only sugar and high-sugar foods.

Most physicians treat diabetes with an approach which is midway between the former two methods. They prescribe the *exchange method* of diet planning, based on standard household measurements. Sugar or high sugar content foods are excluded to prevent rapid blood swings.

The diet is nutritionally adequate and provides enough energy in the form of calories for a 24-hour period. The exchange list is based on milk, vegetables in groups A and B, fruit, bread, and meat. Selections are allowed from each of these groups and patients are allowed to make equivalent substitutions within each group.

Accurate evaluation and reporting of intake is important since insulin administration may be dependent upon your observations.

Sodium-restricted Diet

Sodium-restricted diets may be ordered for patients with chronic renal failure and cardiovascular disease.

Diabetic	Amounts of carbohydrates, fats, and proteins are balanced and prescribed. Concentrated sweets are restricted.
Low Sodium (Sodium Restricted)	Amounts of sodium specifically prescribed such as 500 mg. sodium. Sodium rich foods such as milk and bacon or salted nuts are excluded.
Calorie Restricted	Limits the number of calories while balancing nutrients.
Low Fat	Foods with high fat content restricted such as whole milk and eggs. Eliminates use of fats in preparation of food.
Antianemic	High in protein, iron and vitamins, served in six small meals per day. Hot, spicy foods excluded.
Low Residue	Roughage, fresh fruits and vegetables (except bananas and potatoes), nuts, and whole grains are limited.

FIGURE 23-6.   Special diets

Meat, fish, poultry, milk and milk products, and eggs all contain relatively large levels of sodium. Cereals, vegetables, and fruits have relatively low levels of sodium. Processing foods may add significant levels of sodium. These factors are considered in planning the sodium-restricted diet. Diets may be prescribed which are moderately, mildly, or severely restricted in sodium content. This latter diet is one of the most difficult for patients to follow. Patients need to be taught to read labels and look for "hidden" sources of sodium.

Calorie-restricted Diet

Calorie-restricted diets are prescribed for patients who are overweight. They are planned to meet general nutritional needs and takes into consideration the patient's energy output, general nutritional state, and weight goal.

Providing activity remains constant, a person must take in approximately 500 calories a day less than usual (3,500 calories deficit per week) to lose one pound.

In planning the calorie-restricted diet, 20 percent of the diet should come from protein sources such as lean meat, poultry, fish, and low-fat cheeses. The exact amount of fats and carbohydrates are not uniformly prescribed, but fats may account for 35 percent while 45 percent comes from carbohydrates.

A realistic balance between fats, proteins and carbohydrates is more apt to encourage the formulation of better, more consistent food intake habits.

Some physicians use a factor of 10 calories multiplied by the desired weight in calculating the daily calorie requirements. For example, if the desired weight is 120 pounds, the patient would be placed on a 1200 calorie per day diet.

SUPPLEMENTARY NOURISHMENTS

Serving between-meal nourishments is an important function of the assistant. Milk, juice, gelatin, custard, or plain ice cream is served usually in the midmorning, midafternoon, and before bedtime. Wash your hands before you start.

Check the nourishment list of each patient for any limitations on supplementary nourishments or special dietary instructions. Allow patients to choose from the available nourishments whenever possible. Assist those who are unable to take their nourishment alone. Remember to pick up used glasses and dishes after the patient has finished and return to the proper area. Again, notice what the patient was or was not able to take. Record on I & O sheet if required.

CHANGING WATER

It is important to provide fresh water for patients since water is essential to life. Because patients often do not drink enough water, sometimes the physician will leave orders that fluids are to be *forced*. Forcing fluids means that the patient must be encouraged to take as much fluid as possible. Providing fresh water is one way to encourage the patient to increase his intake of fluids, Figure 23-7. The procedure for providing fresh water varies greatly. In some hospitals the water pitcher and glass are replaced with a new sterilized set each time water is provided. In others, the pitcher and glass are washed, refilled, and returned to the patient's bedside table. In all cases be sure you know whether a patient is allowed ice or tap water.

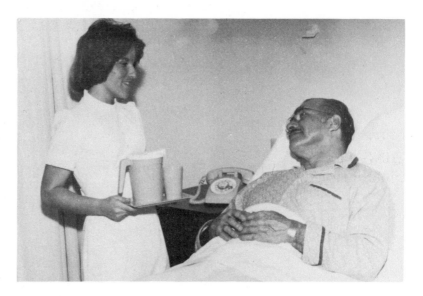

FIGURE 23-7.   Fresh water encourages adequate fluid intake.

Be sure you follow orders in regard to diets, nourishments, and water. Special diets and nourishments are therapeutic, therefore, instructions must be followed carefully.

FEEDING THE PATIENT

In preparing the patient for his food tray, he should be offered the bedpan and assisted to wash his hands and face. The head of the bed should be raised, if permitted, or the patient's position adjusted with pillows. Sitting in a chair often will stimulate the appetite. The overbed table should be cleared. Anything unpleasant, such as emesis basins or bedpans, should be removed from sight. Eating should be an enjoyable experience. After you have washed your hands, assist the patient by cutting meat, pouring liquids, or buttering bread. Allow the patient to do as much for himself as his condition or orders permit. If the patient is blind, explain the arrangement of the tray as items relate to the face of a clock. At times you will be responsible for the entire feeding procedure. It is important that you are pleasant and unhurried in your manner.

Procedure

ASSISTING THE PATIENT WHO CAN FEED HIMSELF

1. Wash hands.
2. Identify patient and explain what you plan to do.
3. Offer bedpan or urinal (if used, follow procedure in Unit 18 Giving and Receiving a Bedpan).
4. If permitted, elevate head of bed or assist out of bed.
5. Provide water, soap, and towel to wash patient's hands and face.
6. Clear overbed table and position in front of patient. Remove unpleasant equipment from sight.
7. Wash hands and obtain tray from dietary area.
8. Check dietary name tag against patient's identification.
9. Place tray on overbed table and arrange food in a convenient manner.
10. Assist in food preparation as needed. Encourage the patient to do as much for himself as permitted.
11. Remove tray as soon as patient is finished. Make sure to note what the patient has and has not eaten. Record fluids on intake record if necessary.

12. Push overbed table out of the way. Assist patient to return to bed or into a comfortable position.
13. Leave call bell and water within reach and the unit tidy.
14. Wash hands.

Procedure

FEEDING THE HELPLESS PATIENT

1. Wash hands and check the diet order.
2. Food trays are prepared in the kitchen with the patient's name card on it. Add nothing to the tray without checking the diet order. Check the name card against the patient's identification.
3. Remove unnecessary articles from the overbed table.
4. Adjust patient to a comfortable position.
5. Place napkin under patient's chin.
6. Butter bread and cut meat. Do not pour hot beverage until patient is ready for it.
7. Use drinking straw to give fluids.
8. Holding spoon at a right angle, give solid foods from point of spoon. Alternate solids and liquids. Describe or show patient what kind of food you are giving him. Test hot foods by dropping a small amount on the inside of your wrist before feeding them to the patient.
9. Allow patient to hold bread or assist to the extent that he is able.
10. Use napkin to wipe his mouth as often as necessary.
11. Remove tray as soon as patient is finished. Make sure you note what the patient has or has not eaten. Wash hands. Record fluids on intake record if necessary.

Summary

The "Basic Four Food Groups" contain the essential nutrients for health. Hospital diets are selected from the basic food groups but are prepared in special ways. The assistant serves trays, special nourishments, and fresh water and feeds those unable to help themselves.

Specific diets are often an essential part of therapy and must be carefully followed.

SUGGESTED ACTIVITIES

1. Plan a day's menu (three meals) based on the Basic Four Food Groups.
2. Discuss differences between the four basic hospital diets.
3. Practice the following:
   a. Serving trays
   b. Preparing patients for meals
   c. Assisting patients with meals
   d. Feeding helpless patients
   e. Serving nourishments
   f. Providing fresh water

VOCABULARY

Learn the meaning and correct spelling of the following words.

carbohydrates	gastrostomy tube	protein
cellulose	intravenous infusion	therapeutic
defecation	mineral	vitamin
fats	nasogastric tube	"withhold"
flow rate	nutrient	
forced fluids	nutrition	

UNIT REVIEW

A. Brief Answer. Answer the following questions.

1. What are the names of the four basic hospital diets?

2. Why is an unhurried attitude important when feeding a patient?

3. What is meant by the order to force fluids?

B. Clinical Situations. Briefly describe how a health care assistant should react to the following situations.

1. Your patient is on I & O and you picked up the lunch tray.

2. You serve a tray to a blind patient who is able to feed himself.

3. Your patient's chart includes an order to force fluids.

C. Classification. Write the names for the four basic food groups at the top of each column below. Write the names of each of the following foods in the column under the proper food group.

flour	rice	apples	milk
beef	cereal	potatoes	ice cream
chicken	cheese	spinach	fish
pears	cottage cheese	liver	macaroni

Group 1	Group 2	Group 3	Group 4
_____	_____	_____	_____
_____	_____	_____	_____
_____	_____	_____	_____
_____	_____	_____	_____
_____	_____	_____	_____

Unit 24 Recording Intake and Output and Collecting and Testing Routine Specimens

OBJECTIVES

As a result of this unit, you will be able to:

- Use the metric system of measurement.
- Record intake and output.
- Explain the importance of accurate measurement in the hospital.
- Collect and label specimens.

INTAKE AND OUTPUT

Because two-thirds of the body weight is water, there must be a careful balance between the amount of fluid taken into the body and the amount that is lost under normal conditions. Generally we do not need to concern ourselves about this balance; it usually takes care of itself.

We generally lose approximately 2-1/2 quarts of fluid each day which must be replaced. When extra fluid is lost, however, because of vomiting, bleeding, diarrhea, or excessive perspiration, the normal relationship may be unbalanced. Excessive fluid loss results in *dehydration.* Retention of fluid in the tissues causes *edema.*

Our intake of fluid comes from liquids we drink, foods we eat, and may come artificially from IVs. Our output of fluids is largely through our kidneys as urine and our skin as perspiration. It also comes from our lungs and bowels.

Recording Intake and Output

An accurate recording of intake and output (often abbreviated I & O) is basic to the care of many patients. The doctor will specify when a record is to be made. Intake and output is usually monitored in most patients with a catheter or IV.

A knowledge of metric measurement is essential in performing the procedure, because (1) most of the scientific work in the United States is done with the *metric system,* and (2) hospitals generally use the metric system in the measurement of fluids.

The container used in hospitals for measuring fluids like urine is marked in metric measurements, for example: cubic centimeters (cc) or milliliters (ml). One cubic centimeter equals one milliliter. There are approximately 15 drops of fluid per ml. For the purpose of general measurements, a drop is approximately equal to a minim. Figure 24-1 shows a comparison of US customary units and metric units.

U.S. CUSTOMARY UNITS	METRIC UNITS
1 minim	0.06 milliliter
16 minims	1 ml
1 ounce	30 ml
1 pint	500 ml
1 quart	1000 ml (1 liter)
2.2 pounds	1 kilogram
1 inch	2.5 centimeters
1 foot	30 centimeters

FIGURE 24-1.   Approximate measurements

Procedure

MEASURING AND RECORDING FLUID INTAKE

1. Wash hands and assemble the following equipment:
   - Intake and output record at bedside
   - Pen
   - Graduated pitcher
2. Identify the patient and explain what you plan to do. Ask the patient to help by recording the amount of fluid taken by mouth; see Figure 24-2.
3. Record intake on the intake-output record at the bedside. Intake includes:
   - Amount of liquid patient takes with meals. This includes anything liquid at room temperature such as ice cream or jello.
   - Amount of water and other liquids taken between meals.
   - All other intake including all fluids given by mouth, intravenously, or by tube feeding. How it is taken should also be recorded.
4. Copy information on the patient's chart from the bedside intake and output record, according to hospital policy. Remember, intake and output (I & O) are recorded in milliliters (ml), which are the same as cubic centimeters (ccs). The total is recorded at the end of each shift and at the end of 24 hours, Figure 24-3.

Coffee/tea cup, 8 oz	240 ml
Water carafe, 16 oz	480 ml
Foam cup, 8 oz	240 ml
Water glass, 8 oz	240 ml
Soup bowl, 6 oz	180 ml
Jello, 1 serving, 4 oz	120 ml
Ice chips, full 4 oz glass	120 ml

FIGURE 24-2.   Approximate liquid amounts of common containers and servings. Note: Sizes of containers vary. Learn the fluid content of the containers used at your health care facility. Remember that there are 30 ml per ounce (240 ml ÷ 30 ml = 8 oz)

INTAKE		OUTPUT	
I.V.	3000 ml	Urine	2000 ml
By mouth	2000 ml	Vomitus	500 ml
		Drainage	600 ml
Total	5000 ml	Total	3100 ml

FIGURE 24-3.   Computing intake and output

Procedure

MEASURING AND RECORDING FLUID OUTPUT

1. Save urine specimen and take to utility room or patient's bathroom. You will need:
   - Graduate pitcher
   - Pen for recording
2. Pour urine from bedpan or urinal into graduate. Measure amount.
3. Record amounts immediately under output column on bedside intake and output record, Figure 24-4. All liquid output should be recorded. Output includes urine, *vomitus*—also called *emesis*, drainage from a wound or the stomach, liquid stool, blood loss, and perspiration. Fluids used to irrigate the bladder or for an enema are *not* included in calculating the output.
4. Empty urine into bedpan hopper. If specimen is accidentally lost, estimate amount and make notation that it is an estimate. Note: In some cases, the physician will request that the totally incontinent patient's diapers be weighed to determine output.
5. Rinse graduate with cold water. Clean according to hospital policy.
6. Clean bedpan or urinal and return to proper place, according to hospital policy.
7. Wash hands.
8. Copy information on chart from intake and output record, according to hospital policy. Perspiration and blood loss may be described as little, moderate, or excessive. Also record on the chart instances in which linens or dressings have been changed or reinforced because of such fluid losses.

ELMSVILLE GENERAL HOSPITAL

FLUID INTAKE AND OUTPUT

Name _____ Ward _____

Date	Time	Method of Adm.	INTAKE			OUTPUT		
			Solution	Amounts Rec'd.	Time	Urine Amount	Others	
							Kind	Amount

Code: Method of Administration: M — Mouth, HC — Hypodermoclysis, IV — Intravenous, R — Rectal, TF — Tube Feeding

FIGURE 24-4. Intake and output record

ROUTINE SPECIMENS

Laboratory tests are frequently performed on body discharges such as *urine*, *feces*, and *sputum*. Results of these tests give the doctors much information about the patient's condition. *All specimens must be carefully cared for, labeled, and sent to the lab as soon as possible.* Mistakes in labeling and preparing the specimens can not only make the test results inaccurate, they could endanger your patients.

Urine Specimens

ROUTINE URINE SPECIMEN. *Urinalysis* is the most common laboratory test made in the hospital. The specimen is usually taken when the patient first *voids* (urinates) in the morning.

Procedure

COLLECTING A ROUTINE URINE SPECIMEN

1. Wash hands and assemble the following equipment:
   • Bedpan or urinal and cover
   • Container and cover for specimen
   • Graduate
   • Laboratory requisition slip, properly filled out
   • Label, including patient's full name, room number, hospital number, date and time of collection, doctor's name, examination to be done, and other information as requested.
2. Identify patient and explain what you plan to do. Tell patient not to discard toilet tissue in the pan with the urine. Provide paper towels or a small plastic sack in which to place the soiled tissue.
3. Screen the unit. Offer bedpan or urinal.
4. After patient has voided, take pan to utility room. Offer wash water to patient.
5. Pour specimen from the bedpan into the graduate. Note the amount if patient's intake and output are to be recorded, Figure 24-5.
6. Pour about 120 ml into the specimen container, Figure 24-6.
7. Wash hands. Do not contaminate outside of container.
8. Cover container. Attach completed label and requisition slip to container.
9. Clean and replace equipment according to hospital policy.
10. Take or send specimen to laboratory.
11. A record of the procedure is made on the patient's chart.

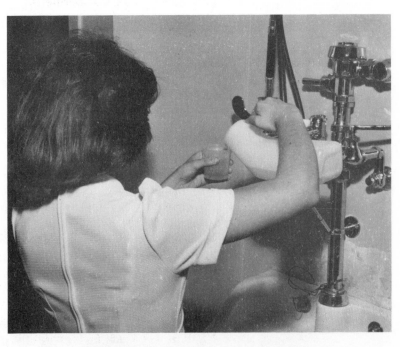

FIGURE 24-5.   Measuring the urine specimen

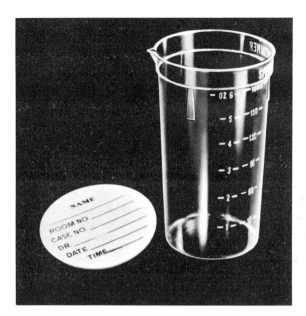

FIGURE 24-6. Urine specimen container

Procedure

COLLECTING A ROUTINE SPECIMEN FROM AN INFANT

1. Wash hands and assemble the following equipment:
   - Clean diapers (2)
   - Disposable urine collection bag
   - Wash basin
   - Specimen container/labels
   - Sterile cotton balls
2. Identify child and explain what you plan to do even if you feel the child is too young to completely understand. Speak in a gentle, calm manner.
3. Fill the basin with warm water and take to bedside.
4. Place child on his back and remove diaper. Dispose according to hospital policy.
5. Flex knees to expose perineum.
6. Using cotton balls, cleanse the perineal area. Each cotton ball should be used only once for a single stroke. Clean directly over the meatus last. Rinse and dry area.
7. Remove paper cover from adhesive portion of collection bag.
   a. If female child, bending the adhesive area slightly on the bottom will help it fit more snugly against the perineum. Position this section first, bringing up against vulva.
   b. If a male child, position penis in opening of bag and secure adhesive area to skin.
8. Apply clean diaper.
9. Offer fluids, if permitted.
10. Make sure child is secure in crib with siderails up before leaving unit.
11. Check child frequently until voiding has been achieved.
12. Wash hands and screen unit.
13. Fill the basin with warm water and take to bedside.
14. Remove diaper and dispose of properly.
15. Gently remove collection bag by lifting the edges and pulling toward perineum. Be careful not to spill urine.
16. Put adhesive edges together and pour urine into the specimen container through drainage port. Be very careful not to lose specimen.
17. Wash and dry perineal area using the same technique as in step 6. Be sure all adhesive is removed.

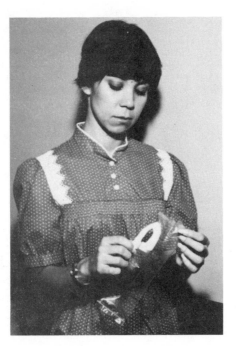 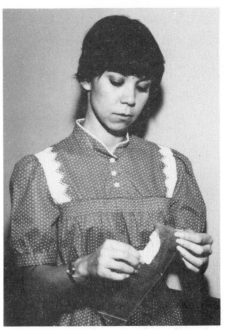

A. Remove the paper cover from the adhesive portion before applying the infant urine collection bag.

B. Slightly bending the opening will help it fit more snugly against the female perineum.

FIGURE 24-7.

18. Apply a fresh diaper.
19. Raise siderails, unscreen unit, and be sure child is secure in crib before leaving.
20. Take equipment to patient's bathroom or utility room and clean according to hospital policy.
21. Wash hands and label specimen properly.
22. Care for specimen per instruction.
23. Report completion of your task to the nurse.

CLEAN-CATCH URINE SPECIMEN. When a urine specimen is needed that is free of contamination from organisms that are found in areas near the urinary *meatus*, the specimen is collected either by inserting a sterile tube (catheter), or the area is cleansed and the patient is instructed to void. After the flow is started, the container is moved into position catching the urine midstream. This specimen is also called a *midstream specimen*. This is the best way to obtain any urine specimen.

Procedure

COLLECTING A CLEAN-CATCH URINE SPECIMEN

1. Wash your hands and assemble the following equipment:
   • Sterile urine specimen container
   • Label for container with patient's full name, room number, date and time of collection, physician's name, type of specimen/test to be performed, and any other information requested.
   • Gauze squares or cotton
   • Antiseptic solution
2. Identify the patient and explain what you plan to do.
3. Wash the patient's genital area properly, or instruct the patient to do so.
   a. For female patients: Using the gauze or cotton and the antiseptic solution, cleanse the outer folds of the *vulva* (folds are also called

labia, or lips) with a front-to-back motion. Discard the gauze/cotton. Then, cleanse the inner folds of the vulva with another piece of gauze and antiseptic solution, again with a front-to-back motion. Discard gauze/cotton. Finally, cleanse the middle, innermost area (*meatus* or urinary opening) in the same manner. Discard the gauze/cotton.

    b. For male patients: Using the gauze or cotton and the antiseptic solution, cleanse the tip of the penis from the urinary meatus (opening) down, using a circular motion. Discard the gauze/cotton.

4. Instruct the patient to void, allowing the first part of the urine stream to escape. Then, catch the urine stream that follows in the sterile specimen container. Allow the last portion of the urine stream to escape. Note: If the patient's I & O is being monitored, or if the amount of urine passed must be measured, catch the first and last part of the urine in a bedpan or urinal.

5. Place the sterile cap on the urine container immediately to avoid contamination of the urine specimen.

6. Allow the patient to wash hands.

7. With the cap securely tightened, wash the outside of the specimen container.

8. Wash hands.

9. Label the container as instructed previously, and attach requisition slip for appropriate test.

10. Clean and replace all equipment according to hospital policy.

11. Take or send specimen to laboratory immediately.

12. Record the procedure on the patient's chart.

Procedure

COLLECTING A FRESH FRACTIONAL URINE SAMPLE

1. About one hour before testing is to be done, wash your hands and assemble the following equipment:
   - Two specimen containers
   - Urinal or bedpan
   - Testing materials if urine testing is to be performed (Clinitese, Ace-test, Ketostix, or Testape)
   - Small plastic bag for used toilet tissue

2. Identify patient and explain what you plan to do. Instruct the patient that two samples will be taken, an initial sample now and a smaller sample in about one hour.

3. Screen unit and offer bedpan or urinal (patient may be assisted to the commode if permitted).

4. Encourage patient to empty his/her bladder.

5. Do not permit tissue to be placed in receptacle. Place in plastic bag and discharge.

6. Take receptacle to bathroom or utility room.

7. Pour sample into one specimen container. Test this sample in case patient fails to void second specimen.

8. Make a note of the test results but do not officially record it.

9. Clean equipment according to facility policy and return to proper area. Measure and record urine if patient is on I & O.

10. Wash hands.

11. Offer wash water for the patient to wash his or her own hands.

12. If permitted, encourage patient to drink water. Be sure to record intake on I & O sheet.

13. Tell patient when you will return for the second sample and then return to the patient's unit at the proper time.

14. Wash hands. Identify patient and explain what you plan to do.

15. Repeat steps 3–11.
16. Report and record findings of the second testing.

TWENTY-FOUR HOUR SPECIMEN. If a 24-hour urine specimen is ordered, all urine excreted by the patient in a 24-hour period is collected and saved in a large, carefully-labeled container. The container is usually surrounded by ice to keep it cool. The patient is asked to void and this first urine is discarded so that the bladder is empty at the time the test begins. All other urine is saved, including that voided as the test time finishes. No toilet tissue should be allowed to enter the specimen. If you or the patient forget to save a specimen during the test period, report it immediately to the nurse.

Procedure

COLLECTING A 24-HOUR URINE SPECIMEN

1. Wash hands and assemble the following equipment:
   • 24-hour specimen container (supplied by health care facility)
   • Label
   • Sign for patient's bed
2. Label the container with the patient's name, room number, test ordered, type of specimen, date, and physician's name, Figure 24-8.
3. Identify the patient and explain what you plan to do. Emphasize the necessity for saving all urine passed.
4. Allow the patient to void. Assist with the bedpan/urinal as needed. Measure the amount of urine passed if the patient's I & O is being monitored. Discard the urine specimen. Note the date and time of voiding; this time will mark the start of the 24-hour collection. Note: A 24-hour urine specimen requires that the patient start the 24-hour interval with an empty bladder. This is the reason this first specimen is discarded.
5. Place a sign on the patient's bed to alert other health care team members that a 24-hour urine specimen is being collected. (Sign may read "Save all urine—24-hour specimen.")
6. From this time on, all urine is voided into the specimen container for a period of 24 hours. Often, the container is refrigerated when not in use. Check hospital policy regarding handling of the specimen container. Note: If any urine is accidentally discarded, the test must be discontinued and started again for another 24 hours.

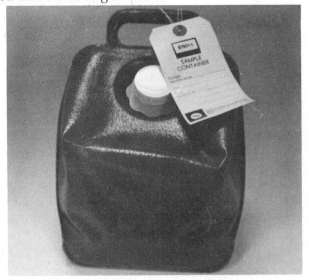

FIGURE 24-8. Many agencies use disposable containers for 24-hour urine specimen collections. The urine is preserved by the use of chemicals or cold storage. (*From Simmers,* Diversified Health Occupations, *1983, Delmar Publishers Inc.*)

7. At the end of the 24-hour period, ask the patient to void one last time. Add this urine to the specimen container.
8. Remove sign from patient's bed. Check label for accuracy and completeness and attach the appropriate requisition slip.
9. Clean and replace all equipment used, according to hospital policy.
10. Wash hands.
11. Take or send specimen to laboratory immediately.
12. Record the procedure on the patient's chart.

OTHER TYPES OF URINE SPECIMENS AND TESTING. Urine testing for diabetic conditions will be discussed in Unit 34.

Stool Specimens

A specimen of stool is a sample of fecal material (solid body waste or bowel movement) collected in a special container. The specimen is then sent to the laboratory for examination. In the laboratory, stools may be examined for pathogenic microorganisms (germs), *parasites, occult blood* (hidden blood, or blood that cannot be seen by the naked eye), and chemical analysis.

Procedure
COLLECTING A STOOL SPECIMEN

1. Wash hands and assemble the following equipment:
   • Bedpan and cover
   • Specimen container and cover
   • Toilet tissue
   • Tongue blades
   • Label including: patient's full name, room number, date and time of collection, doctor's name, examination to be performed, and other information as it is requested.
2. Collect stool from daily bowel movement. Offer wash water to patient. Take covered pan to utility room.
3. Use tongue blades to remove specimen from bedpan and place in specimen container, Figure 24-10.
4. Wash hands. Do not contaminate the outside of the container.
5. Cover container and attach completed label. Make sure cover is on container tightly. Label the container appropriately.
6. Clean and replace equipment according to hospital policy.
7. Take or send specimen to laboratory promptly.
8. A record of the procedure should be made on the patient's chart.

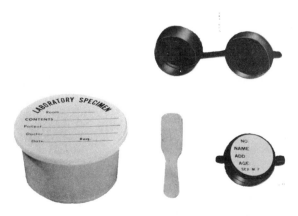

FIGURE 24-9. Two types of disposable containers available for the collection of stool specimens

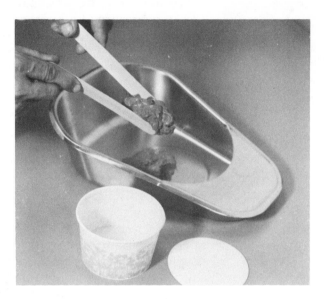

FIGURE 24-10. Use tongue blades to transfer the stool specimen from the bedpan to the specimen container. *(From Simmers,* Diversified Health Occupations, *1983, Delmar Publishers Inc.)*

The following advanced procedures are included in Unit 39.

- Testing for Occult Blood Using Hemoccult® and Developer
- Testing for Occult Blood Using Hematest® Reagent Tablets
- Testing Urine With the Hemacombastix®

These procedures are to be carried out only after adequate practice and supervision, and only in accord with specific hospital policy.

Sputum Specimens

Sputum refers to matter which is brought up by mouth, usually after coughing. This matter comes from the lungs. Sputum specimens are frequently taken from patients who have chest conditions. Some tests on specimens may be done by the health care assistant in the utility room.

Procedure
COLLECTING A SPUTUM SPECIMEN

1. Wash hands and assemble the following equipment:
   - Container and cover for specimen
   - Glass of water
   - Tissues
   - Emesis basin
   - Label including: patient's full name, room number, hospital number, date and time of collection, doctor's name, examination to be done, and other information as it is requested.
2. Identify the patient and tell what you plan to do. Screen the unit.
3. Have the patient rinse his mouth. Use emesis basin for waste.
4. Ask patient to cough deeply to bring up sputum and *expectorate* (spit) into the container. Have patient cover his mouth with tissue to prevent spread of infection. Collect 1 to 2 tablespoonfuls of sputum unless otherwise ordered.
5. Wash hands. Do not contaminate the outside of the container.
6. Cover container tightly and attach completed label.
7. Clean and replace equipment according to hospital policy.
8. Take or send specimen to laboratory promptly.

9. A record of the procedure should be made on the patient's chart. Be sure to include a description of the specimen such as odor and color. Note: If a 24-hour specimen is being collected, leave the container at the patient's bedside.

Summary

Fluids in the hospital are measured in cubic centimeters or milliliters. It may be necessary to convert from ounces to milliliters to add the totals. All fluids consumed by or lost from the patient must be included in the totals. Intake and output totals are very important and must be carefully measured.

The composition of urine reflects the chemistry of the blood. Many tests are done on urine samples which have been collected in specific ways.

Careful collecting, handling and labelling of urine, stool, and sputum specimens protects your patient and assures accuracy in results.

SUGGESTED ACTIVITIES

1. Make an intake and output chart like that in Figure 24-4. Put the following information in the proper column and total the figures as explained in this unit. The information covers the waking hours.

7:30 AM	urine	500 ml
8:00 AM	grape juice	90 ml
	milk	120 ml
9:30 AM	water	180 ml
11:30 AM	coffee	120 ml
	soup	180 ml
1:00 PM	urine	500 ml
1:15 PM	water	90 ml
3:00 PM	orange juice	120 ml
3:15 PM	vomitus	120 ml
4:20 PM	tea	120 ml
	milk	60 ml
5:30 PM	urine	400 ml
6:00 PM	water	150 ml
9:00 PM	ginger ale	150 ml
9:30 PM	urine	300 ml
10:00 PM	water	90 ml

2. Look at samples of specimen containers, labels, and requisition slips used in your hospital. Be sure you know what kind of specimen is put in each container and the information asked for on the labels and requisition slips.

3. Practice collecting specimens in the classroom. Use water and gelatin for specimens.

4. Familiarize yourself with the size of usual containers in your facility.

VOCABULARY

Learn the meaning and correct spelling of the following words.

dehydration	labia	restricted fluids
edema	meatus	sputum
emesis	metric system	urinalysis
expectorate	NPO	urine
feces	midstream specimen	void
force fluids	occult blood	vomitus
intake and output	parasite	vulva

UNIT REVIEW

A. Brief Answer. Answer the following questions.

1. What does intake include?

2. What does output include?

3. In what unit of measurement are intake and output recorded?

4. For what period of time are intake and output totalled?

5. Why must all specimens be labeled and handled carefully?

6. How is the fecal matter transferred from bedpan to container?

7. Why should you wash your hands before putting a cover on the specimen container?

8. What are the three common specimens collected for examination in the hospital?

B. Clinical Situations. Briefly describe how a health care assistant should react to the following situations.

1. You accidentally spill a urine specimen that was to be measured.

2. Your patient consumed 6 ounces of fluid and you need to record the amount in ml.

C. Completion. Below is a label which is attached to specimen containers. Fill it out correctly, using the following information: Mr. James Brown is a patient in room 604. His hospital number is 689473. Dr. Smith has ordered a urine specimen to be taken today for routine examination.

Name _____	Room _____
Date _____	Hospital Number _____
Doctor _____	
Specimen _____	Examination _____

Section Nine
Self-evaluation

A. Match Column I with Column II.

Column I

1. Gastrostomy tube
2. Carbohydrates
3. Proteins
4. Roughage
5. I & O Record
6. f.f.
7. Edema
8. Gavage
9. Feces
10. Fats

Column II

a. tube feeding
b. important nutrient for body building and repair
c. measure of fluids taken into and lost from the body
d. stored form of energy
e. solid body wastes
f. artificial tube leading directly into the stomach
g. encourage fluid intake
h. accumulation of excess fluid in the body
i. called "energy" foods
j. cellulose

B. Select the one best answer.

11. Foods which contain the greatest amount of carbohydrates come from
    a. eggs.
    b. milk.
    c. fruits.
    d. nuts.
    e. pork.

12. Your patient has an order for a regular diet. This means
    a. rich pastries will be included.
    b. more calories than usual must be supplied.
    c. only liquids may be consumed.
    d. a basic normal diet will be provided.
    e. salt must be omitted.

13. Your patient has been nauseated and has been placed on a clear liquid diet. You would
    a. feed your patient once a day.
    b. offer coffee with cream and sugar.
    c. offer 7-Up or gingerale.
    d. offer tomato juice.
    e. offer vegetable soup.

14. Your patient has poorly-fitting dentures. His nutritional needs would best be met with a
    a. regular diet.
    b. full liquid diet.
    c. salt free diet.
    d. clear liquid diet.
    e. soft diet.

15. Your patient is on a full liquid diet. When the tray arrives and you check it, you discover one of the following which does not belong.
    a. Soup (strained)
    b. Sherbert
    c. Eggnog
    d. Crackers
    e. Strained grape juice

16. You are assigned to "pass" nourishments. One patient's name has a "withhold." You will
    a. offer him only solids.
    b. remember to measure his intake.
    c. offer him an extra portion of juice.
    d. refuse to give him juice.
    e. give him a choice of nourishments.

17. Your patient is blind but able to feed herself. You will
    a. feed her, it's faster.
    b. explain the tray arrangement related to the face of clock.
    c. place all food in a straight line across overbed table.
    d. place the tray with no explanation.
    e. explain the tray arrangement by putting all hot foods toward the tray top and cold toward the tray bottom

18. You're assigned to record your patient's I & O. Which of the following should be counted?
    a. 500 ml IV D/W
    b. 700 ml urine
    c. 200 ml of vomitus
    d. 300 ml gavaged nutrients
    e. All of the above.

19. Your patient has had a twenty-four hour specimen collected. You know you will
    a. collect the first specimen after 24 hours of hospitalization.
    b. send each individual specimen of urine to the lab immediately after voiding.
    c. you must collect the first specimen of urine every twenty-four hours for three days.
    d. report immediately to your nurse if a specimen is lost, since the test will be discontinued.
    e. leave the urine collection jar on the open table in the dirty utility room.

20. Your patient took in 240 ml of juice and 180 ml of sherbert. The total intake would be
    a. 8 ounces.
    b. 320 ml.
    c. 10 ounces.
    d. 410 ml.
    e. 14 ounces.

21. Your patient put out 16 ounces of urine. You might record this as
    a. 460 ml.
    b. 480 ml.
    c. 500 ml.
    d. 520 ml.
    e. 556 ml.

C. The daily servings from each of the basic four food groups should include:

Groups	Servings
22. Vegetables and fruits	a. 1 or more
23. Dairy foods (Adults)	b. 2 or more
24. Bread and cereals	c. 3 or more
25. Meat groups	d. 4 or more
	e. 5 or more

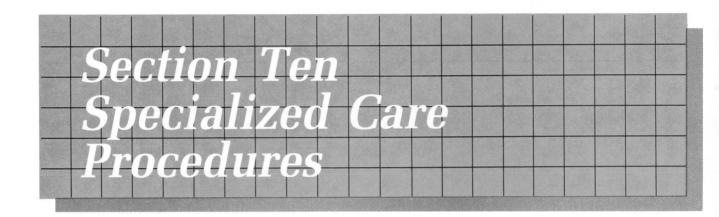

Section Ten
Specialized Care
Procedures

Unit 25 Heat and Cold Applications

OBJECTIVES

As a result of this unit, you will be able to:

- Name types of hot and cold applications and list the conditions requiring their use.
- Describe the effects of hot and cold applications and demonstrate the various procedures involved.

The physician frequently orders the use of hot or cold applications to relieve pain, combat local infection, check bleeding *(hemorrhage)*, and to reduce body temperature. Some facilities limit the application of heat and cold to professional personnel. Health care assistants who have been specially trained are permitted to carry out these procedures under the supervision of the nurse in other facilities. Be sure you follow the policy of your facility and are adequately prepared and supervised. Local applications of hot and cold are made with ice bags or hot water bags applied to a small area of the body.

Standard ice bags and hot water bottles are being replaced in many areas by the electronically operated Aquamatic K-Pad®. K-Pads come in many shapes and sizes. They can be used for the application of dry heat and, by use of an attachment, they can be used for cooling.

Prepackaged, single-use units for the application of hot and cold are now available also, Figure 25-1. A single blow to the surface activates the contents, providing a controlled temperature.

General treatments of hot and cold consist of special baths such as *Sitz baths* and alcohol sponge baths. The Sitz bath is a means of providing moist heat to the genital and anal area. The alcohol sponge bath is used to reduce an elevated temperature; thermal mattresses known as *hypothermia blankets* are also widely used for this purpose. Hot and cold applications are used only on written orders of the doctor.

TYPES OF COLD AND HEAT

There are two kinds of cold and heat: dry and moist. Dry cold is provided by ice bags, ice caps, and ice collars. Dry heat is produced by the use of hot water bags, electric heating pads, and heat lamps. Moist hot and cold applications are more penetrating than dry types. Wet compresses,

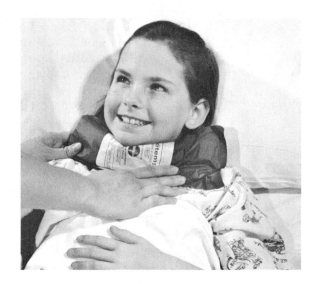

FIGURE 25-1.   A single-use cold pack *(Photo courtesy of Wyeth Laboratories, Philadelphia, PA)*

soaks, and packs provide moist heat or cold depending on the temperature of the moist application. Remember that moisture intensifies the application of heat so extra care must be taken.

BODY RESPONSE

Cold causes blood vessels to constrict or become smaller *(vasoconstriction)*. Intense cold numbs the sensation of pain. It also slows all life processes and slows down inflammation. Heat *(diathermy)* has the opposite effect. It speeds inflammation and reduces itching. It makes blood vessels larger *(vasodilation)* and increases the blood supply to the area. The additional blood supply promotes healing and can be soothing.

CAUTIONS

Extreme watchfulness must be used when cold or hot applications are used on young children, the aged, or patients who are uncooperative or unconscious.

An electric heating pad must not be used with moist dressings unless a rubber cover is placed over the pad. If the wires should become damp, a short circuit will result. The patient must not lie on the pad since severe burns can result. Sensitivity to heat varies, so patients receiving heat treatments must be checked frequently.

Heat cradles are sometimes used to stimulate the circulation in the legs and feet, and sometimes the perineal area. A bed cradle is equipped with ordinary light bulbs of 25 watts placed three feet from the area to be treated to provide continuous dry heat. The bulbs are hung under the top of the cradle and encased in wire frames to avoid burning the patient. The length of treatment is always specified. Other lamp treatments, such as *infrared* and *ultraviolet,* are given by experts because of the danger involved since these produce penetrating heat.

Procedure
APPLYING AN ICE BAG

1. Wash hands. Assemble and prepare the following equipment in the utility room:
   - Ice bag or collar
   - Spoon or similar utensil
   - Cover (usually muslin)

- Ice cubes or crushed ice
- Paper towels

2. If ice cubes are used, rinse them in water to remove sharp edges.
3. Fill ice cap half full, using ice scoop or large spoon. Avoid making ice bags too heavy.
4. Expel air by resting ice bag on table in horizontal position with top in place but not screwed on. Squeeze the bag until air has been removed.
5. Fasten top securely.
6. Test for leakage.
7. Wipe dry with paper towels.
8. Place muslin cover on ice bag. Never permit rubber or plastic to touch patient's skin.
9. Take equipment to bedside on tray.
10. Identify patient and explain what you plan to do.
11. Apply to the affected part with the metal cap away from patient.
12. Refill bag before all ice is melted.
13. A record of the procedure is made on the patient's chart.
14. Check skin area with each application. Report to supervising nurse immediately if skin is discolored or white or if patient reports skin is numb.
15. When ice bag is removed after use, wash with soap and water, drain, dry, and screw top on. Leave air in ice bag to prevent sides from sticking together.
16. If a reusable cold pack is used, wash thoroughly with soap and water and return to the refrigerator. Discard a disposable pack.

Procedure

APPLYING A DISPOSABLE COLD PACK

1. Wash your hands and assemble the following equipment:
   - Disposable cold pack (commercially prepared). Read directions.
   - Cloth covering (towel, hot water bag cover)
   - Tape or rolls of gauze
2. Identify the patient and explain what you plan to do. Screen unit.
3. Expose area to be treated. Note condition of area.
4. Place cold pack in cloth covering.
5. Strike or squeeze cold pack to activate chemicals.
6. Place covered cold pack on proper area. Note time of application.
7. Secure with tape or gauze.
8. Leave patient in comfortable condition with signal cord within easy reach.
9. Return to bedside every 10 minutes. Check area being treated for discoloration or numbness. If these signs and symptoms occur, discontinue treatment and report to your supervisor.
10. If no adverse symptoms occur remove pack in 30 minutes. Note condition of area. Continuous treatment requires application of a fresh pack.
11. Remove pack from cover and discard according to hospital policy. Return unused gauze and tape.
12. Put cover in laundry.
13. Leave patient comfortable and unit tidy.
14. Wash hands. Record and report:
    - Type of treatment
    - Length of treatment
    - Any observations you have made

Procedure

APPLYING A HOT WATER BAG

1. Wash hands. Assemble and prepare the following equipment in the utility room:
   - Hot water bag
   - Container for hot water

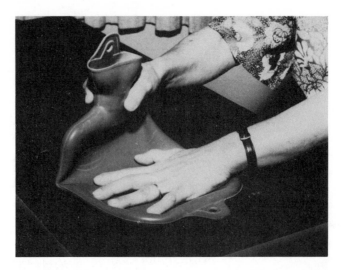

FIGURE 25-2. Force air out of the bag by pressing with your hand against a flat surface and holding the neck of the bag upright. Note: Some hospitals have discontinued use of hot water bottles because of the risk of burns.

- Paper towels
- Cover
- Thermometer

2. Fill container with water and test for correct temperature, which should be approximately 115°F unless otherwise ordered.
3. Fill hot water bag 1/3 to 1/2 full to avoid unnecessary weight.
4. Expel air by placing hot water bag horizontally on flat surface, holding neck of bag upright until water reaches neck, Figure 25-2. Close the top when all air has been expelled.
5. Wipe hot water bag dry with paper towels and turn bag upside down to check for leakage.
6. Place cover on hot water bag so that patient's skin does not come in contact with rubber or plastic.
7. Take equipment to bedside on tray. Identify patient and explain what you plan to do.
8. Apply to the affected area as ordered. Never allow patient to lie on the hot water bag.
9. Check patient's condition at intervals.
10. Clean and replace equipment according to hospital policy. Place cover in laundry hamper. Wash hands.
11. Repeat procedure as necessary. Check condition of skin with each reapplication. Report any unusual observations immediately to supervising nurse.
12. A record of the procedure is made on the patient's chart.

Procedure
APPLYING THE AQUAMATIC K-PAD

1. Wash hands and assemble the following equipment:
   - K-pad and control unit
   - Covering for pad
   - Distilled water
2. Screen unit. Identify patient and explain what you plan to do.
3. Place the control unit on the bedside stand, Figure 25-3.
4. Remove the cover and fill the unit with distilled water to the fill line.
5. Screw the cover in place and loosen it one-quarter turn.
6. Note time of application. Turn on the unit. The temperature, usually 95 to 100 degrees F, is set by a key which is removed after setting.

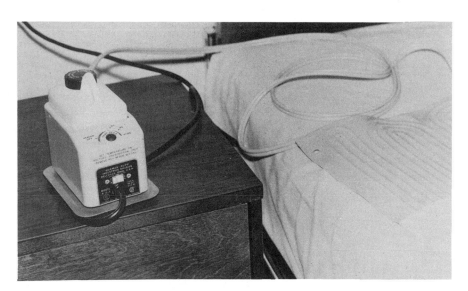

FIGURE 25-3. The Aquamatic K-pad and control unit in position *(Photo courtesy of Gorman-Rupp Industries, Inc.)*

7. Cover pad and place it on the patient. Secure with tape. Never use pins. Be sure that the tubing is coiled on the bed to facilitate the flow, as shown in the figure. Do not allow it to hang below the level of the bed.
8. Check the control unit periodically and refill the unit if the water drops below the fill line.
9. Remove after prescribed period of time.
10. Clean equipment and return to proper area.
11. Make patient comfortable and leave unit tidy.
12. Wash hands. A record of the procedure is made on the patient's chart. Include:
    - Procedure: Application of K-pad
    - Time applied and removed
    - Your observations

Procedure

ASSISTING WITH THE HOT FOOT SOAK

1. Wash hands and assemble the following equipment on a tray:
   - Bath thermometer
   - Solution as ordered in container
   - Extra pitcher of hot water
   - Place the tray on the overbed table.
   Also bring the following equipment to the bed:
   - Large rubber or plastic sheet
   - 2 bath blankets
   - 2 bath towels
   - Tub or basin of appropriate size
2. Screen the unit. Identify the patient and explain what you plan to do.
3. Have patient flex knees. Loosen the top bedclothes at the foot of the bed and fold them back, just below patient's knees.
4. To make bed protector, place the rubber sheet across the foot of the bed. Place bath blanket folded in half, top half fanfolded toward foot of bed, over rubber sheet. Place towel on blanket and a hot water bottle at lower edge of towel.
5. Raising patient's feet, draw rubber sheet, blanket, and bath towel up under the legs and feet of patient. Bring upper half of bath blanket over feet.

6. Fill tub half full of water and place it lengthwise at the foot of bed. Temperature should be 105 degrees F unless otherwise ordered.
7. Raising the feet with one hand, draw tub under them and gradually immerse feet. Place a towel between the edge of the tub and the legs.
8. Draw the bath blanket up over the knees and fold it over from each side. Bring top covers over foot of bed to retain heat.
9. Replenish water as necessary to maintain desired temperature.
10. Discontinue treatment within 15 or 20 minutes.
11. Remove the patient's feet from tub and move them to the towel with hot water bottle under towel. Cover feet.
12. Remove tub to table or chair.
13. Dry and powder feet. Remove hot water bottle if desired.
14. Remove bath blanket, rubber sheet, and towel.
15. Draw down top covers and tuck in at foot.
16. Clean and replace equipment according to hospital policy. Wash hands.
17. A record of the procedure is made on the patient's chart. Include:
    - Area treated
    - Length of treatment
    - Your observations

Procedure

ASSISTING WITH THE HOT ARM SOAK

1. Wash your hands and assemble the following equipment on a tray:
   - Bath thermometer
   - Pitcher
   - Armsoak basin
   Also collect and bring to bedside:
   - A large plastic sheet
   - Bath blanket
   - Bath towel
2. Bring equipment to bedside. Identify the patient and explain what you plan to do.
3. Screen the unit and place equipment on overbed table.
4. Cover patient with bath blanket.
5. Fanfold bedding to foot of bed.
6. Expose arm to be soaked.
7. Elevate the head of the bed to a sitting position, if permitted.
8. Help patient to move to far side of bed, opposite the arm to be soaked. Be sure siderail is up and secure.
9. Cover bed with plastic sheeting and towel.
10. Fill armsoak basin half full with water at prescribed temperature (usually 100 degrees F). Check temperature with bath thermometer.
11. Take armsoak basin from overbed table and position on bed protector.
12. Assist patient to place arm gradually in basin.
13. Check temperature every 5 minutes. Use pitcher to get additional water and add to armsoak basin to maintain normal temperature.
14. Discontinue procedure at end of prescribed time. Lift patient's arm out of basin. Slip basin forward and allow arm to rest on bath towel. Place basin on overbed table and gently pat the arm dry with the towel.
15. Remove plastic sheeting and towel.
16. Adjust bedding and remove bath blanket. If treatment is to be repeated, fold bath blanket and place in bedside table. Leave unit tidy and call bell within reach.
17. Lower head of bed and make patient comfortable.

18. Take equipment to utility room. Clean and store according to hospital policy.
19. Record and report procedure and include:
    • Area treated
    • Length of treatment
    • Your observations

Procedure

APPLYING A MOIST COMPRESS

1. Wash hands and assemble the following equipment on a tray:
   • Asepto syringe
   • Basin with prescribed solution at temperature ordered
   • Bath thermometer
   • Bed protector
   • Binder or towel
   • Compresses
   • Pins or bandage
2. Identify patient and explain what you plan to do.
3. Bring equipment to the bedside. Screen the unit.
4. Expose only the area to be treated.
5. Protect bed and patient's clothing with bed protector (Chux®).
6. Moisten the compresses; remove excess liquid. Apply to treatment area.
7. Secure the dressings with bandage or binder. Dressing must be in contact with skin.
8. Help patient to maintain a comfortable position throughout the treatment. Practice good body mechanics.
9. If dressings are to be kept hot, a hot water bag or K-pad may be applied. If dressings are to be kept cool, an ice bag may be applied. An Asepto bulb or syringe, or a 50 cc syringe may be used to apply the solution to keep the dressing wet, Figure 25-4.
10. Remove dressings when ordered. Change once in 24 hours. Check skin several times each day.
11. Discard compresses.
12. Clean and replace equipment according to hospital policy. Wash hands.
13. A record of the treatment is made on the patient's chart.

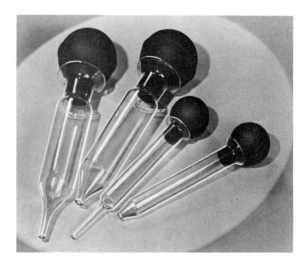

FIGURE 25-4.   Asepto or bulb syringes

Procedure
APPLYING A HEAT LAMP

1. Wash hands and assemble the following equipment:
   - Bath blanket
   - Heat lamp
   - Tape measure
2. Identify patient and explain what you plan to do.
3. Screen unit. Position patient and drape with bath blanket so only the area to be treated is exposed.
4. Position the lamp at a safe distance from the patient. Distance is determined by the wattage of the electric bulb. A 40-watt bulb is usually used and the light positioned 18 inches from the patient's body.
5. Check distance with the tape measure.
6. Turn lamp on, noting time.
7. Check patient every 5 minutes. Observe the skin carefully for signs of redness or burning.
8. Discontinue procedure after prescribed time.
9. Assist patient to a comfortable position.
10. Adjust bedding and remove drape.
11. If procedure is to be repeated, fold and leave bath blanket in bedside table.
12. Leave unit tidy.
13. Clean and return equipment according to hospital policy.
14. Wash hands.
15. Report and record procedure and include:
    - Time started
    - Length of treatment
    - Any observations you have made

Procedure
ASSISTING WITH THE SITZ BATH

1. Wash hands, assemble equipment, and take to the bathroom:
   - Bath thermometer
   - Bath towel
   - Bath blanket
   - Clean gown
   - Face towel
   - Safety pin
2. Temperature of bathroom should be 78 to 80 degrees F. Clean or rinse tub. Go to patient's room.
3. Identify patient. Explain what you plan to do and take patient to bathroom.
4. Fill tub half full. Level of water should extend only to patient's abdomen.
5. Check temperature with bath thermometer. It should be 105–110 degrees F.
6. Remove patient's robe and slippers and assist her into tub. A special tub is in common use in most hospitals, Figure 25-5. If a special tub is used, the patient's feet will remain on the floor and, therefore, she will wear her slippers. Figure 25-6 shows a portable unit.
7. Cover her shoulders with the bath blanket. Hold in place with a safety pin.
8. Place cool compresses on patient's forehead to prevent headache.
9. Patient should be watched throughout the procedure. Discontinue if patient shows signs of fatigue or faintness.
10. Allow some water to run out of tub; replace it to maintain constant temperature.

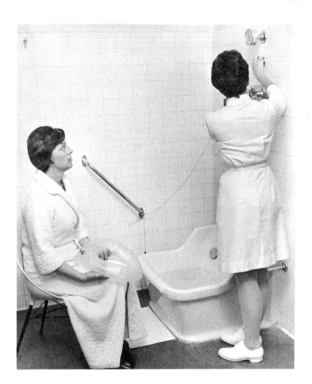

FIGURE 25-5.   Preparing for the sitz bath. This sitz bath is the stationary type.

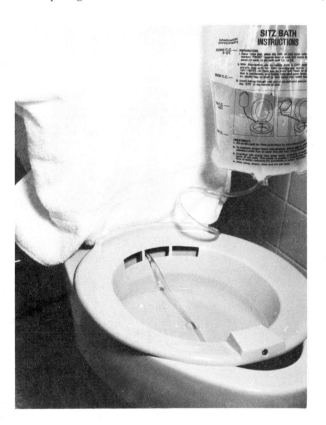

FIGURE 25-6.   The portable sitz bath fits on the toilet. (*From Simmers,* Diversified Health Occupations, *1983, Delmar Publishers Inc.*)

11. Assist patient from tub after 10 to 20 minutes.
12. Help patient to towel-dry and put on clean gown.
13. Assist patient to return to bed.

14. Clean tub. Clean and replace equipment according to hospital policy. Wash hands.
15. A record of the procedure is made on the patient's chart.

Procedure

ASSISTING WITH THE COOLING BATH (ALCOHOL SPONGE BATH)

1. Wash hands and assemble the following equipment:
   - 2 bath towels
   - Basin of tap water (ice cubes if ordered)
   - 2 bath blankets
   - Covered, filled icecap
   - 1 wash cloth
   - 5 covered, filled hot water bottles
   - Alcohol (70%)
2. Identify patient and explain what you plan to do.
3. Screen unit for privacy and to prevent drafts.
4. Take the patient's temperature.
5. Cover the patient with a bath blanket. Remove gown. Fanfold top bedding to foot of bed.
6. Position bath blanket under patient.
7. Add alcohol to water. The temperature should be about 70 degrees F.
8. Apply ice cap to head.
9. Apply hot water bags to the feet, groin and axilla.
10. Sponge with washcloth. Expose only one area at a time. Cover and allow to air dry. Sponge strokes should be in direction of heart. Continue procedure for approximately 20 minutes.
11. Bathe entire body. Avoid the eyes and genitals.
12. Replace gown and top bedding. Remove bath blankets and discard.
13. Clean equipment according to hospital policy. Wash hands.
14. Vital signs should be taken 10 minutes following sponge bath. Procedure may be repeated if temperature is still elevated.
15. Report and record:
    - Time
    - Cooling bath and solution used
    - Vital signs at beginning and termination of procedure
    - Patient response

Summary

Hot and cold applications are only given when there is a written order by the doctor. Care must be exercised in following the procedure accurately. The patient must be observed closely for signs of undesired reaction to the procedure. Carelessness will result in a patient being injured. Constantly keep in mind the cautions about these treatments that you have learned.

SUGGESTED ACTIVITIES

1. Practice carrying out procedures for hot and cold applications, using a Chase mannequin.

2. Practice properly filling a hot water bag.

VOCABULARY Learn the meaning and correct spelling of the following words.

diathermy   infrared   vasoconstriction
hemorrhage   sitz bath   vasodilation
hypothermia blanket ultraviolet

UNIT REVIEW **A. Clinical Situations.** Briefly describe how a health care assistant should react to the following situations.

1. You found the cover of the Aqua K-pad unit screwed on tightly.

2. You found an icebag without a cloth cover being used on a patient.

3. The patient receiving a cold treatment complained of numbness in the part being treated.

4. The patient receiving a sitz bath appears fatigued or dizzy.

B. Completion. Complete the following sentences.

1. Two types of hot and cold applications are _____ and _____.
2. Examples of hot applications are _____, _____, and _____.
3. Examples of cold applications are _____, _____, and _____.
4. A sitz bath provides _____ heat.
5. a. An ice bag or hot-water bag, should be filled _____.
   b. When filling the hot-water bag, pressing the hand against the flat surface expels the _____.
6. No application of heat or cold can be given without _____ _____.
7. The Aqua K unit should be filled with _____ water.
8. After securing the cap on an Aqua K unit, the cap must be loosened _____ turn.

Unit 26 Assisting with the Physical Examination

OBJECTIVES

As a result of this unit you will be able to:

- Name the positions for the various physical examinations.
- Drape patient for the various positions.
- Name the basic instruments necessary for physical examinations.

POSITIONING THE PATIENT

Physical examinations are done by the physician either in his office or after the patient's admission to the hospital. You will assist the doctor by preparing the equipment he will use, draping and positioning the patient, and remaining available during the examination, Figure 26-1.

The doctor may ask you to hand him equipment or to assist in providing additional lighting. Try to anticipate his needs. The gown may be removed and sheets used to *drape* (cover) the patient. Only the area being examined should be exposed. Be prepared to readjust drapes as needed to assure patient privacy. After completion of the examination, make sure the patient is comfortable and all equipment has been cleaned and returned to its proper location.

Some of the following positions may also be used for purposes other than the physical examination.

Dorsal Recumbent Position

The patient is flat on his back. Knees are bent (flexed) and slightly separated with feet flat on the bed. Loosen the gown at the neck. Cover the patient with a sheet. Place a small pillow under the head. This is the basic examination position.

Horizontal Recumbent Position

The patient is flat on his back; the legs are slightly separated. A pillow is placed under the head.

Knee-chest Position

The patient is placed on her abdomen. Head is turned to one side on a small pillow. Arms are bent and rest on either side of head. Knees are flexed and drawn up to meet chest. This is a difficult position to maintain, so the patient must never be left alone. Draping may be done with either one or two sheets. This position is used to examine the anal and vaginal area and to relieve pain following childbirth.

Prone Position

The patient is placed on his abdomen. Head is turned to one side on a small pillow. Arms are at sides or positioned on either side of head. One sheet is used for draping.

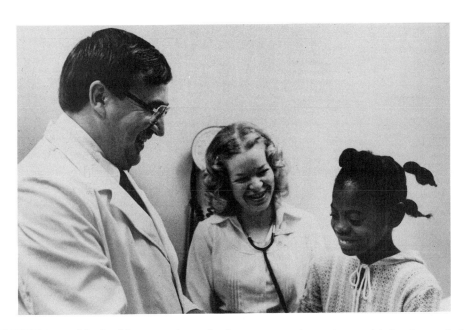

FIGURE 26-1.   The health care assistant lends support to the patient and helps her to feel comfortable.

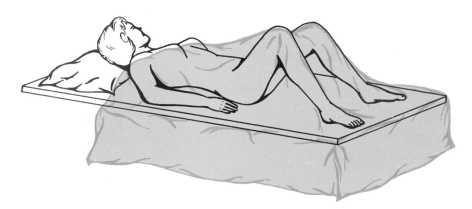

FIGURE 26-2.   The dorsal recumbent position

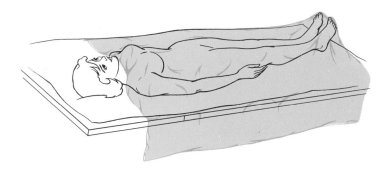

FIGURE 26-3.   The horizontal recumbent position

Sims' Position

The patient is positioned on his left side. Head is turned to one side on a small pillow. Left arm is placed behind the body. Right arm is comfortably positioned in front. The left leg is slightly bent while the right leg is sharply flexed on abdomen. One drape is usually adequate. Sims' position is used for vaginal and rectal examinations and for giving enemas.

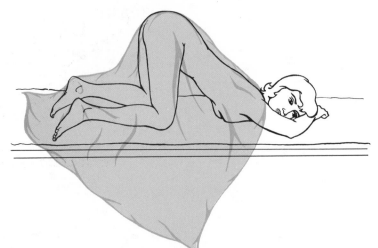

FIGURE 26-4.   The knee-chest position

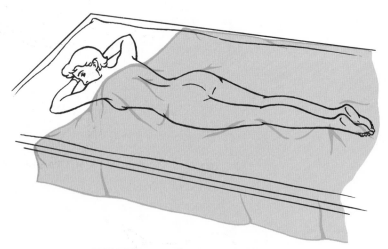

FIGURE 26-5.   The prone position

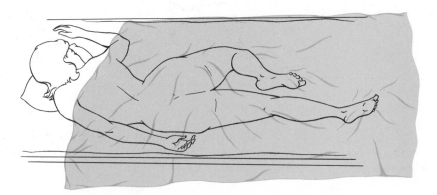

FIGURE 26-6.   Sims' position

Semi-Fowler's Position

The patient is positioned on his back with backrest elevated at a 45-degree angle to the bed. The knees are supported in a slightly bent position. The arms rest on the abdomen. One drape is usually adequate.

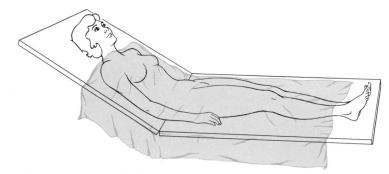

FIGURE 26-7.   Semi-Fowler's position

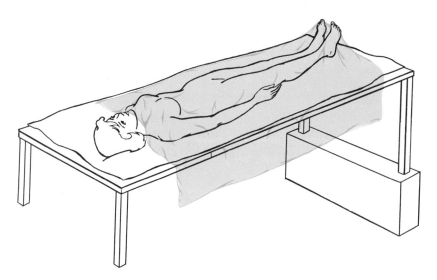

FIGURE 26-8.   Trendelenburg position

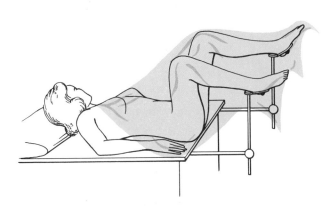

A. The patient's feet are placed in stirrups for the dorsal li-thotomy position so that the knees are well flexed and separated.

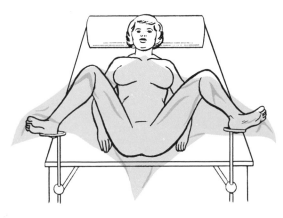

B. The patient may be draped with one sheet placed so that the corners fall at the patient's neck, pelvis, and feet.

FIGURE 26-9.

Trendelenburg Position

The patient lies flat on his back with the head lower than the rest of the body. If possible, the lower half of the bed or table is broken so the legs are flexed. In an emergency, the entire bed frame may be supported on blocks tilting the bed to a 45 degree plane, Figure 26-8. Beds that are electrically powered may be adjusted to this position. Shoulder braces may be needed to prevent the patient from slipping. This position encourages circulation to the patient's heart and brain.

Dorsal Lithotomy Position

The patient is positioned on her back. The knees are well separated and flexed. Usually, this position is achieved by placing the feet in stirrups. One or two drapes may be used to cover the patient, Figure 26-9A and B. The draping may be similar to draping for the knee-chest position. Remember the patient who "feels" covered and comfortable will be able to cooperate with the doctor more fully.

The dorsal lithotomy position is frequently used for the pelvic examination of female patients. The special equipment which you will assemble for the pelvic examination is shown in Figure 26-10.

MODIFICATIONS. Some of the positions discussed may be modified and used for other purposes such as to change the position of a patient confined to bed or to perform specific procedures. Adequate support with pillows must be provided if a position is to be maintained in any position for a period of time.

EQUIPMENT FOR PHYSICAL EXAMINATION

Some hospitals have examining instruments and equipment collected on trays. At other hospitals the assistant will gather the necessary equipment and assemble it, Figure 26-11. The basic equipment includes:

- Flashlight
- Gloves
- Percussion hammer
- Tongue depressors
- Cotton balls in antiseptic solution
- Emesis basin (lined with paper towel)
- Vaginal speculum
- Tissues

- Lubricant
- Skin pencil
- Tape measure
- Nasal speculum
- Otoscope
- Ophthalmoscope
- Blood pressure cuff
- Stethoscope

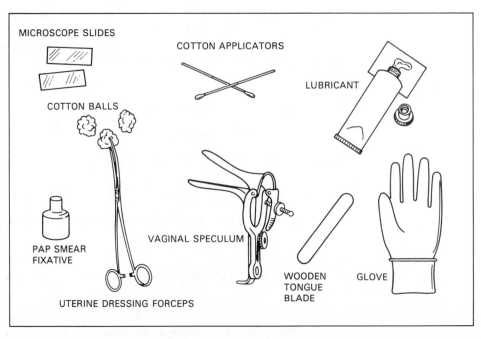

MICROSCOPE SLIDES

COTTON APPLICATORS

LUBRICANT

COTTON BALLS

PAP SMEAR FIXATIVE

UTERINE DRESSING FORCEPS

VAGINAL SPECULUM

WOODEN TONGUE BLADE

GLOVE

FIGURE 26-10.   Equipment for pelvic examination

Fig. 26-10 Equipment for pelvic examination

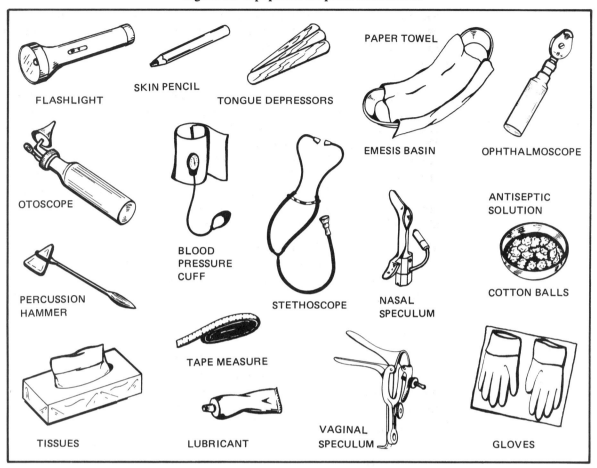

FIGURE 26-11.   Basic equipment for the physical examination

Summary

The physical examination is performed by the physician. Provide privacy while the doctor discusses the patient's history. Be ready to assist during the examination and to provide proper lighting. Avoid overexposing the patient as you adjust the drapes. Remember, most patients feel *apprehensive* (frightened) about physical examinations. It is very important for the assistant to know the equipment to be used. A quiet, assured approach can do much to help the patient at this time.

SUGGESTED ACTIVITIES

1. Practice positioning and draping.

2. Set up a tray of examination equipment.

3. Assist with a physical examination.

UNIT REVIEW

A. Brief Answer.

1. Name the instruments and equipment used in a pelvic examination.

2. Explain how the health assistant assists during a physical examinaton.

B. Clinical Situations. Briefly describe how a health care assistant should react to the following situations.

1. The patient seems very apprehensive before a physical exam.

2. The physician wants to do a pelvic examination.

C. **Completion.** Complete the following sentences.
   1. When in the lithotomy position the knees are _____.
   2. When in the dorsal recumbent position, the patient lies on his _____.
   3. When in the knee-chest position, the patient should never be _____.
   4. When in the prone position, the patient lies on his _____.
   5. When in the Sims' position, the patient lies on his _____ side.

Unit 27 The Surgical Patient

OBJECTIVES

As a result of this unit, you will be able to:

- Assist patients in preopertive care.
- Assist patients in postoperative care.
- Prepare the patient's unit for his return from the operating room.
- List the various types of anesthesia.
- Prepare a recovery bed.
- Shave the operative area.

The care of the surgical patient can be divided into three parts: *preoperative* (before surgery), *operative* (in the operating room), and *postoperative* (following surgery). During the immediate postoperative period, the patient recovers from *anesthesia;* frequently in a special area, the *recovery room*, which is located right next to the operating room.

Anesthesia is medicine given to patients so that they will not be uncomfortable during the operation. It keeps them from feeling the pain. There are several ways that anesthesia may be given.

Patients facing any surgical procedure tend to be fearful. It is well to remember that these patients require great emotional as well as physical support.

PREOPERATIVE CARE

Preoperative care begins at the moment when surgery is planned by the doctor with the patient. Your responsibilities begin when the patient is admitted to the hospital. Remember that you may answer general questions that the patient asks but you must refer specific questions about the surgery, its possible outcome, and anesthesia to your team leader.

Frequently, patients wish to talk with their clergymen before undergoing surgery, Figure 27-1. Transmit requests of this kind to the proper person. When the clergyman arrives, provide privacy by screening the unit. A spiritual visit can be of great emotional support and should not be neglected if requested.

The Evening Before Surgery

Part of the final preparation is done the evening before surgery. It usually includes: a bath with surgical soap, enemas, surgical prep (shaving of the operative site), medication to ensure a good night's rest, and the insertion of special tubes for draining body cavities. The patient is usually put on NPO (nothing by mouth) after midnight, and the water pitcher is removed from the bedside table. An NPO notice should be posted on the bed and bedside table.

THE SURGICAL PREP AREA. The area to be washed and shaved will be greater than the surgical incision, Figure 27-2. Make sure you know exactly

271

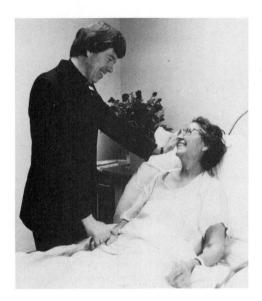

FIGURE 27-1. A visit from the patient's clergy can be very comforting preoperatively.

what area is to be shaved. Usually, female patients do not have their neck or face shaved. The preparations for cranial surgery are usually performed after the patient has been medicated and taken to the operating suite. Doctors have special preferences in this regard. Most hospitals also have routine prep areas. If a spinal anesthesia is given, the back may be shaved also.

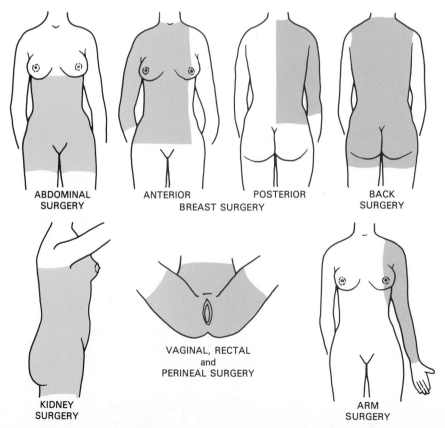

ABDOMINAL
SURGERY

ANTERIOR
BREAST SURGERY

POSTERIOR

BACK
SURGERY

KIDNEY
SURGERY

VAGINAL, RECTAL
and
PERINEAL SURGERY

ARM
SURGERY

FIGURE 27-2. Shaded areas indicate areas usually shaved preoperatively.

Procedure

SHAVING THE OPERATIVE AREA

1. Wash hands and assemble the following equipment:
   - Bath blanket
   - Individual prep pack
       OR
   - Tray with razor and new razor blades
   - 2 small bowls
   - Applicators
   - Cleansing soap
   - 4 × 4 sponges
   - Paper towels
   - Towels or disposable Chux
2. Determine the exact area to be prepped.
3. In utility room, fill small bowls with warm water. Add cleansing soap to one. Adjust razor and blade. Make sure they are tight.
4. Cover tray and take to bedside.
5. Identify the patient and explain what you plan to do. Screen the unit. Provide adequate lighting.
6. Drape patient with bath blanket. Place towel under area to be shaved, Figure 27-3.
7. Holding skin taut with one hand, lather area to be shaved. If hair is very long, such as on the pubis and axilla, it may be clipped with scissors before shaving.
8. Shave area with strokes in same direction as the hair grows. Be careful not to cut the skin or to remove any warts or moles. Work carefully around this area.
9. Using the applicators, clean the *umbilicus* (navel) and shave it if it's in the operative area.
10. Check carefully for hairs after shaving is complete. Unattached hairs are easily removed by gently pressing a piece of tape against the area. Discard hair in paper towel.
11. Cleanse the skin with warm soapy water. Rinse and dry thoroughly.
12. Remove towel from under patient. Make sure linen is dry. Change if necessary. Leave patient in a comfortable position.
13. Return equipment. Clean and store in accordance with hospital policy. Wash hands.

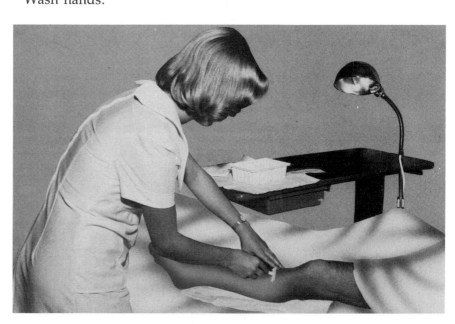

FIGURE 27-3.   Prepping the operative area

14. Record:
   • Date and time
   • Procedure, surgical prep (area shaved, any unusual observations)

Immediate Preoperative Care

Approximately one hour before surgery, the patient will be given additional medication by the nurse. All your responsibilities regarding the patient must be completed before this time. You may be asked to do the following:

• Take and record vital signs (see Section Three).
• Take care of valuables according to hospital policy.
   Remove dentures and other *prostheses* (artificial parts) and see that they are safely cared for, Figure 27-4.
• Remove nail polish, makeup, hairpins, and jewelry. Long hair should be neatly braided.
• Dress the patient in a hospital gown and cover the hair with surgical cap or towel.
• See that the patient voids and measure the urine.
• Make sure that the room is quiet and comfortable.

As soon as the nurse gives the medication, the siderails must be in place for safety. All unnecessary equipment is removed, and the bedside table, overbed table, and chair are pushed out of the way to make room for the stretcher when it arrives from surgery.

You may have a surgical checklist which must be completed, Figure 27-5. You are responsible for checking off those duties to which you were assigned. Be sure also to note the time your patient leaves for surgery. The nurse and surgical attendant will check the patient's identification and surgical checklist before the patient is moved. A staff member, and sometimes a family member, accompanies the patient to the doors of the operating

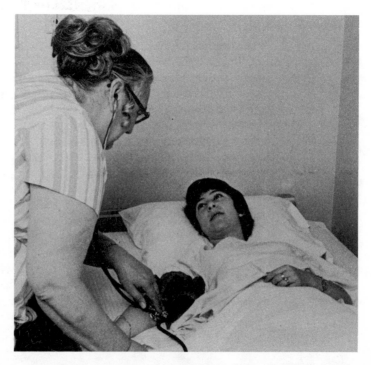

FIGURE 27-4. Immediate preoperative care includes taking vital signs. Jewelry will be removed and properly cared for. Dentures should also be removed.

☐ Admission sheet

☐ Surgical consent

☐ Sterilization consent (if necessary)

☐ Consultation sheet (if necessary)

☐ History and physical

☐ Lab reports (pregnancy test also if necessary)

☐ Surgery prep done and charted, if required

☐ Latest T.P.R. and blood pressure charted

☐ Preoperative medication has been given and charted (if required)

☐ Name tape on patient

☐ Fingernail polish and makeup removed

☐ Metallic objects removed (rings may be taped)

☐ Dentures removed

☐ Other prostheses removed (such as artificial limb or eye)

☐ Bath blanket and head cap in place

☐ Bed in high position and siderails up after preop is given

☐ Patient has voided prior to surgery and voiding charted

FIGURE 27-5.   Surgical checklist

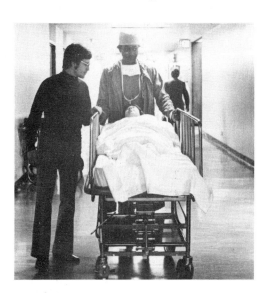

FIGURE 27-6.   Sometimes, a family member is allowed to go to the doors of the OR with the patient and a staff member.

room, Figure 27-6. You will probably be asked to assist in transferring the patient from the bed to the stretcher and after surgery, from the stretcher to the bed. Review Procedure in Unit 14.

DURING THE OPERATIVE PERIOD

While the patient is in the operating room, Figure 27-7A and B, you will prepare the room for the patient's return. A special *surgical bed* will be made. This was covered in Unit 15. The surgical bed is also called a postop or recovery bed. Everything should be removed from the bedside stand except an emesis basin, tissue wipes, tongue depressors, and equipment to check vital signs. A pencil and small pad to record the signs should be available also. Check with your team leader for any special equipment such as oxygen, IV poles, suction or drainage bags that might be necessary for your patient. Be watchful while carrying out your other assignments for the return of your patient from surgery.

ANESTHESIA

Anesthesia is given to prevent pain and induce forgetfulness. The choice of anesthetic agent (drug) and method of administration will be de-

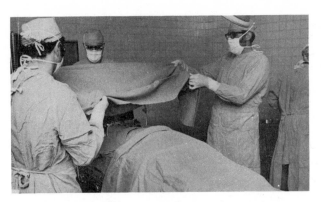

A. In surgery, the patient is draped with sterile linen.

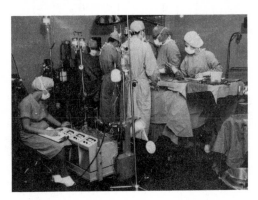

B. During the surgery, all team members work
with absolute precision and cooperation.

FIGURE 27-7.

termined by the location and type of surgery to be performed, the length
of time needed for the surgery, and the patient's physical condition. There
are two main types of anesthetics: *general* and *local*.

General Anesthesia

GASES. Some anesthetics like ether and other gases are inhaled. The patient loses total consciousness during the procedure. Since inhaled anesthetics are apt to make the patient secrete more mucus and be nauseated,
special attention must be given during the postoperative period to keeping
the respiratory tract clear. There is real danger that vomitus may be drawn
into the respiratory tract. This is called *aspiration.*

INTRAVENOUS ANESTHETICS. Drugs may be given directly into the veins.
They act rapidly, and the patient is soon unconscious. IV anesthetics are
often used for short operations or in addition to other anesthesia.

Local Anesthesia

Drugs such as procaine hydrochloride may be injected into the area
around the operative area. These drugs stop the sensation of pain only in
that area and are called locals. The patient remains awake but free from
pain during the operation.

Spinal Anesthesia

A drug is injected into the spinal canal which prevents feeling from
any point below the level of the injection. The patient remains awake. Spinal
anesthesia is commonly used for abdominal surgery because it produces
good relaxation of the muscles.

Following this type of anesthetic, the patient is unable to feel or move the legs for a period of time. If not prepared ahead of time, the patient may be frightened by this experience. Since the patient will be unable to move independently until sensation returns, extra care must be given to frequent turning and proper alignment.

There is an exception, however. Some physicians require that the patient remain flat on the back and without a pillow for 8 to 12 hours following a spinal to avoid headaches. Any complaints of a headache following spinal anesthesia should be reported promptly.

POSTOPERATIVE CARE

Immediate postoperative care takes place in the recovery room of the hospital. When the patient's condition is stabilized, he or she is returned to the unit. Upon the patient's return from the recovery room, the health care assistant should identify the patient and assist in the transfer from the stretcher to the bed (see Unit 14). Unconscious patients must not be left alone at any time. Your team leader will inform you of any special instructions. The following are routine instructions to be followed unless otherwise ordered.

- Take vital signs of the patient upon arrival on the unit and every 15 minutes for four readings (see Section Eight). The patient's temperature may not always be taken at this time. If signs are *stable* (approximately the same) at the end of this time, repeat in one hour. Note the patient's state of consciousness (unresponsive, drowsy, alert).
- Check dressings for amount and type of any drainage. The nurse may reinforce them as necessary.
- Check IV solution for flow rate. Restrain infusion site whenever necessary (prn). Remember the flow rate is ordered by the doctor.
- Encourage the patient to breathe deeply, cough, and move in bed. Position should be changed every 2 hours.
- Turn the patient's head to one side and support if vomiting. Have emesis basin ready, as well as tissues and wet cloth. If patient is conscious, allow him to rinse mouth with water after vomiting. Note type and amount of vomitus.
- Be sure all drainage tubes have been connected (the nurse will usually attend to this). If you notice a tube clamped shut, check with your team leader.

Patients often return from surgery with a variety of tubes and drains in place. Some tubes may deliver materials into the patient: oxygen tubes or intravenous tubes. Other tubes may have been placed in the patient to provide drainage from wounds or body cavities. The following are some special precautions to be taken:

1. Learn the type, purpose, and location of each tube.
2. Check drainage for character and amount.
3. Check for obstructions to the tube system.
4. Check flow rate of infusions from intravenous lines.
5. Keep *orifices* (body openings) clear of secretions and discharge.
6. Never disconnect tubes or raise drainage bottles above the level of the drainage site.
7. Never lower infusion bottles below the level of infusion site.
8. Never put stress on the tubes when moving patient or giving care.
9. Restrain infusion sites as necessary to prevent dislocation.
10. Monitor levels of infusions and report to the nurse before they run out.

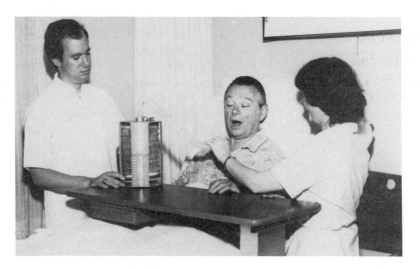

FIGURE 27-8.   The health care assistant may assist the patient with the equipment, but the incentive spirometer is a self-administered treatment.

11. Report any signs of leakage or disconnected tubes at once.
12. Report pain, discoloration or swelling at sites of drainage and infusion.

When the patient has responded sufficiently and his vital signs are stable, he may be refreshed by washing his hands and face, changing his linen, and giving him a light back rub.

At this time, the physician may write orders for an *incentive spirometor* or *respirator,* Figure 27-8, to help the lungs to fully expand, thereby preventing collapse of the alveolar air sacs, called *atelectasis,* or pneumonia.

The patient is instructed how to use the incentive spirometer by a respiratory therapist or nurse. The idea is to exhale normally and then, with the lips placed tightly around the mouthpiece, to inhale through the mouth sufficiently to raise the balls in the chambers. The deep breath should be held as long as possible (or as ordered) thereby keeping the balls suspended. The patient then removes the mouth piece and exhales in the normal manner. The exercise is repeated as many times as is ordered. This procedure may be carried out with the patient in bed, with head and shoulders well-supported if permitted. The patient may be taught this procedure before surgery.

Although this procedure is started by the professional, you too, have responsibilities. Observe the patient for correctness of procedure and be sure the patient does not become overly fatigued. Encourage the patient to cough and clear the respiratory passageways. Report to your team leader if the patient seems overly fatigued during the procedure. Carefully observe and report any unusual responses such as pain, dizziness or throat and airway irritation.

When the patient has completed the pulmonary exercise, the mouthpiece should be washed in warm water, dried, replaced in the plastic bag and left at the bedside.

Some time after surgery, a patient is permitted to sit up with his legs over the edge of the bed. This position is called *dangling.* He must be watched carefully for signs of fatigue and dizziness *(vertigo).* The patient should be assisted to assume the dangling position slowly. The first *ambulation* (walking) is usually short and preceded by a brief period of dangling. It is an important part of post-operative care since it stimulates circulation and helps prevent the formation of blood clots (emboli).

Procedure

ASSISTING THE PATIENT TO DANGLE

1. Wash hands and assemble the following equipment:
   • Bath blanket
   • Pillow
2. Identify patient and explain what you plan to do. Check the pulse (see Unit 21).
3. Provide privacy as needed. Lock bed in the down position.
4. Drape patient with bath blanket and fanfold top bedcovers to foot of bed.
5. Gradually elevate head of bed.
6. Help patient to put on bathrobe.
7. Place one arm around patient's shoulders and the other under the knees.
8. Gently and slowly turn patient toward you. Allow patient's legs to hang over the side of the bed.
9. Roll pillow and tuck firmly to patient's back for support.
10. After putting slippers on patient give an instruction to swing the legs. A chair may be placed to support the patient's feet for a few minutes.
11. Have the patient dangle as long as ordered. If he becomes dizzy or faint, return him to bed position. Report to the supervising nurse immediately.
12. Check the patient's pulse.
13. Rearrange pillow at head of bed. Remove patient's bathrobe and slippers.
14. Place one arm around patient's shoulders and the other under his knees. Gently and slowly swing the patient's legs onto the bed.
15. Lower head of bed and rearrange top bedcovers. Check the patient's pulse. Make sure he is comfortable before leaving him. Wash hands.
16. Record:
    • Date and time
    • Procedure, dangling (observations, duration, pulse)

Procedure

ASSISTING THE PATIENT IN INITIAL AMBULATION

1. Follow the procedure for dangling. Make sure bed is not elevated. Have a chair available in case patient becomes fatigued.
2. After patient has dangled without ill effects, assist to stand. Check pulse. (If patient becomes dizzy or faint, return to bed position. Have the patient take deep breaths and look around the room rather than closing his eyes. Talk to and reassure the patient.)
3. Transfer your arm behind the patient's waist, and turn so you face the same direction.
4. Walk slowly for a short distance and return to bedside. If patient appears tired or faint, or if there is a marked change in his pulse, allow him to rest.
5. Assist patient back to bed and make him comfortable. Check pulse.
6. If patient should faint during procedure, gently lower to the floor, protecting head. Do not attempt to hold the patient up. Signal for help.
7. Record:
   • Date and time
   • Procedure, ambulation (special observations, duration, pulse)

Binders

Binders are pieces of cotton material that are applied to different parts of the body to hold surgical dressings in place and provide support, Figure 27-9. The binder should be clean and be applied smoothly to prevent pressure areas. It should fit snugly, but it should not be so tight that it causes discomfort.

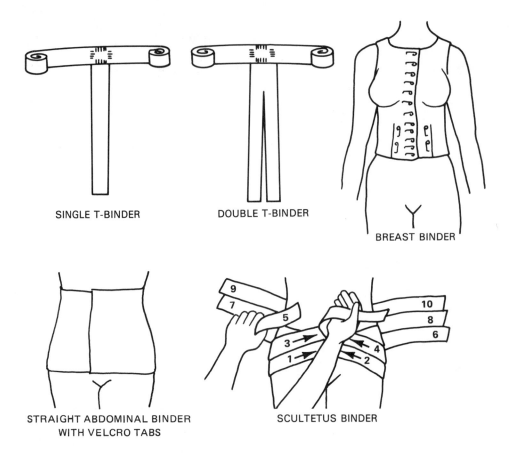

SINGLE T-BINDER   DOUBLE T-BINDER   BREAST BINDER

STRAIGHT ABDOMINAL BINDER
WITH VELCRO TABS   SCULTETUS BINDER

FIGURE 27-9. Types of binders

The straight abdominal binder, the *scultetus* (many tailed) binder, and single and double T-binders may be used postoperatively. Figure 27-10 shows the application of the scultetus binder. As a rule, the binder is applied from the bottom to the top in alternating layers. The top two tails are crossed over the abdomen and pinned or fastened at the hips.

T-binders are used to hold dressings on the rectal and perineal areas

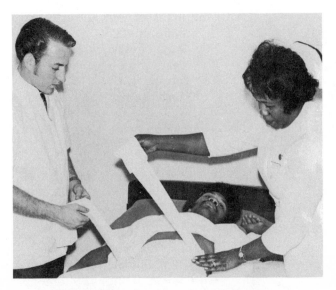

FIGURE 27-10. Applying the scultetus binder

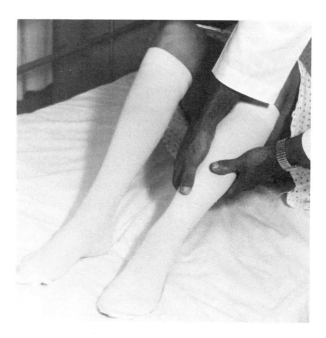

FIGURE 27-11. Both hands are used to smooth the hose into place and to remove any wrinkles. *(From Simmers,* Diversified Health Occupations, *1983, Delmar Publishers Inc.)*

in place. The single T-binder is usually used for female patients; the double T-binder for male patients. The binder is placed around the patient's waist, and the tail is passed between the patient's legs and fastened at the waist with a pin. The split tails of the double T-binder are brought up on either side of the scrotum. The straight binder or a special halter type may be used to support the breasts of female patients.

Elasticized Stockings

Elasticized stockings, called TED Hose or anti-embolism hose, or Ace bandages which extend from the ankle or foot to calf or mid-thigh, are often applied during the postoperative period to support the veins of the legs. This reduces the incidence of *thrombophlebitis,* which is inflammation of the veins with blood clots. They must be applied smoothly and evenly before getting the patient out of bed, Figure 27-11. They should be removed and reapplied at least every 8 hours; more often if necessary.

Procedure
APPLYING ELASTICIZED STOCKINGS

1. Wash hands and assemble:
   • Elasticized stockings of proper length and size
2. Identify patient and explain what you plan to do.
3. With patient lying down, expose one leg at a time.
4. Grasp stocking with both hands at the top and roll toward toe end.
5. Adjust over toes, positioning opening at base of toes (unless toes are to be covered). Remember that the raised seams should be on the outside.
6. Apply stocking to leg by rolling upward toward body.
7. Check to be sure stocking is applied evenly and smoothly and there are no wrinkles.
8. Repeat procedure on opposite leg.
9. Report and chart:
   • Date and time
   • Any unusual observations
   • Procedure: application or reapplication of elasticized hose

Drainage

When a body cavity is the operative site, it may be necessary to drain fluid, such as blood, pus, or gastric juice from it before or after surgery. The drainage outlet may be a catheter, T-tube, Penrose drain or cigarette drain. When such a drain is in place, the drainage accumulates on the dressing. The health care assistant should note the amount and character of the drainage. The dressing will be reinforced or changed by the nurse as needed.

At times the withdrawal of fluids is controlled by attaching the drainage tube to a connecting tube and then a suction apparatus. The drainage accumulates in a bottle which is emptied and the contents measured at the completion of each shift. A record of the amount and character of the drainage is entered in both the output chart and the nurses' notes.

It is the responsibility of the health care assistant to report either excessive or diminished drainage, or a change in the character of the drainage. The assistant must also make sure that the flow of drainage is not blocked by kinking of the tube. The assistant must never assume responsibility for chest drainage or attempt to empty chest bottles. Chest bottles and irrigations require professional attention.

Summary

The surgical patient requires continuous care before, during, and after surgery. The health care assistant helps in preoperative and postoperative care: preparing the operative site, readying the patient on the morning of surgery, helping in the transfer of the patient to and from the stretcher, and preparation of the surgical bed.

Immediate postoperative care is given in the recovery room by professional personnel. Once the patient's condition has stabilized, he or she will be returned to the unit. Be sure you are available to assist in transferring the patient into bed and have all equipment needed in readiness.

Carefully observe the patient for levels of consciousness, complaints of pain, amount and type of drainage, infusion flow, dressings, and vital signs. Report all observations to your supervising nurse.

SUGGESTED ACTIVITIES

1. Using the mannequin, practice the technique of shaving the operative site.

2. Under direct supervision, give care to preoperative and postoperative patients.

3. With your instructor, investigate the policies in your hospital in regard to areas to be shaved for different operations.

VOCABULARY

Learn the meaning and correct spelling of the following words.

ambulation	incentive spirometer	recovery room
anesthesia	local anesthetic	respirator
aspiration	operative	surgical bed
atelectasis	orifice	thrombophlebitis
dangling	postoperative	umbilicus
emboli	preoperative	vertigo
general anesthetic	prosthesis	

UNIT REVIEW

A. Clinical Situations. Briefly describe how a health care assistant should react to the following situations.

1. You are assigned to do a pubic prep and your patient's pubic hair is very long.

2. You are assisting a patient with initial ambulation, and the patient faints.

3. You find that the antiembolism stockings your patient is wearing are wrinkled and have slipped down his leg.

B. Completion. Complete the following sentences.
1. The three phases of care required by the surgical patient are: _____, _____, and _____.
2. The purpose of anesthesia is _____.
3. Gaseous anesthetics are _____.
4. When patients have general anesthesia, they are apt to _____ postoperatively.
5. Gaseous anesthetics keep the patient _____ during surgery.
6. During a local anesthetic, the patient may remain _____ during surgery.
7. When a spinal anesthetic is given all sensations _____ the level of the injection are _____.
8. Intravenous anesthetics make the patient fall asleep _____.
9. Seven duties the assistant may be assigned in regard to the preoperative patient are:

10. Equipment left on the bedside table after the recovery bed is made includes: _____.
11. When a patient vomits, his head should be _____ to prevent _____.
12. Spinal anesthesia is often given for abdominal surgery because it produces good _____.
13. Postoperatively, the assistant should check the _____ of the IV solution.
14. The patient's position should be changed every _____ hours following surgery.
15. You should always check the patient's _____ frequently as the patient dangles or ambulates for the first time.
16. Three kinds of binders used postoperatively are _____, _____, and _____.
17. Elasticized stockings or Ace bandages are applied postoperatively to help support the _____ of the legs.

Unit 28 Long-term Care of the Elderly and Chronically Ill

OBJECTIVES

As a result of this unit, you will be able to:

- List the signs of aging.
- Define various types of extended-care facilities.
- Describe ways of communicating more effectively with hearing-impaired patients.

Health assistants function in the acute-care institution in a variety of useful ways, giving care under the direct and careful supervision of a professional health provider. They also function in long-term care facilities providing for those activities of daily living (ADL) that patients are no longer able to carry out themselves.

Many of the same health care skills that were previously discussed are needed in this setting; sometimes these skills need to be modified and adapted to the chronic conditions of the patient in long-term care facilities, however. The health assistant still will be supervised and guided by the professional nurse who is responsible for carrying out the physician's orders.

LONG-TERM CARE FACILITIES

Long-term care facilities provide housing and care for about 5% of the elderly population. The older a person becomes, the greater the likelihood he or she will become part of the long-term care population.

These institutions, monitored by state and federal agencies, vary both in size and in the type of services which they provide. They are identified by a variety of names which often indicate the extent of the nursing care provided.

All long-term or extended-care facilities are equipped to provide for dietary and housing needs and most provide some degree of assistance in helping the occupants carry out their activities of daily living and in meeting their various health needs.

Skilled Nursing Care Facilities

These facilities, also called *convalescent homes*, provide for nursing service needs that do not require acute hospitalization. These extended-care facilities usually provide rehabilitation and social services. Specific nursing care plans are formulated for each patient, establishing both short- and long-term goals. As conditions improve, patients may move to their own homes or to one of the other long-term care facilities. Some families prefer to have their members continue under this care when other satisfactory alternatives are not feasible.

Intermediate Care Facilities

These facilities provide less nursing care, and many of these patients are ambulatory or able to help with their own care to some degree.

Personal Care Homes

These homes, called personal care or residential bed and board, are sometimes also referred to as homes for the aged. The amount of care in these facilities is varied. Most of these patients need little supervision or help with their activities. Most are older and have chronic conditions but are able to remain active. One requirement in some is that the tenant be able to get to the dining room for at least one meal a day.

The work of the health care assistant is very important to the patients in each of these types of care facilities, Figure 28-1. He or she may become the most significant person in the lives of the old or dependent person for whom he or she cares.

ROLE OF THE HEALTH CARE ASSISTANT IN LONG-TERM CARE

As in the acute care hospital, the assistant carries out the procedures that have been taught, assisting in the health care of elderly patients under the direct supervision of a professional nurse. Basic physical care, as well as special procedures, will be carried out to help these patients reach their maximum degree of well-being.

The health care assistant who is successful in this setting must be patient and kind. The assistant must be able to derive satisfaction from being part of slow progress and small, if any, gains. A sense of humor is vital, as is the ability to communicate. These are attributes that are important in any health setting, but in the long-term care facility they become *paramount*.

Many of the patients will remain under your care for long periods of time, even for years. You will develop growing relationships which will become important to both care giver and care receiver. In those circumstances, communications take on greater importance. Greater significance may be attached to the attention to care or even the way thoughts are expressed in words.

Thus, the long-term care giver is a *very special person* working, perhaps, in a less dramatic but equally important area of health care.

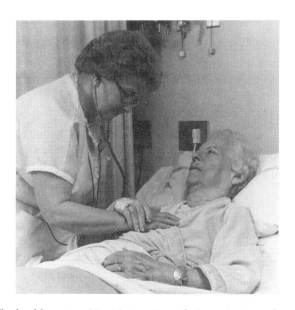

FIGURE 28-1. The health care assistant is an extremely important member of the health care team in a long-term care facility.

EFFECTS OF AGING

The patient in the long-term facility is usually advanced in age with one or more chronic, somewhat *debilitating* conditions. Some are mentally alert while others are confused and disoriented.

There are, however, some features of aging which are characteristic for most elderly clients. Do not expect every client to exhibit the same characteristics at the same *chronologic* age, but remember that aging is a natural, progressive process that begins at birth and extends to death. Remember also, that every patient is unique and must be treated with dignity and respect.

Physical Changes in Aging

Some investigators believe we are born with a biologic time clock, programmed for a specific life span, barring accidents and disease process. As we move toward old age, changes which have been taking place gradually become more evident. For example, the elderly person may lose vitality, sleep less at night, and benefit from rest periods during the day. Tissues in the body lose fluids and become more dehydrated, resulting in a loss of elasticity and resiliency. Fibrous changes decrease tone, mass, and strength of both skeletal and smooth muscles. Secretory and endocrine cells become less functional and nerve sensitivity is reduced.

Response to sensory stimuli is slower and less accurate. Pain and awareness of injury are not always perceived with the same intensity and serious situations may be ignored.

Smell and taste are less acute, influencing appetite which tends to lag.

Eyes undergo changes which limit peripheral vision and near vision: *accommodation*, making additional lighting necessary. Hearing diminishes, sometimes so slowly that hearing loss is significant before being recognized. Lessening or loss of sight and hearing may make the older person feel isolated and frustrated in their ability to communicate.

Joints become less flexible and some *degeneration* or breakdown is evident. Reaction time may be prolonged, and muscles lose strength and tone. Bones become more brittle and *porous*. These changes often combine to make falls more common and serious. Muscular walls may become less functional, leading to protrusion of organs through restraining walls, called *herniations*, and making elimination more difficult. Changes in the bones of the vertebral column result in loss of height, as well as postural changes, Figure 28-2.

Getting up to void during the night: known as *nocturia*, may become a problem when the kidneys lose some of their ability to concentrate urine. You know that the amount of urine that is produced and eliminated is affected by loss of smooth muscle tone and loss of *vascular* pathways. In the same way, emptying the bladder incompletely *predisposes* the elderly to urinary infections. Enlargement of the prostate, frequently seen in elderly men, complicates the problem of urinary retention.

Changes within the cardiovascular system are reflected throughout the entire body. Atherosclerotic changes narrow vessels, increasing blood pressure and diminishing blood flow throughout the body. The changes increase the stress on the heart, further accelerating its natural degenerative changes.

Adequate nutrition is often hampered in the elderly by loss of tastebuds, decreased digestive enzymes, and poor dentition.

Perhaps the most obvious changes are seen in the *integumentary* system, as loss of fat and water lead to wrinkling and sagging. The skin color

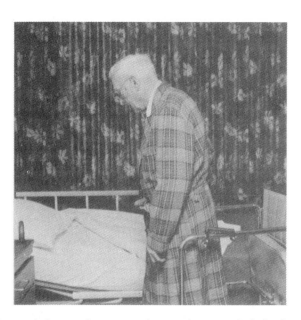

FIGURE 28-2. Postural changes become evident as the musculoskeletal system undergoes changes associated with aging. *(From Caldwell and Hegner,* Geriatrics: a Study of Maturity, *1981, Delmar Publishers Inc.)*

becomes more sallow as capillaries recede; fingernails and toenails thicken and become more brittle. Areas of *pigmentation* become more pronounced, resulting in elevated patches of yellowish or brown spots, known as *senile lentigines* or liver spots. *Senile keratoses*, which are roughened, scaly, wart-like lesions, develop. These must be considered potentially dangerous since they may become malignant.

The amount and color of the hair undergo changes that are indicative of the normal aging process. Hair usually becomes both thinner and lighter in color. Decrease in oil production makes the hair dull and lifeless.

Changes in the functioning of the reproductive organs are closely related to changes in endocrine levels. Nevertheless, the older person's ability to engage in successful, satisfying intercourse is not precluded. Some *accommodation* (adjustment) for slower erectile response and for thinning and less *lubrication* of the vagina must be made, but with adequate care, sexual response can continue.

Some physical changes associated either with aging or other causes will necessitate the use of a *prosthesis*, which is an artificial body part. It replaces a part of the body that has been lost or severely impaired. Dentures are prosthetic devices, as are artificial legs and eyes. Each prosthetic device is expensive and is designed to meet the needs of a particular patient. You must learn how each prosthesis is applied, how it is cared for, and how it should be stored. Your team leader or the patient himself are excellent sources for this information.

Emotional Adjustments to Aging

Emotional adjustments in aging are basically extensions of the adjustments the individual has made throughout life to the many changes in a person's circumstances. Personality characteristics and ways of reacting to stress are developed fairly early in life and tend to become a constant in the personality of the individual. In fact, as a person ages, personality traits become even more pronounced. The stress produced by the circumstances and illnesses that accompany old age do not drastically alter the individual's personality, but they do tend to enhance and, in some cases, distort the basic traits.

Old people have the same emotional needs and require the same supports for good mental health as young people, Figure 28-3. They need to be loved, to feel a sense of achievement and recognition, and to have a degree of economic security. Although these needs are common to all human beings, regardless of age, the avenues for achieving satisfaction and gratification of these needs, however, are narrowed greatly for older people. The opportunities for social exchange and sexual expression, the two major means of gratification, are greatly reduced as the years advance and end by being practically nonexistent for those confined to homes for the aged.

The attitude of the Western world toward old people is such that it tends to *relegate* them to a position of lesser and lesser significance. The older people become, the more their self-image is *depreciated* both in their own eyes and in the eyes of others.

Physical ailments, far more common in the elderly because of slowed body processes, are *superimposed* upon the changes brought about by the natural aging process. Change of body image and loss of the vigor and *vitality* of former years are major losses the older person must accept—losses that further alter their self-image and self-esteem.

In old age, some accommodations must be made in the attitudes or psychological outlooks of all persons. The most healthy emotional responses are based on philosophies that accept aging as a natural progressive stage, in life-attitudes that recognize the strengths as well as the limitations of the body, and on a form of behavior that demonstrates interest in living here and now. Healthy psychological adjustments mean both a realistic appraisal of the present circumstance and building on the positive values while coming to terms with the negative aspects.

Some of your long-term care patients will have already made these adjustments. Some will be in the process. Your supportive caring will be important and helpful to each.

SPECIFIC EMOTIONAL RESPONSES. Frustration is a common emotion experienced by the elderly; frustration at physical limitations and at having less control over their own lives. That is why it is important to allow the elderly the opportunity to make as many decisions as possible for themselves.

Signs of frustration are often demonstrated in aggressive behavior: anger, hostility, demanding behavior, and complaining. Some patients even resort to bullying families, staff, or other patients in an attempt to relieve their feelings of helplessness, Figure 28-4. Crying, complaints of self-pity, and whining represent more ways patients *overtly* respond to their anxieties and fears.

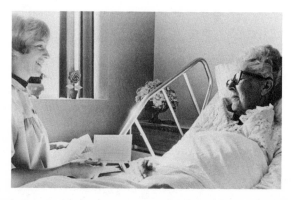

FIGURE 28-3.   Older people have the same basic need for love and respect as do younger persons.

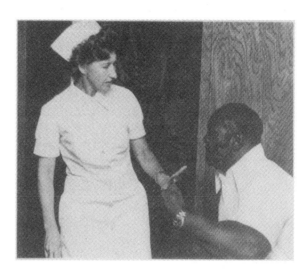

FIGURE 28-4. Feelings of helplessness are sometimes relieved by striking out at others. *(From Caldwell and Hegner,* Geriatrics: A Study of Maturity, *1981, Delmar Publishers Inc.)*

Anxiety and fears may also be expressed in periods of depression and withdrawal. The depression experienced by the elderly is easily understood. In many instances, they are cut off from their social support systems and, in large measure, have had to make major adjustments in their lifestyles. Loved ones and friends may be gone and finances very limited. They may truly feel that they no longer have any control of their destiny or even of their day-to-day activities. Physical weakness and disease stresses their coping ability to the breaking point.

Withdrawal, a common frustration response, is shown by lack of communication, temporary confusion, hallucinatory states, and general emotional disorientation as to time and place. These people need to be reassured that they will not be abandoned now that they are no longer able to care for themselves.

You need to calmly help your patients keep in touch with reality while conveying your own feelings of compassion and caring.

Be sure to report changes in behavior, mood swings and emotional responses to your supervisor.

NUTRITIONAL NEEDS

Malnutrition is a problem for the aged because, in general, the older person frequently develops an apathy toward food which becomes progressive. Decreased activity, inadequate dentition, decreased saliva, diminished smell and taste, and poor oral hygiene all contribute to the lack of appetite, Figure 28-5. Obesity, which increases the stress of existing pathologies, does not assure that adequate proteins and vitamins are being consumed. In fact, obesity is a major nutritional problem that is seen among the elderly.

The diet for the elderly person should be (1) easy to chew and (2) contain decreased amounts of refined sugars, fats, and cholesterol. Complex carbohydrates found in fruits, vegetables, and grains should be increased. These foods also provide good sources of vitamins and minerals which tends to be deficient in the elderly diet. Weight control is important now and calories are generally limited to about 2,000 calories for the average woman and 2,400–2,500 calories for the average man.

Because of the loss of muscular tone, constipation, *flatulence* (gas), and *diverticulosis:* which are small pockets, or diverticula, of weakened in-

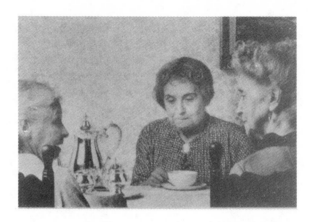

FIGURE 28-5. Loss of tastebuds and teeth make appetites lag and chewing difficult. *(From Caldwell and Hegner,* Geriatrics: A Study of Maturity, *1981, Delmar Publishers Inc.)*

testinal wall, are common. Soft bulk foods, such as cooked whole grain cereals and cooked fruits and vegetables, are helpful in overcoming the constipation. Skins and seeds should be avoided to prevent *diverticulitis,* which is an inflammation of the diverticula.

Proteins and vitamins need to be adequate to provide for optimum function and repair.

The presentation and service of the food are important in stimulating appetites. Additionally, several smaller meals seem to be more easily tolerated than three large meals.

Patients should be allowed to feed themselves as much as possible. You may assist by cutting up the food into bite-sized morsels but even if you must do most of the feeding, allow the patient to participate to the fullest extent possible.

Adequate liquid is absolutely essential. This is an area which is frequently neglected, leading to dehydration. Encourage fluid intake and be alert that the fluid is actually consumed. Fruit and vegetable juices, eggnogs, and soups can serve the dual purpose of providing nourishment and fluids.

EXERCISE AND RECREATIONAL NEEDS

Patients in rest homes need the stimulation of planned recreation and exercise, but the type of activity must be carefully tailored to the needs and abilities of the patients, Figure 28-6. Health workers in these facilities are often responsible for coordinating this aspect of care.

Recreation

It is important for those who do the activity planning to keep in mind the age and possible physical limitations of the participants. Planning must also take into consideration the fact that older people have less coordination and are more apt to have hearing and vision deficiencies. The fact that recreation with a purpose must also be considered as being the most stimulating and enjoyable form to mature people. Activities that are planned by the participants are generally the most successful. Shows and skits call for many different talents; exhibits, sales, and making gifts for others are some other examples of activities that combine recreation with purpose, and are usually enjoyed by everyone.

With care, activities can be planned which even meet special rehabilitation objectives. For that reason, the occupational therapist is a valuable person to serve in a consultant capacity, both in care facilities and recreational centers. Recreational planning can thus combine physical and reha-

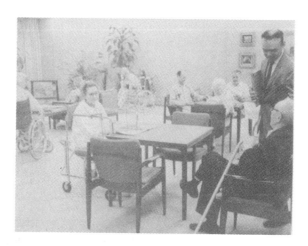

FIGURE 28-6.   The day room in a facility offers a place for social exchange and rehabilitative activities. *(From Caldwell and Hegner,* Geriatrics: A Study of Maturity, *1981, Delmar Publishers Inc.)*

bilitative activities with enjoyment. Exercising, singing, and handclapping to music can be enjoyed to some degree by bed patients, wheelchair patients, Figure 28-7, and even those who are confused. For those patients who are ambulatory, marching can be a stimulating as well as an enjoyable activity. Simple handicrafts and games, and even television and conversation, offer a measure of entertainment to the less active. Most care facilities have a special room where out-of-bed patients can gather.

Exercise and Lack of It

Patients should be encouraged to move about on their own and handle as much of their own personal care as they can, because one of the greatest threats to the well-being of the chronically-ill or geriatric patient is immobility. Muscle tone is quickly lost when muscles are unused. This is especially true of the ankles, hips, knees, and abdomen. Even *vital capacity*

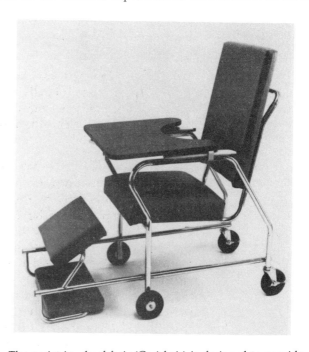

FIGURE 28-7.   The geriatric wheelchair (Gerichair) is designed to provide position changes for nonambulatory patients. The tray provides support and an area to eat and carry on activities. *(Photo courtesy of Invar Care Corporation)*

is 10 percent less in the supine position. Immobility may also cause respiratory problems.

Confinement with little activity predisposes the patient to constipation, renal calculi, and metabolic disturbances. Circulation is not stimulated, and bones lose minerals. There is usually a decrease in weight since lagging appetite lowers food consumption.

Inactivity causes serious muscle and joint problems. Stiffness develops into *atrophy*: shrinking, loss of strength, *contractures*: muscle shortening,

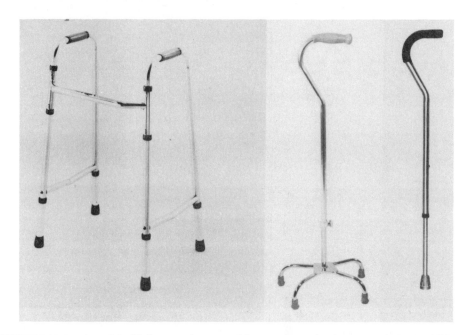

FIGURE 28-8.   A and B. Walkers and canes add a measure of safety to ambulation. *(Photos courtesy of Invar Care Corporation)*

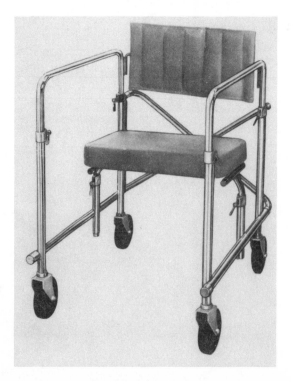

C.   This type of walker has a seat which lifts for ambulation and which may be lowered for sitting if the patient becomes tired. *(Photo courtesy of Invar Care Corporation)*

and permanent disability. Continuous lack of activity is dangerous and may ultimately lead to pneumonia. When walking and active ambulation are not feasible, range-of-motion exercises for all healthy joints should be carried out. The bath is one of the best opportunities to carry out passive range-of-motion (ROM) exercises and to encourage active ROM by the patients (see Unit 33).

Muscle tone can be maintained through a regular program of planned *setting exercises* when joints cannot, or should not, be moved because of existing pathology. Setting exercises tighten muscle groups without actually moving the joints. Muscles are alternately contracted and relaxed for short periods. Carried out frequently and regularly, these exercises help maintain muscle tone. You must understand exactly the type and amount of exercise to be performed, and the extent of your responsibility.

AMBULATION. Patients should be encouraged to ambulate as much as possible according to their physical condition and stamina.

Safety rails along corridor walls assist in ambulation; walkers, canes and crutches can be important aids too, Figure 28-8. Be sure they are being properly used. Check for worn rubber or insecure attachments.

Braces are specially constructed to meet individual patient needs. Be sure you know how each appliance is secured. Check for worn straps and loose screws. Inspect the patient's skin for signs of irritation and breakdown. If braces are secured to shoes, check these as well. Shoes should be well fitting and in good condition and shoelaces must be securely tied.

Any irregularities in equipment or patient mobility should be promptly reported.

Procedure

ASSISTING THE PATIENT WHO AMBULATES WITH A CANE OR WALKER

1. Wash hands and assemble either of the following pieces of equipment:
   - Cane
   - Walker
2. Check appliance for worn areas or loose parts.
3. Identify patient and explain what you plan to do.
4. Lower bed to lowest horizontal position.
5. Raise head of bed and assist patient to a sitting position.
6. Assist patient with robe and slippers. Swing legs over edge of bed to allow feet to rest on floor.
7. If necessary, apply a transfer belt around patient's waist.
8. Place walker or cane within easy reach.
9. Assist patient to standing position.
10. Have patient grasp walker or cane to maintain balance.
11. Walk beside patient grasping transfer belt for additional support.
12. After ambulation, return patient to bed by reversing the procedure.
13. Leave patient in comfortable position with side rails up.
14. Wash hands.
15. Chart:
    - Date and time
    - Procedure: ambulation with cane/walker
    - Patient reaction

GENERAL HYGIENE

Skin Care

Aging skin has two main characteristics: (1) it has less oil, so dryness from too-frequent bathing causes itching, which is sometimes referred to as "bath itch," and (2) the skin of an elderly patient is easily hurt and takes a long time to heal because general circulation is less efficient.

Lotions should be applied to dry areas to protect them. Bath oils lubricate the skin but are dangerous because they make a bathtub slippery. It is better to apply lotions directly to the areas that are dry.

Skin areas that touch must be kept free from perspiration and should not be allowed to rub together. Any time moisture, perspiration, urine, or feces are present, skin breakdown is imminent. After gently washing and drying local areas, a light dusting of powder is sufficient; too much powder tends to cake and cause irritation.

Cleanliness of the skin is essential but a daily bath for the older person is neither necessary nor advisable. Although a daily overall bath is unnecessary, frequent local bathing is. The face, groin, underarms, and other body creases need regular cleaning, inspection, and care. Elderly people tend to be sensitive to deodorants, so care should be used when applying them. Many soaps are very drying, but super-fatted soaps are not only less drying but are less irritating. Pat the skin dry gently, do not rub.

Tubs or shower baths given two or three times a week are preferable. General safety factors and the patient's physical limitations should be considered before giving a tub or shower bath. Placement of handrails and availability of tub and shower seats or hydraulic lifts are aids that enhance safety, Figure 28-9 and 28-10.

Facial Hair

Elderly women tend to have an increase in the growth and coarseness of the hairs on their chin and upper lips. The excess hair is very distressing to many women who feel it *defeminizes* them. The hairs can be removed periodically with tweezers or more permanently by a professional with an electric needle. A mild bleach is used by many women to lighten the hairs, making them less noticeable.

Men need to shave or be shaved regularly, usually daily. Sometimes it is only necessary to provide the equipment; at other times, it is necessary to shave the patient. A safety razor or electric razor is far safer than the straight razor that many elderly men are accustomed to using.

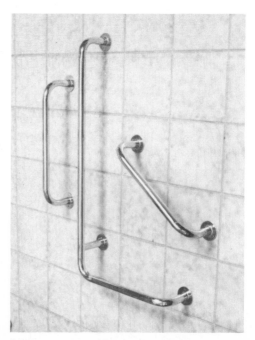

FIGURE 28-9. Tub and shower rails add to the overall safety of patient bathing. (*Photo courtesy of Invar Care Corporation*)

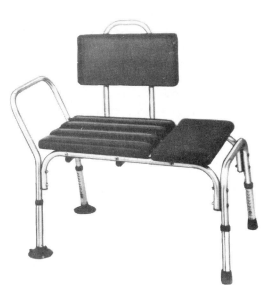

FIGURE 28-10. The shower chair allows the patient to sit safely while bathing. *(Photo courtesy of Invar Care Corporation)*

Hand and Foot Care

Fingernails can be cleaned during the morning care period and should not be neglected. A soft brush and blunt-edged orange wood stick will clean the nails without causing injury. The hands can be soaked in warm water and the cuticles pushed back gently with a towel. Softening creams and olive oil soaks help to soften the cuticles. Fingernails should be cut and filed, following the contour of the fingertips. Care should be taken not to injure the corners since improper cutting of fingernails and toenails is the biggest single cause of infections.

Foot care should also be a routine part of the morning care. This should include careful washing and drying of the feet plus close inspection for any abnormalities. Olive oil, lanolin, cocoa butter, hand cream, or lotion can be applied to dry, scaly skin and a very light dusting of powder given to perspiring feet. Toenails should be cut straight across.

Thickened nails which are difficult to cut or nails of diabetic patients that need to be cut should always be reported to your supervisor. Be sure slippers/shoes are well fitting and in good repair.

Hair Care

Hair care is important in maintaining the client's overall personal appearance. Hair should be styled and neatly arranged. Recognition of the relationship between neat appearance and high morale leads many care facilities to incorporate the services of a beautician and a barber into the cost of basic care. If the services of a beautician or barber are not available, sometimes a family member or a volunteer can provide this service.

An order is required for a shampoo to be given once or twice a month. A mild conditioning shampoo is best. A dryer will dry the hair quickly, decreasing the chance of chilling. The patient must be kept out of drafts while the hair is drying. Shampoos are more safely given in bed; or if the person is seated, a shampoo board can be used. Bending is difficult for older persons and their decreased sense of balance is apt to result in a fall.

Mouth Care

The condition of the teeth affect the aged person's total health. Poor oral hygiene can result in loss of appetite and weight, and may be the focus of any infection. Even if teeth are missing, the remaining teeth should be cleaned regularly. Dental checkups should be given the same amount of attention as in younger years.

False teeth, called *dentures*, must be cleaned daily under running water with a brush especially made for this purpose. Be sure to fill the washbowl half full of water so that if the teeth are dropped accidentally, there is less chance of breakage. Hot water and strong antiseptic solutions may injure dentures and should not be used. A place should be provided where they can safely be stored in solution so they will not warp while out of the mouth. Check the mouth and gums routinely for signs of irritation. Periodic dental examinations should be made to have the teeth checked and polished. Lips should be inspected for excessive dryness or *fissures*. These hygienic routines and observations are the responsibility of the health care worker when an individual is no longer able to do these things for herself. See Unit 18 for specific care procedures.

Mouth care is especially important for the bed patient who is no longer able to maintain dentures in the mouth. A commercial mouthwash, a warm wash of saline, or baking soda used before and after meals, and glycerine and lemon applied with applicators between meals are very refreshing. Creams, petroleum jelly, or glycerine applied to the lips can prevent fissures from developing into deep sores and infections.

Eyes, ears, and nose should also be surveyed daily for any signs of irritations, redness, or excess dryness of the skin that could lead to breaks and fissures. Observations of this nature by staff members should be part of routine care.

ELIMINATION NEEDS

Urinary Incontinence

Urinary incontinence may be due to one or a combination of causes; it is not unusual to find more than one factor present at the same time. Any interruption of *cerebral* control, such as a stroke, brain damage which destroys the control centers or pathways, confusion and decreased awareness due to general cerebral degeneration, or *aphasia* and the patient's inability to communicate the need for help to others will lead to incontinence.

Incontinence may occur simply because the patient is unable to reach the proper facilities in time. The condition may be related to fecal impaction which acts as a mechanical obstruction, causing the urine to be retained. The incontinence in this case is actually overflow. Perhaps the most common reason for incontinence is infection. Inflammation irritates sensory nerve endings in the bladder. Mucosal and bladder contractions are increased, causing the incontinence.

Incontinence may be temporary, lasting only a few days. For example, after a period of illness continence may improve as the patient becomes more able to respond to the environment. Attention to the underlying causes and the temporary use of incontinence pads may be all that is needed. Every effort should be made to help the patient become continent soon as possible with little reference to the temporary incontinence. You can do much to give emotional support and reassurance to the patient.

Incontinence of an established nature continues even though the patient is ambulant. This is a more difficult, but still not impossible, form of incontinence to treat. Drugs are sometimes used to achieve bladder control, but retraining may also be needed.

RETRAINING. The first step in retraining is to enlist the patient's cooperation. Keep in mind, though, that not all patients are able to cooperate to the same degree. The second step is to provide the patient with the opportunity to void. Nocturnal incontinence, commonly called *nocturia*, can be helped by making sure a urinal is kept at the bedside in an easily accessible spot, by taking the patient to the bathroom, or by offering the bedpan at midnight. When the record shows a specific time that incontinence occurs the patient should be awakened routinely one hour in advance of that time.

Some authorities advocate the control of fluids as an aid to continence; the fluids are forced during daytime hours and restricted at night. Others believe the limitation of fluids is inadvisable because this presents a very real danger to the elderly of *dehydration*, increased confusion, and even *uremia*.

Retraining usually takes from six to eight weeks of continuous effort, so during these weeks the importance of emotional support cannot be overemphasized. The entire staff must present a confident attitude, helping to assure the patient that new habits can be established. Developing new habits and achieving appropriate responses to them requires diligence, patience, and time. Successes should be praised, and lapses accepted as a natural part of the training process. The attitude and reactions of all staff members must be consistently positive.

At times, difficulty initiating the flow of urine is encountered. Sitting upright, with hips and knees flexed, and feet flat for support is the optimal position.

A bedside commode, Figure 28-11, may be used or the patient may sit on a bedpan on the edge of the bed with the feet resting on a footstool. The height of the regular toilet seat can be raised for maximum comfort, and fitted with handrails for safety and support, Figure 28-12A and B. A height of twenty inches is usually the most satisfactory. Wheelchairs that can be pushed over the commode are more convenient for many patients, Figure 28-12C. Men find it easier to void in the standing position, but they may require support. When patients must remain in bed, the bedpan should be padded and the body supported with pillows. Use of an orthopedic bedpan may provide additional comfort.

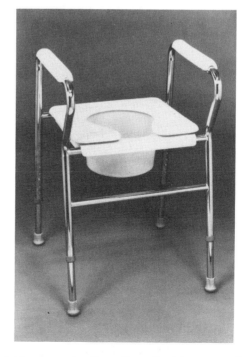

FIGURE 28-11.   A bedside commode allows the patient to assume the best position during the retraining period. *(Photo courtesy of Invar Care Corporation)*

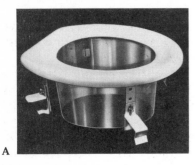

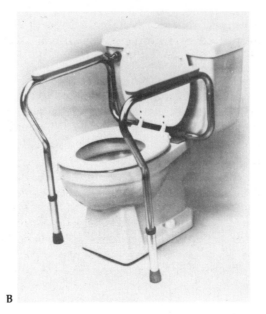

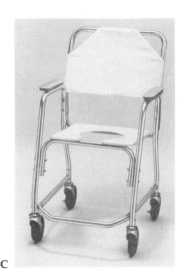

A   B   C

FIGURE 28-12. *(Photos courtesy of Invar Care Corporation)*

Attention to position, a glass of water to drink, or a measured amount of water poured over the perineum may act as a stimulus. Helping the patient to lean forward, gently stroking the inner thigh, or tickling the side of the urinary meatus with a wisp of cotton can be tried. Patients should be encouraged to bear down at the end of voiding to completely empty the bladder. Slight pressure over the abdomen may aid the process. Regular, routine cleansing of the skin of an incontinent patient must be meticulous if breakdown is to be avoided. Carefully used heat lamps and a fine dusting of zinc oxide powder help to heal *excoriated* areas.

Fecal Incontinence and Constipation

Fecal incontinence is less common than urinary incontinence but is more easily controlled. It is most commonly caused by fecal *impaction*, the severest form of constipation. The fecal mass gradually loses water if it is not eliminated from the bowel. This dehydrated mass acts as an irritant to the mucosa, and mucus production is increased. Some of the outer mass is dissolved by the mucus and there is evidence of apparent diarrhea. Any time you note diarrhea in the elderly patient, especially in one who is bedridden, you should suspect fecal impaction.

The cause of constipation is not always evident, but certainly improper diet, lack of exercise, and inaccessibility of the lavatory are contributing factors. Bowel retraining aims at establishing continence and preventing impaction. Oil-retention enemas may be helpful when followed by a soapsuds enema. (See Unit 36 for information on administering enemas.)

Regularity is the key to bowel retraining and proper sitting helps considerably. The patient should be comfortably and safely positioned. Guard rails on either side of the toilet will increase the feeling of security. Privacy and an unhurried atmosphere are important.

COMMUNICATION NEEDS AND SENSORY ABILITIES

Communications are a two-way interaction between a sender and receiver. Elderly persons may have difficulty sending messages when a stroke hampers their ability to speak or form thought properly, or when hearing or vision are impaired. They may have difficulty in receiving messages when mental deterioration clouds cerebral awareness.

Aphasia

The term *aphasia* means a language impairment, and involves either an inability to express through speech or to understand speech. Some patients have no remaining useful language after a stroke and for them the prognosis is very poor. Other patients have retrained to some degree of useful language ability.

For the first group of patients, the outlook is indeed bleak. They have no useful means of communication through reading, writing, or speaking. These patients might be unable to even gesture meaningfully.

The prognosis for the second group of patients, who still have some basic skills that can be developed, is better. Their degree of aphasia means that they may make errors in reading and writing, misuse words, and show confusion over related expressions. Words that sound alike and number and time concepts might confuse them also. Their *visual fields* may be imperfect, so those items in certain sections of their visual fields are disregarded when reading. Automatic speech, or words—frequently sprinkled with profanity—which have no real meaning or relationship to each other are not unusual either.

Your approach to the aphasic patient is very important and can contribute greatly to the patient's recovery; patience is essential. Short, precise sentences must be used, speaking slowly to give the patient time to comprehend. Raising one's voice is of no value; the problem is one of comprehension. Gestures can be used to help convey meaning. Too often, the staff fails to talk to aphasic patients because of the lack of significant response. The aphasic patient needs examples to *emulate*, so you must talk to the patient.

Actual speech therapy requires the service of a competent speech therapist, but your cooperation is very important. For further information, see Unit 32.

Hearing Deficits

Elderly persons who are hard of hearing may have suffered ear infections or ear diseases in childhood or middle life and, as a result, have carried this socially incapacitating handicap into their later years. Other elderly people are victims of the most common problem as a result of aging: *otosclerosis*. In otosclerosis, the tissues of the labyrinth and middle ear become hardened, and hearing is gradually diminished. Extreme tones are lost first, with the greatest loss in the low-pitched range. Patients with otosclerosis may also be disturbed by distressing inner sounds.

Hearing aids, which amplify sounds, can help these people. Hearing aids must be properly fitted to the individual and the patient should be carefully instructed in their use and care.

Presbycusis, known commonly as senile deafness, or eight-nerve-damage deafness, is caused by damage to the eighth cranial, or *auditory*, nerve which is responsible for conducting sound waves. *Senescent* (aging) changes in this nerve, probably due to degeneration, make perception and conduction more difficult. Since hearing aids essentially increase the sound which still must be carried by the auditory nerve, they are of little value when the auditory nerve itself no longer functions.

Communication with a deaf person takes skill and practice, but is well worth the effort. The technique suggested here is based on patience. Since the deaf person must use the sense of sight for help, health workers must stand directly in front of the patient to be clearly viewed. The sug-

1. Speak slowly and distinctly.
2. Form words carefully; keep sentences short.
3. Rephrase words as needed.
4. Face the listener.
5. Make sure any light source is behind the listener.
6. Use facial expressions or gestures to help express meanings.
7. Encourage lip reading.
8. Diminish outside distractions.

FIGURE 28-13. Guidelines for communicating with patients who are hearing impaired

gestions in Figure 28-13 are helpful in establishing successful communication.

Impaired Vision

Aged persons may also experience a decline in their ability to see. This can result in a loss of peripheral vision, or disease conditions such as glaucoma or cataracts. These specific conditions are discussed more fully in Unit 35, but briefly, many elderly persons wear glasses or a prosthesis (artificial eye) as a result of vision problems. The variety of eye problems experienced by the elderly is wide. Drugs that the elderly person is taking for a condition, as well as the aging process itself, will affect visual ability. Any redness, burning, blurring or excess watering may also be early indications of more serious eye involvements. These signs and symptoms must be noted and reported promptly.

Farsightedness in the elderly is called hyperopia; presbyopia (nearsightedness) is an impaired vision due to only the aging process. For the person who has worn glasses for nearsightedness all their lives the changes may make glasses no longer necessary or require a new prescription for near work. The presbyopia is due to a loss of elasticity in the crystalline lens of the eye. The crystalline lens of the eye changes its shape to bend light rays which emit from objects being seen. When the lens is less functional, the object must be moved further away to be clearly seen.

Procedure
CARE OF EYEGLASSES

1. Wash hands and assemble the following equipment:
   • Patient's eyeglasses
   • Cleaning solution
   • Clear water
   • Soft cleaning tissues
2. Explain what you plan to do.
3. Handle glasses only by frames.
4. Clean with cleaning solution or clear water.
5. Dry with tissues.
6. Return eyeglasses to case and place on bedside stand or return to patient.

Procedure
CARE OF PATIENT WITH AN ARTIFICIAL EYE

1. Wash your hands and assemble the following equipment:
   • Eyecup lined with gauze
   • Cotton balls
   • Washcloth
   • Lukewarm water
   • Cleansing solution, if ordered
2. Identify the patient and explain what you plan to do.
3. Assist patient into bed and draw curtains.
4. Have patient close the eyes and turn head to the side of the prosthesis.

Wash external eye with warm water. Use one cotton ball at a time. Stroke once only from medial eye to outer eye with each cotton ball.

5. Remove eye by depressing lower eyelid with your thumb while lifting upper lid with your finger. Collect eye in your hand and place in eyecup. Place eyecup and prosthesis in center of overbed stand or beside stand.

6. Clean eye socket in the same manner using warm water and cotton balls. Dry area around eye gently.

7. Carry eyecup to bathroom and half fill sink with lukewarm water. Place folded wash cloth in bottom of sink as added precaution against breakage. Remove all secretions from the prosthesis. Use no abrasives or general solvents.

8. Empty water from eyecup. Place a fresh gauze square on the bottom and place the wet eye on the gauze. Add water if eye is to be stored in the drawer of the beside stand.

9. Wash your hands and return to the bedside to reinsert the eye.

10. Raise the upper lid with one finger and insert the eye into the socket with notched edge toward the nose.

11. Depress lower lid and slip over prosthesis.

12. Wash hands and clean, replace, or dispose of equipment per hospital policy.

13. Chart:
    • Date and time
    • Procedure: Prosthetic eye cleaned and reinserted/stored
    • Type of solution used
    • Patient reaction

PSYCHOLOGICAL NEEDS

Mental deterioration may stem from physical (organic) or emotional causes. Frequently a combination of both are exhibited in the very old patients in your care.

Many times periods of emotionally confused behavior are transient and temporary, perhaps due to unusual stress such as an underlying infection or a transfer to an unfamiliar setting. At other times the excess emotionalism signifies a progressive deterioration of mental abilities, Figure 28-14. Organic brain changes include those associated with arteriolosclerosis and senile dementia of the Alzheimer's disease type.

Arteriorclerosis results in a decrease in circulation, inhibiting normal cerebral functioning. Periods of confusion and incoherence gradually increase in frequency.

Recent memory is limited, and errors in judgment may be made. Lightheadedness and so-called "drop attacks" in which the patient falls suddenly, are attributed to *hypoxia*. Reflex responses to danger are lessened, and so the patient is usually admitted to custodial care for protection.

This is the type of patient one frequently sees in a facility for the aged. Such patients may shuffle as they walk, and have a tendency to maintain balance by leaning backwards.

In some cases, there seems to be a decline in moral standards. This type of patient may be seen exposing himself.

The patient with arteriosclerotic brain changes appears restless, spending the days walking or rocking to and fro. Since these actions are disturbing to other patients, and since the patient with cerebral arteriosclerosis tends to have little emotional control, aggressiveness and irritability can lead to frequent quarrels with others.

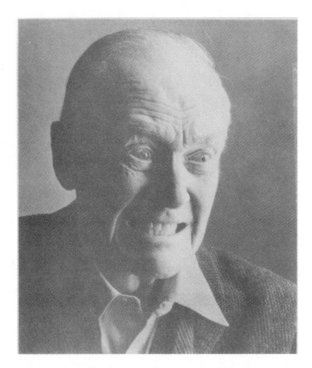

FIGURE 28-14. A change in behavior may signal a breakdown *(From Caldwell and Hegner,* Geriatrics: A Study of Maturity, *1981, Delmar Publishers Inc.)*

Fifty percent of nursing home admissions suffer from *senile dementia* of the Alzheimer's type. The patient gradually becomes severely impaired mentally, requiring constant care and supervision. The cause of this unfortunate condition is unknown, but a great deal of research is currently being conducted. Whatever the cause, the process results in destruction of the nervous cells, resulting in loss of mental functioning and control.

The physical changes are usually accompanied by a change in behavioral response. Confusion of a progressive nature is most prominent. Recent memory is decreased and the person is not able to reason accurately. Although forgetful of recent happenings the patient may remember, in detail, some episode in the distant past. The patient with this condition is very self-centered and tends to repeat himself over and over. You may explain that it is too early for a patient's daughter to visit, only to be asked the same question again within five minutes. The patient is just unable to retain the information.

Adjustment to new situations is particularly difficult. The stress of admission can bring about a rather severe regression which tends to improve with the supportive orientation by the staff.

Reality Orientation

You have a real task in helping to reorient the patient, and a calm, unhurried approach will help in this respect. Glasses, dentures, and hearing aids should be returned to the patient as soon as possible. These aids are designed to keep a person in touch with reality, yet often they are taken away and their return is neglected.

Sensory stimulation can be provided. As the *sensorium*, which is that portion of the brain which functions as a center of sensations, begins to clear you can talk with the patient, giving him an opportunity to verbalize about familiar subjects. Short, concrete sentences should be used and the patient should be told the time and day while given care. It should be repeated patiently when necessary. A calender and clock are helpful in the

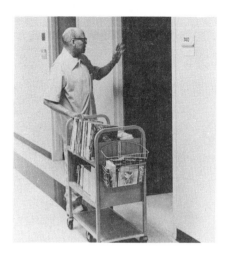

FIGURE 28-15. Continuous and consistent interactions with staff are essential if patients are to remain reality-oriented.

reorientation process. Familiar objects from home also help in the reorientation process. Color coding of corridors and communal areas help patients find their way more easily.

One of the most significant factors in improvement of mental status is the *consistent* interaction between staff and patient, Figure 28-15. Prompt attention to the patient's needs can do much to relieve the confusion and prevent further deterioration. It is the staffs' job to carry out three important objectives: (1) to limit the patient's disorientation by preventing those factors known to precipitate an episode; (2) to provide protection for the patient during periods of abnormal behavior; and (3) to help the patient become better oriented to reality.

Restraints

Despite this consistency, the patient's condition may make temporary restraints necessary, since patients need to be protected when they are disoriented. They should be placed in an area where they can be closely observed, and should be isolated only if absolutely essential for the well-being or protection of others. When isolation is necessary, frequent contact must be made with the patient; simple observation is not enough.

Restraints should be used only after all other previously mentioned methods have been tried, and *only* if the policies of both your health care agency and state regulations permit their use. Two things about restraints should be clearly understood: (1) the use of restraints contributes more often than not to an increase in agitation, and the struggle against these restraints frequently leads to exhaustion; and (2) even the confused and disoriented patient interprets their use as punitive, and the degree of communication is very likely to be decreased accordingly.

Restraints, by their very nature, tend to immobilize patients, increasing the risk of pneumonia, problems with blood circulation, and skin breakdown. There are times, however, when restraints are the only way to keep a patient from dislodging intravenous needles or pulling out tubes. Soft restraints are best, Figure 28-16, but they should be removed just as soon as possible. Explain the necessity for their use and reassure the patient even if it is thought that the patient cannot understand.

Restraints must be removed periodically and areas carefully inspected for signs of irritation and circulatory impairment. You must watch positioning and alignment carefully and give careful attention to the skin. The

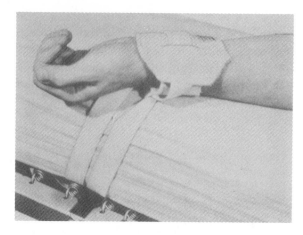

FIGURE 28-16. If restraints are necessary, soft ones are best. *(From Caldwell and Hegner, Geriatrics: A Study of Maturity, 1981, Delmar Publishers Inc.)*

basic physiologic needs of hydration and elimination must also be anticipated since a patient who is restrained cannot provide for himself.

It if often possible to remove the restraints when someone is with the patient. If a member of the family can stay with the patient, use of restraints can sometimes be avoided altogether.

Summary

The patient being cared for in the long-term health care facility is often elderly, and may have chronic conditions that limit his or her mental and physical abilities. You will carry out many of the basic care procedures you have already learned, but you will need to adjust them to meet the greater dependency of this group of patients.

SUGGESTED ACTIVITIES

1. Under supervision, give care to patients in a long-term care facility.

2. Practice carrying out procedures of ambulation under supervision.

3. Practice communicating with patients who are hard of hearing or are visually impaired.

VOCABULARY

Learn the meaning and correct spelling of the following words.

accommodation	diverticulosis	presbycusis
ADL	excoriated	prosthesis
Alzheimer's disease	fissures	relegate
aphasia	flatulence	senescence
atrophy	herniations	senile aeratoses
automatic speech	hypoxia	senile dementia
bed and board residence	impaction	senile lentigines
chronologic	incontinence	sensorium
convalescent home	integumentary	setting exercises
debilitating	nocturia	skilled care facility
defeminize	otosclerosis	superimpose
degeneration	overtly	visual field
dentition	pigmentation	vital capacity
depreciate	porous	vitality
diverticulitis		

UNIT REVIEW   **A. Clinical Situations.** Briefly describe how a health care assistant should react to the following situations.

1. You found a patient crying and feeling sorry for himself.

2. Your patient reported drinking a lot of water, but the water carafe was still almost full.

3. You are about to ambulate a patient who uses a cane and you find that the rubber tip is partially broken.

B. Multiple Choice. Select the best answer to complete the following statements.

1. Skilled nursing care facilities
   a. are known as intermediate care homes.
   b. are bed and board facilities.
   c. provide nursing care of a less acute nature.
   d. employ only registered nurses.

2. Most patients in extended-care facilities
   a. are very young.
   b. have temporary acute conditions.
   c. require very little health care and supervision.
   d. have chronic, progressive conditions.

3. Characteristics of the health care assistant that are specially important while caring for older patients include
   a. patience.   c. a sense of humor.
   b. kindness.   d. All of the above.

4. Characteristics of the elderly include the fact that
   a. vitality is increased.
   b. night sleep is decreased.
   c. appetite is increased.
   d. mobility and agility is increased.

5. Nocturia refers to
   a. wandering at night.   c. frequent napping.
   b. frequency of urination at night.   d. increased appetite.

6. Senile lentigines are
   a. malignant tumors.
   b. related to greying of the hair.
   c. roughened, scaly, wart-like lesions.
   d. areas of increased pigmentation.

7. Which of the following changes should be made in the diet of the older person?
   a. Increase fats.
   b. Increase vegetables and whole grains.
   c. Roughage needs to be increased.
   d. Calories need to be increased.

8. Which of the following applies to the bath of the elderly?
   a. Full daily baths are essential.
   b. Use large amount of soap to rid the skin of dead cells.
   c. Frequent local bathing is essential.
   d. Use deodorants liberally.

9. Which of the following are true of nail care?
   a. Toenails should be cut straight across.
   b. A stiff brush should be used to clean nails.
   c. Fingernails should be cut straight across.
   d. Thick, dry toenails can be safely filed.
10. Fecal impaction is best treated by
   a. high-bulk foods.   c. oil-retention enemas.
   b. decreasing exercise.   d. manual extraction.

C. **True/False.** Answer the following questions true (T) or false (F).
   _____ 1. Sexual appetites are lost as people age.
   _____ 2. Old people have the same emotional needs for good mental health as young people.
   _____ 3. Frustration is a common emotion experienced by the elderly.
   _____ 4. Calories should be generally increased in the diet of the elderly.
   _____ 5. Elderly people may not be aware of their need for fluids.
   _____ 6. Recreation and exercise should be handled at different times to prevent fatigue in the elderly.
   _____ 7. The patient's mouth should be carefully inspected each time dentures are cleaned and replaced.
   _____ 8. Shampoos should be given at least once a week.
   _____ 9. Bladder retraining usually takes a period of one to two weeks.
   _____ 10. Aphasia means language impairment.

Section Eleven
Self-evaluation

A. Choose the phrase which best completes each of the following sentences by encircling the proper letter.

1. When applying a hot-water bag, remember
   a. fill the bag to the top.
   b. the water should be 115 degrees F.
   c. the bag need not be covered.
   d. None of the above.

2. A sitz bath is given principally to
   a. relax the patient.
   b. provide moist heat to the anal and genital area.
   c. stimulate the patient.
   d. provide moist heat to the upper part of the body.

3. If you are assigned to surgically prep the patient, remember
   a. always use a safety razor.
   b. shave hair opposite to the direction of growth.
   c. do not use soap because a dry shave is best.
   d. do not wash the shave area.

4. When a patient is allowed to dangle or ambulate for the first time, remember to
   a. help him sit up rapidly.
   b. watch closely for signs of vertigo or fatigue.
   c. stay with him as he walks a long way.
   d. take his temperature before assisting him up.

5. When a patient returns from surgery, you should check
   a. for drainage tubes.
   b. vital signs.
   c. the dressing.
   d. All of these.

6. After which type of anesthesia is a patient most apt to be nauseated?
   a. Local
   b. Spinal
   c. Intravenous
   d. Inhalation

7. The best binder to use to hold the dressing after rectal surgery on a male patient would be a
   a. single-T binder.
   b. scultetus binder.
   c. double-T binder.
   d. straight abdominal binder.

8. Patients are often required to lie flat following spinal anesthesia in order to reduce the chance of
   a. nausea.
   b. headache.
   c. blood clots.
   d. abdominal pain.

9. The skilled nursing care facility
   a. provides care for premature babies.
   b. provides the same care as acute hospitals.
   c. cares mostly for the aged.
   d. provides only bed and board.

10. Elderly persons are characterized by
    a. loss of vitality.
    b. graying of the hair.
    c. less sensibility to pain.
    d. All of the above.

11. Foot care for the elderly should include
    a. daily washing and inspection.
    b. heavy use of powder to keep dry.

      c. cutting toenails on a curve.

      d. ignoring thick nails since they are too difficult to cut.

  12. Continence retraining requires

      a. that the patient be ambulatory.

      b. that the patient consume large amounts of water.

      c. that the patient be wakened every hour during the night.

      d. the cooperation of all staff members.

B. Answer the following questions.

  13. List the equipment you would need to assist the doctor to perform a routine physical on a female patient.

  14. List the early signs and symptoms of cancer.

  15. Name three natural defenses of the body.

  16. Write a brief statement concerning the preoperative care of a patient the morning of surgery.

C. Name the following examination positions.

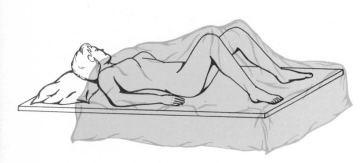
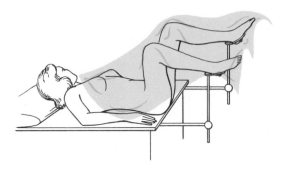

17. _____ 18. _____

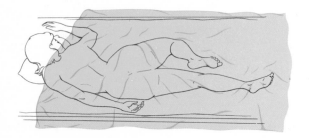
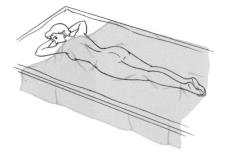

19. _____ 20. _____

D. Name the piece of equipment pictured below.

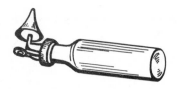

21. _____

Unit 29 The Integumentary System

OBJECTIVES

As a result of this unit, you will be able to:

• List the functions of the skin.
• Name and describe the most common skin lesions.
• Demonstrate the special nursing procedures for the various skin conditions.

The skin tells us much about the general health of the body. A fever may be indicated by a hot dry skin. Unusual redness: *rubra*, or flushing of the skin often follows strenuous activity. *Pallor*, which is less color than normal, is a sign associated with many conditions. The oxygen content of the blood can be noted quickly by the color of the skin. When the oxygen content is very low, the blood is darker and the skin appears bluish or *cyanotic*.

STRUCTURE AND FUNCTION

The skin is one of the most important organs in the body, Figure 29-1. The integumentary system includes the skin and accessory structures: the hair, nails, nerves, and the sweat and oil glands. The *epidermis* is constantly being washed or worn away as it is renewed from the *dermis*. *Subcutaneous* tissue lies directly under the dermis. Functions of the skin include:

• Protection: the intact skin is a mechanical barrier to injury and disease.
• Heat regulation: many small blood vessels are present in the deeper part of the skin: *dermis*. When they *dilate* with blood, heat is brought to the surface where it escapes from the body. When heat needs to be conserved, these vessels *constrict*, thereby preserving heat within the body.
• Storage: energy in the form of fat as well as some vitamins are stored in this vital area.
• Elimination: some waste products as well as excess water are cast off *(excreted)* as perspiration through the activities of the sweat glands.
• Sensory perception: many nerve endings are found in the skin. They tell us much about our *environment*. They respond to heat, cold, pain, and pressure. This is called our sense of touch or *tactile sense*.

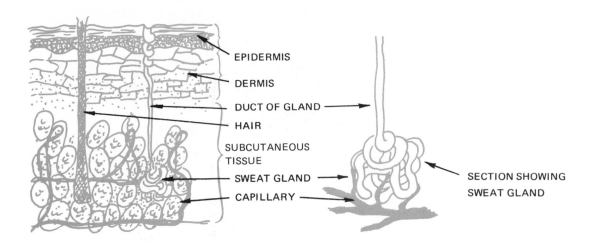

EPIDERMIS

DERMIS

DUCT OF GLAND

HAIR

SUBCUTANEOUS
TISSUE

SWEAT GLAND

CAPILLARY

SECTION SHOWING
SWEAT GLAND

COMMON CONDITIONS

Skin Lesions

Injury or disease causes changes in areas of the skin. These changes are called lesions. Some of the most common skin lesions are:

- Macules: flat, discolored spots as in measles, Figure 29-2
- Papules: small, solid, raised spots as in chickenpox
- Pustules: raised spots filled with pus as in acne, Figure 29-3
- Vesicles: raised spots filled with serous fluid such as a blister, Figure 29-4
- Wheals: large, raised, irregular areas frequently associated with itching, as in hives
- Excoriations: portions of the skin appear scraped or scratched away
- Crusts: areas of dried body secretions such as scabs

Skin lesions may be a result of communicable diseases or allergies. Communicable diseases are those which are easily transmitted, directly or indirectly, from person to person. Measles and chickenpox are two such diseases. Each has characteristic skin lesions.

Allergies, also called sensitivity reactions, may have associated skin lesions—the vesicles of poison ivy are well known. The material causing the sensitivity is called an *allergen*. Individuals respond to allergens in different ways. *Anaphylactic shock* is a severe, sometimes fatal, sensitivity reaction. Observation of the skin and accurate descriptions of what you see must be carefully charted.

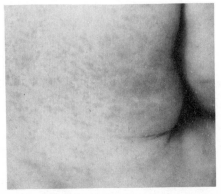

FIGURE 29-2.   The macules of German measles (*Photo courtesy of the Center for Disease Control, Atlanta, GA*)

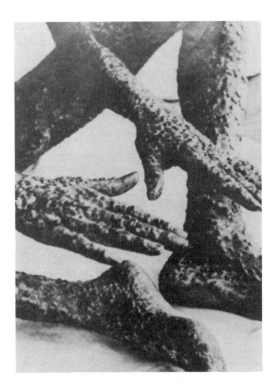

FIGURE 29-3.   Pustules are raised areas filled with pus and debris *(Photo courtesy of the World Health Organization)*

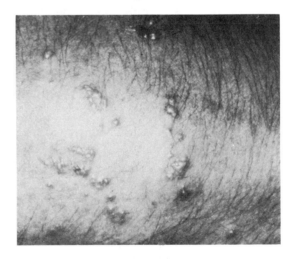

FIGURE 29-4.   The fluid-filled vesicles of poison ivy—a form of allergy *(Photo courtesy of the Center for Disease Control, Atlanta, GA)*

CARE OF SKIN LESIONS. When skin lesions are present, certain general nursing care is indicated. The assistant should take the following precautions when caring for these patients.

- Closely observe the patient's skin on admission, but do not remove any dressings.
- Soap and water and rubbing lotions are often *contraindicated* (not permitted). Check the nursing care notes before bathing the patient or giving a back rub.
- Do not attempt to remove any crusts from skin lesions without special instruction from your supervisor.
- Handle the patient gently. Avoid rubbing the skin.

Special baths may be ordered to soothe and treat the condition. These baths are called *emollient* or *colloidal* baths. Emollient baths are given in tepid water to which a medication such as baking soda, cornstarch or oatmeal has been added.

Procedure **GIVING AN EMOLLIENT BATH**	1. Wash hands and assemble the following equipment: • Bath mat • Slippers and robe • 2 bath towels • Bath thermometer • Gown • Medication as ordered 2. Be sure tub is clean. 3. Fill tub with tepid water (95–100 degrees F). Check temperature with bath thermometer. 4. Add medication if ordered. Stir well. 5. Have patient lie in tub for 30 minutes to 1 hour as ordered. Gently sponge areas not covered with water. Make sure patient does not become chilled. Add warm water as needed. 6. Dry the skin by patting with a soft towel. Do not rub. 7. Apply lotion by patting if ordered. 8. Assist patient to bed and encourage him to rest. 9. Clean tub and replace equipment according to hospital policy. Wash hands. 10. Chart: • Date and Time • Procedure, emollient bath (kind of medication, temperature of water, length of treatment) • Effects of treatment/patient reaction

Pressure Sores

Pressure sores, commonly called bedsores or *decubitus ulcers*, may occur in patients of any age. They are particularly common in the elderly, the very thin, the overweight *(obese)*, and those unable to move. Decubiti result from extended pressure on one area of the body so that there is an interference with circulation. The tissue first becomes reddened. As the cells die from lack of nourishment, the skin breaks and an ulcer forms, Figure

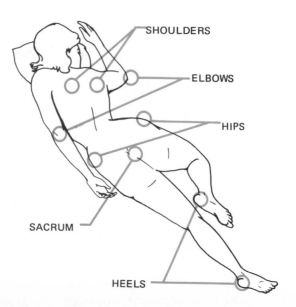

FIGURE 29-5.   Common sites for decubiti

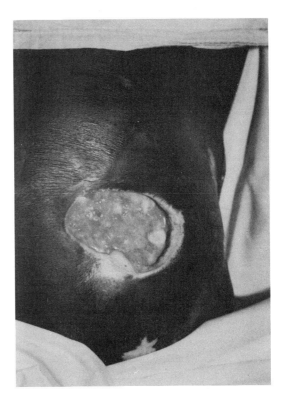

FIGURE 29-6. Decubitus ulcer involving skin area over patient's right hip

29-5. The resulting bedsore may become very large and deep, Figure 29-6. They occur most frequently over areas where bones come close to the surface. The elbows, heels, shoulders, and sacrum are the most common sites.

Obese patients tend to develop pressure sores where body parts rub, causing friction. Common sites are between the folds of the buttocks, legs, and under the breasts. Because pressure sores are far more easily prevented than cured, everyone participating in the patient's care has a responsibility to prevent skin breakdown and, if already formed, to promote decubitus healing. The assistant should take the following precautions to prevent and treat decubiti:

- Change the patient's position every 2 hours. Remember that even the patient who is sitting up may develop decubiti.
- Keep linen dry and free from wrinkles and hard objects such as crumbs and hairpins.
- Massage reddened areas frequently with rubbing solution. Do not use lotion on broken skin areas.
- Keep friction areas lightly dusted with talcum powder, but do not allow talcum powder to accumulate.
- Bathe patient frequently. Pay particular attention to potential pressure or friction areas.
- Use foam padding, sheepskin or alternating pressure mattress to relieve pressure, Figure 29-7.
- The open areas are covered with dry sterile dressings. This is a procedure done by the doctor or nurse only.

Burns

Any time that large sections of skin are destroyed, the body loses fluids and chemicals called *electrolytes*, and is unprotected from infection. Burns are a common cause of loss of large sections of skin, Figure 29-8.

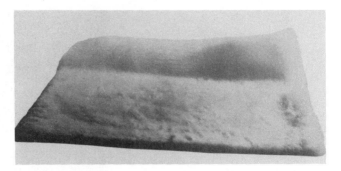

A. Pad of synthetic fur (sheepskin) *(Photo courtesy of J. T. Posey Co.)*

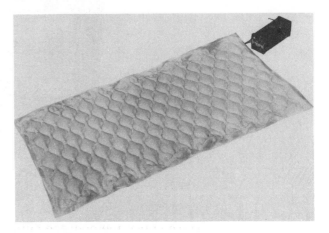

B. Alternating pressure air mattress and motor unit. *(Photo courtesy of Gaymar Industries, Inc.)*

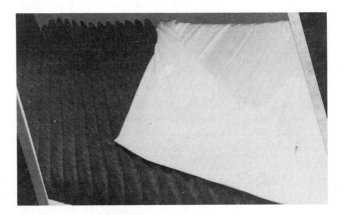

C. Egg-crate foam mattress

FIGURE 29-7.   Means of relieving pressure

CLASSIFICATION. Burns are classified according to how deeply skin tissue is destroyed.

- First-degree burns affect only the epidermis. The skin is reddened but not broken.
- Second-degree burns cause injury to both the epidermis and dermis. Vesicles form, but there is usually little permanent damage or scarring.
- Third-degree burns destroy both layers of skin and the underlying tissues, such as muscle, bones, and nerves. Scarring and deformity are common.

TREATMENT. The first-aid treatment for burns is ice and cold water. Immediate medical attention is essential in third-degree burns and when very large areas are burned.

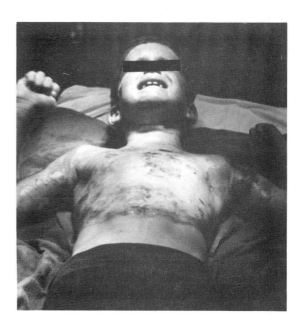

FIGURE 29-8. This child with severe second- and third-degree burns is in extreme pain.

Some hospitals have established special burn centers where specially trained personnel care for burn cases. One of two approaches are in common use and may be used:

- The open method: the burns are left uncovered. Sterile technique, also called reverse isolation technique, is used to care for the patient. (See Unit 6.)
- The closed method: the burns are wrapped in sterile petroleum jelly or nitrafurazone dressings and then completely covered with large compression dressings.

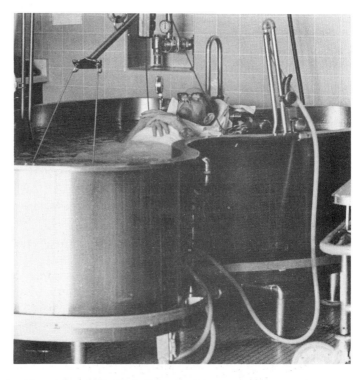

FIGURE 29-9. The patient with severe burns on the lower half of the body is submerged to aid debridement (removal of dead tissue).

New techniques such as keeping the patient submerged in a silicone solution are also being used, Figure 29-9. Each method has its advantages and disadvantages. There are three goals of treatment, whatever method is selected:

- Replacement of lost fluids and chemicals to combat shock
- Relief of pain and anxiety
- Prevention of *contractures*, deformities, and infections. Contractures are shortening of muscles which limits motion and causes deformities. Plastic surgery may also be required.

CARE. Special nursing care emphasizes the accurate recording of intake and output, positioning the patient gently but frequently to prevent contractures, encouraging a high-protein diet, and giving emotional support.

Summary

The condition of the skin gives indication of the general health of the body. Many conditions produce characteristic skin lesions. The health assistant should become familiar with the most common ones. Decubiti are difficult to treat and cure. All members of the nursing team must direct their efforts toward eliminating those conditions which predispose their development.

Burns are classified according to the degree of damage that is done to the skin and deeper tissues. The treatment of serious burns requires special care and is provided in burn centers. Therapy includes pain and infection control and replacement of lost fluids and minerals. Both the open and closed method may be employed in dealing with the actual burn site.

SUGGESTED ACTIVITIES

1. Discuss the procedures in your hospital for giving an emollient bath and caring for pressure areas.

2. Describe how decubiti occur and the methods used to prevent them.

3. Investigate the care given to burn patients in your agency.

VOCABULARY

Learn the meaning and correct spelling of the following words.

allergen	decubitus ulcers	lesions
allergies	dermis	obese
anaphylactic shock	dilate	pallor
colloidal	electrolytes	pressure sores
constrict	emollient	rubra
contractures	environment	subcutaneous
contraindicated	epidermis	tactile sense
cyanotic		

UNIT REVIEW

A. Clinical Situations. Briefly describe how a health care assistant should react to the following situations.

1. You burned your finger.

2. You found a reddened area over the patient's coccyx.

3. You are assigned to give a bedbath and find the patient has skin lesions.

B. **Completion.** Complete the following sentences.
1. Four functions of the skin are _____.
2. The first-aid care for burns is _____.
3. a. A first-degree burn damages _____ tissue.
   b. A second-degree burn damages _____ tissue.
   c. A third-degree burn damages _____ tissue.
4. Nursing care for burns includes _____.
5. The temperature of emollient baths should be _____ degrees F.
6. Bedsores are easier to _____ than _____.
7. Three items used to relieve pressure on bony areas are _____, _____, and _____.

Unit 30 The Respiratory System

OBJECTIVES

As a result of this unit, you will be able to:

- Locate the organs of the respiratory system.
- Describe the structures and function of the respiratory system.
- Name the most common diseases of the respiratory system.
- List five safety measures for the use of oxygen therapy.
- Name and demonstrate two positions for respiratory patients.

The respiratory system is sometimes referred to as the lifeline of the body. Without the oxygen it carries, life cannot be maintained. Diseases of the respiratory tract that interfere with the vital exchange of oxygen and carbon dioxide bring acute distress. All nursing care is directed toward making breathing easier.

STRUCTURE AND FUNCTION

The respiratory system extends from the nose to the tiny air sacs or *alveoli* which make up the bulk of the lungs, Figure 30-1. Organs of the system include the nose, *pharynx* (throat), *larynx* (voice box), *trachea* (windpipe), *bronchi*, and lungs. The sinuses, *diaphragm*, and *intercostal* muscles between the ribs are called auxiliary structures. The nasal cavity is the normal route of air flow for breathing. When there is an obstruction to nasal breathing, people breathe through their mouth. Mouth breathing is very drying to the oral cavity. Special mouth care is absolutely essential in these cases.

The air is warmed, moistened, and filtered as it passes through the nasal cavities which are separated by the nasal *septum*. It passes through the pharynx, a common passageway for air and food, into the larynx, trachea, bronchi, and alveoli. It is at the level of the alveoli that the exchange takes place. The carbon dioxide, brought to the lungs by the pulmonary artery, passes through tiny capillaries which surround the alveoli. The carbon dioxide escapes through the walls of the alveoli and is exhaled. The oxygen absorbed by the blood is carried back to the heart by the pulmonary vein and then is pumped through the general circulation.

The two lungs are found in the *thoracic*, or chest, cavity. They resemble cones. The pointed surface is called the apex; the broad surface, the base. Double-thick *pleura* cover the lungs, and are separated from the lungs by a small amount of fluid. The base of the lungs is attached to the diaphragm.

When the diaphragm and intercostal muscles contract, this creates a vacuum in the thoracic cavity, causing air to rush into the lungs—*inspiration*. When these muscles relax, the thorax becomes smaller, making the space within the lungs smaller and forcing the air out—*expiration*. Inspiration plus expiration equals respiration.

The contraction of the diaphragm is under the automatic control of

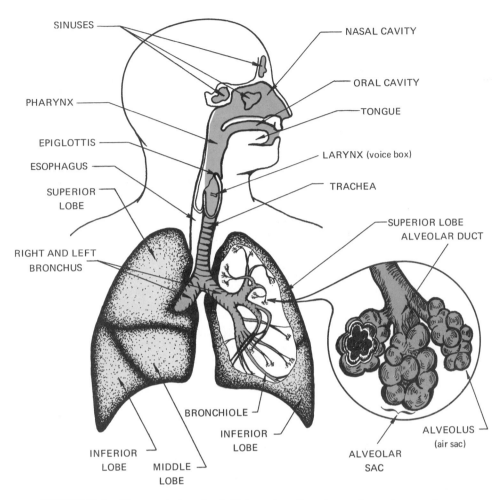

FIGURE 30-1. The respiratory tract. Enlarged section shows the exchange of gases.

the *phrenic nerve*, which responds to the amount of carbon dioxide in the blood. Thus the breathing *rate* depends on the amount of carbon dioxide in the blood. Exercise such as running makes the body cells work faster and put out more waste products, such as carbon dioxide. Therefore, the faster you run, the faster and more deeply you must breathe.

Voice Production

Expiration rids the body of excess carbon dioxide. As it passes through the larynx, it may also be used to produce sound. Two folds of tissue known as the vocal cords extend across the inside of the larynx. Changes in the length of these folds and of the opening (*glottis*) between them, as air passes outward, produce the sounds we use to speak. These sounds are further changed by being bounced against the walls of the sinuses and being shaped by the tongue and lips. When you have a cold, the sinuses often become filled with mucus and cannot function properly. The changes in your voice are easy to detect.

COMMON CONDITIONS

Emphysema

Almost 20,000 Americans die of *emphysema* every year, and the number of cases is increasing. In this disease, the tiny little alveoli lose some of their elasticity. This loss of elasticity means that they cannot become smaller

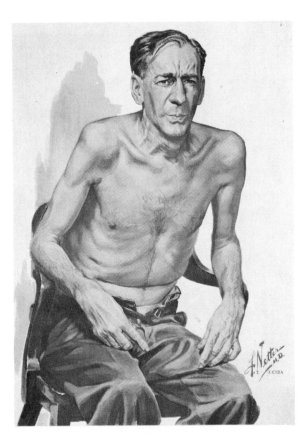

FIGURE 30-2.   Characteristic posture of patient with emphysema (© *Copyright 1968, CIBA-GEIGY Corporation. Reproduced with permission, from the CLINICAL SYMPOSIA, illustrated by Frank H. Netter, M.D. All rights reserved.*)

as they should during expiration, and so a portion of the carbon dioxide is trapped.

Patients with emphysema characteristically lean forward with shoulders raised as they try to force the carbon dioxide out of their lungs, Figure 30-2. This condition develops gradually, usually over a period of years. Interference with the exchange in the lungs puts additional strain on the blood vessels and heart. The heart may enlarge under the strain and then fail. Also, these patients are very *susceptible* to infections. Although the disease is sometimes fatal, it is not contagious. With proper training, in the not-so-severe cases, patients can be taught to live with restricted activity.

Tuberculosis

Tuberculosis, one of the oldest known diseases, still ranks high as a cause of death. It is caused by a microorganism that is easily transmitted to others by sneezing and coughing. Fatigue, fever, weight loss, and *hemoptysis* (spitting of blood) are common in tuberculosis.

The organisms usually attack the lungs, but other parts of the body may also be invaded. If the number of invading organisms is not too great, they may be surrounded by white blood cells and either be destroyed or walled off. A walled-off area is called a *tubercle*; and the organisms are still alive within the tubercle. Sometimes bodily resistance lowers because of fatigue or strain, and the organisms again become active.

Not all cases of tuberculosis make a person feel ill. A tubercle may be formed without the person ever realizing he has come in contact with the disease. The organisms are there, however, and that is why it is important to learn if infection is present through a regular TB checkup consisting of an X-ray or tuberculin test. Today tuberculosis is treated with drugs, although hospitalization is also necessary. When the patient can no longer spread the germs, his case is said to be *arrested*.

Asthma

An asthma attack is the result of sensitivity to an allergen. The body responds to the presence of this allergen by:

- Increased production of mucus in the bronchi and the tiny branches of the bronchi known as *bronchioles*.
- A swelling of the mucous membrane that lines the respiratory tract.

The flow of air is obstructed and the patient experiences *dyspnea* (difficult breathing) and wheezing. Emotional anxiety may also bring about an attack in the asthmatic person. Long term treatment consists of determining the allergen and eliminating it. To relieve the attack, the patient is given medication to decrease the swelling and enlarge (dilate) the bronchioles. Oxygen is also generally administered.

Upper Respiratory Infections (URI)

An upper respiratory infection follows invasion of the upper respiratory organs by microbes. A common cold which is caused by a virus is an example of an upper respiratory infection. It is one of the most ordinary ailments afflicting people. Symptoms include elevated temperature, runny nose, and watery eyes. This usually self-limiting disease is best treated by rest, aspirin, and increased fluid intake. URIs, at times, move down into the chest and develop into bronchitis or even *pneumonia* (an inflammation of the lungs). Today, most pneumonias, though still very serious conditions, respond favorably to antibiotic therapy.

GENERAL CARE

Remember that the special focus in caring for patients with respiratory conditions is to ease their breathing. Since these patients are prone to infection, it is also wise to pay special attention to proper techniques.

Oxygen Therapy

Oxygen is often ordered by the physician. Patients may receive oxygen by:

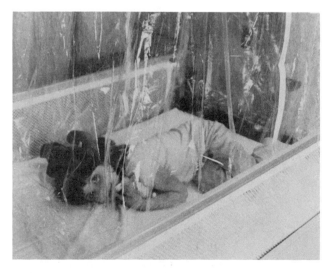

FIGURE 30-3. Oxygen may be administered via a tent.

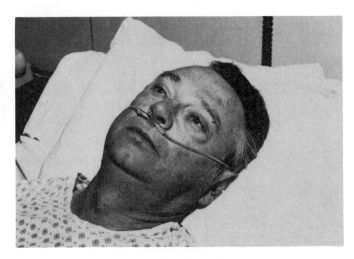

FIGURE 30-4.   Oxygen administration by nasal cannula

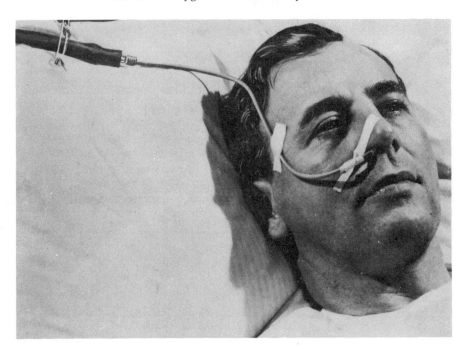

FIGURE 30-5.   Oxygen administation by nasal catheter *(Photo used with permission of the Linde Division, Union Carbide Corporation)*

- The tent method, Figure 30-3.
- Nasal cannulas: small tubes placed at the entrance to the nose, Figure 30-4.
- Nasal catheter: a small plastic or rubber tube that is inserted into the nose, Figure 30-5.
- Mask: cuplike mask held in place over the nose and mouth by hand or by straps around the head, Figure 30-6.
- Intermittent Positive Pressure Breathing (IPPB): Oxygen is administered intermittently under pressure by professional personnel, respiratory therapists, for instance. This technique helps to expand the lungs, Figure 30-7.

PREVENTING FIRE. Although oxygen doesn't explode, burning is more rapid and intense when it is present. Therefore, anything that might result in fire must be eliminated when oxygen is in use. The following safety measures must be taken:

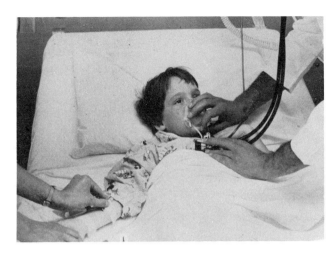

FIGURE 30-6.   Oxygen, delivered by an oxygen mask, may be used to relieve an asthmatic attack.

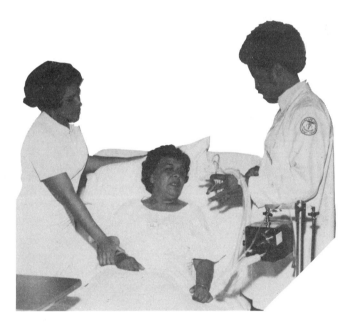

FIGURE 30-7.   Oxygen administration by intermittent positive pressure breathing (IPPB)

- No smoking is allowed in an area of oxygen use. Signs should be posted.
- Provide a hand callbell instead of an electric one. Do not use woolen blankets.
- Before using electrically-operated equipment at the bedside such as an electric razor, discontinue the flow of oxygen.
- No open flames, such as matches or ritual candles are permitted.

IN CASE OF FIRE. If a fire breaks out, safety of the patient is paramount. Sound the alarm by using the call board which connects the patient's unit to the switchboard. Manual alarms close by may also be activated but do not leave the unit to *find* one. If you have been trained in the use of a fire extinguisher, it may be used on small fires, Figure 30-8.

Next, move the patients out of the area as quickly as possible. Bed patients are moved in their beds; ambulatory patients need to be escorted and directed to safety.

Be prepared to follow instructions when a nurse or someone in au-

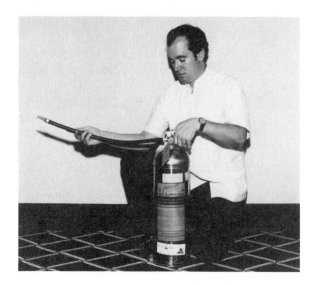

FIGURE 30-8.   Learn the location and method of operation of the fire extinguisher.

thority assumes control, but in the meantime carry out the policies of your facility.

Once the patients are safe, go back to the unit and check to be sure oxygen is shut off and electrical equipment is disconnected. Shut doors and fire doors if they are part of the safety equipment. Be sure to keep all exits accessible.

In all situations get patients to safety, follow hospital policy and keep calm.

MAINTAINING AN OXYGEN SOURCE. Some hospitals have oxygen piped from wall units directly into the patient's room, Figure 30-9. In others the oxygen source is a tank which is brought to the patient's room when therapy is ordered. If a tank is used, be sure that:

- There is sufficient oxygen. Check gauge each time you go to the bedside.
- An additional oxygen tank is readily available for the exchange.

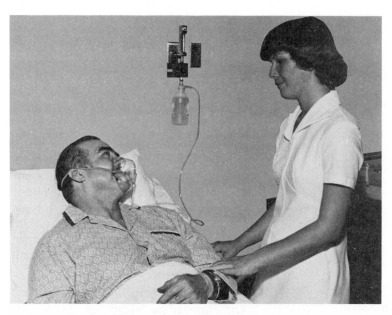

FIGURE 30-9.   Receiving oxygen from wall unit

- Empty tanks are marked and returned to the proper area for refilling promptly.
- The tank is secure and cannot fall. Straps may hold it to the bed or it may be held in a tank holder.

MAINTAINING MOISTURE. Because pure oxygen is very drying, it is damaging to tissues. Oxygen should therefore be moisturized by passing through water before reaching the patient; distilled water is used for this purpose. Be sure the level of water is maintained in accord with your hospital policy. The amount of oxygen (rate of flow measured in liters) is ordered by the physician. You should know the rate that has been ordered and set for your patient. Notify the nurse immediately if you find a change. Since many patients with respiratory difficulty breathe through their mouth, special attention to mouth care is essential.

Special Care During Oxygen Therapy

Note: The oxygen tent is usually used today only when cooling, in addition to oxygen, is needed.

The Oxygen Tent:

- Place a rubber cover over the mattress to prevent loss of oxygen through mattress.
- Check plastic canopy for leaks.
- Be sure oxygen is turned on before the patient is covered with the canopy.
- Tuck the canopy in under the mattress to prevent leakage.
- Secure the canopy across the front of the bed:
  1. Place an additional sheet folded lengthwise over the bed with the opening of the fold toward the patient.
  2. Place the open end of the canopy between the folds.
  3. Tuck the edges of the sheet under the sides of the mattress.
- Work quickly through zippered openings.

The Mask:

- Be sure the straps are secure but not too tight.
- Remove the mask periodically. Wash the area under it. Dry carefully and lightly powder the area.

The Nasal Catheter:

- Keep the patient's face free of any nasal discharge.
- Make sure that there are no kinks or undue pressure on the tubing. Tapes are used to secure the catheter at the nose and temple. A pin tunnel around the tube allows for patient mobility.

Mistogen Units (Croupettes)

Mistogen units are small portable units similar to the oxygen tent. These croupettes are used to provide oxygen and a high degree of humidity at cool temperatures for children and babies. The unit may cover the entire baby or just the head and shoulders of an older child, Figure 30-10.

The same precautions in regard to all oxygen therapy are true of Mistogen unit use. Mistogen units may or may not have a canopy across the top. Oxygen, being heavier than air, accumulates in the bottom of the unit. Ice is kept in the back of some units to maintain a lowered temperature.

Respiratory Positions

Positions permitting expansion of the lungs and a straightened airway are helpful to patients with respiratory distress.

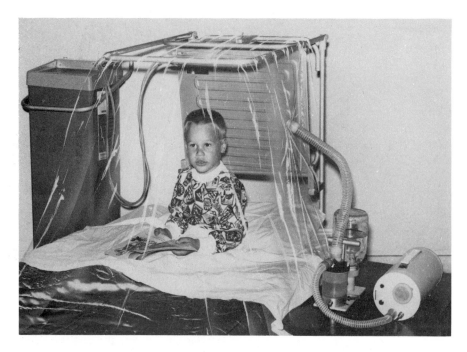

FIGURE 30-10.   The Mistogen unit

HIGH FOWLER'S POSITION. The patient is in a sitting position with the backrest elevated, Figure 30-11. Three pillows may be positioned behind his head and shoulders. The knee rest may be adjusted. The feet should be kept in proper alignment with pillows or footboards.

ORTHOPNEIC POSITION. The orthopneic position may be used as an alternate to the high Fowler's position, Figure 30-12. The position of the bed remains the same. The bedside table is brought across the bed and a pillow or two placed on top. The patient leans forward across the table with his arms on or beside the pillows. Another pillow is placed low behind the patient's back for support.

Incentive Spirometer

Incentive spirometers are used to improve ventilation. For a complete discussion of this therapy, see Unit 27.

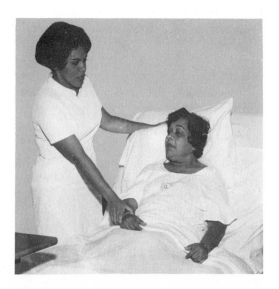

FIGURE 30-11.   Note patient in high Fowler's position.

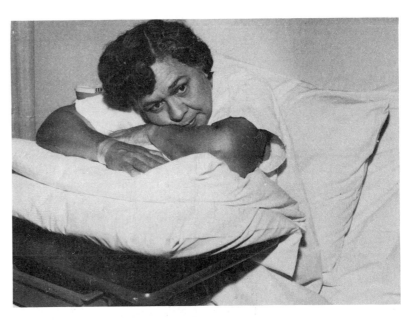

FIGURE 30-12. The orthopneic position

Summary

The organs of respiration function in the intake and exchange of oxygen and the output of carbon dioxide. Diseases which affect the respiratory tract make breathing difficult. Special measures such as positioning and the use of oxygen can make breathing easier. Emphysema, tuberculosis, asthma, and upper respiratory infections are all commonly encountered.

SUGGESTED ACTIVITIES

1. Examine a torso model and locate the organs of the respiratory system.
2. Discuss the source of oxygen and the methods of administration as they relate to your hospital or agency.
3. Under supervision, give care to patients with respiratory conditions.

VOCABULARY   Learn the meaning and correct spelling of the following words.

alveoli	expiration	pleura
arrested	glottis	pneumonia
asthma	hemoptysis	septum
bronchi	inspiration	spirometer
bronchioles	intercostal	thoracic cavity
diaphragm	larynx	trachea
dyspnea	pharynx	tubercle
emphysema	phrenic nerve	tuberculosis

UNIT REVIEW   **A. Brief Answer.** Answer the following questions.

1. What are the organs of respiration?

2. What are the two purposes of respiration?
   a.
   b.

3. What is another name for the larynx?

4. Name three diseases that affect the respiratory system.

5. List five general safety measures for oxygen therapy.

6. Describe and demonstrate two positions which might be used for a patient in respiratory distress.

B. **Clinical Situations.** Briefly describe how a health care assistant should react to the following situations.
   1. You enter a patient's room and find the patient receiving a higher level of O_2 than is ordered.

   2. Your patient complains of mouth dryness while receiving oxygen therapy.

   3. Your patient receiving oxygen therapy wants to shave with an electric razor.

Unit 31 The Circulatory System

OBJECTIVES

As a result of this unit, you will be able to:

- Describe the functions of the circulatory system.
- Locate organs in the circulatory system.
- Name the most common diseases of the circulatory system.
- Name the three kinds of blood cells.

The circulatory system may be thought of as a transportation system. It takes nourishment and oxygen to the cells and carries away waste products. The system is kept in motion by the force of the heartbeat. Diseases which attack any part of this system interfere with the overall function.

STRUCTURE AND FUNCTION

The circulatory system is made up of the heart (central pumping station), blood vessels, lymphatic vessels, lymph nodes, spleen, and the blood itself. It is a continuous network.

The Heart

The heart is a muscular organ, Figure 31-1. It is hollow inside and divided into four chambers: the right and left *atrium*, and the right and left *ventricle*. It is separated into these right and left sides by a wall called a *septum*. One-way valves separate the different chambers and guard the exit point of the pulmonary artery and aorta. The pulmonary artery, which exits from the right ventricle, carries blood high in carbon dioxide to the lungs for oxygenation. The aorta carries the freshly oxygenated blood, via the left ventricle, away from the heart and through its many branches to the cells of the body. Nerve impulses make the heart contract regularly according to body needs. When you run, the cells need more oxygen, and so the heart beats faster.

THE CARDIAC CYCLE. The heart pumps blood through the body by a series of movements known as the *cardiac cycle*. The upper chambers of the heart; called *atria*, relax and fill with blood as the lower chambers; called *ventricles*, contract, forcing blood out of the heart through the aorta and pulmonary arteries. The lower chambers then relax, allowing blood to flow into them from the upper chambers. Then the cycle is repeated.

The systolic blood pressure reading indicates the period when the pressure within the arteries is the greatest during contractions. The diastolic reading indicates the lowest point of pressure between contractions. The coronary arteries, which are branches of the aorta, carry nourishment and oxygen to the heart muscle itself.

Major Vessels

Many big *arteries* and *veins* take their names from the bones they are

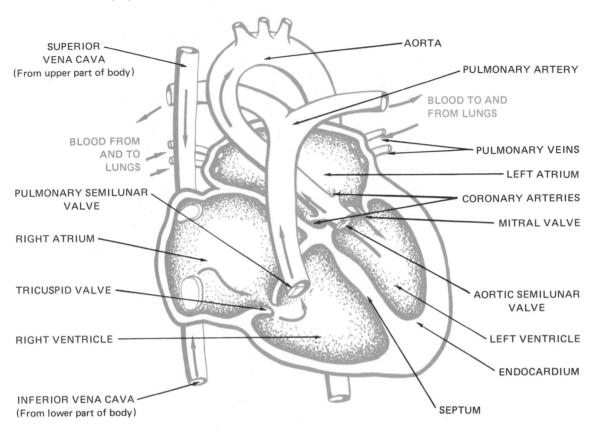

FIGURE 31-1. In this schematic representation of the heart, the red arrows show circulation of blood.

near; others are named after the part of the body they serve, Figure 31-2. For example, the *femoral artery* and vein run close to the femur (thigh bone). Arteries have muscular, elastic walls, and their linings are smooth. They branch, first to form smaller vessels *(arterioles)* whose walls are not as thick and then to form *capillaries* whose walls are only one cell thick. The exchange of nutrients and waste products takes place through the capillary wall. Fluid called *serum* carrying nutrients and oxygen bathes the cells. Waste materials and products of cellular activity pass from the cells into this "tissue fluid."

The capillaries merge to form tiny veins *(venules)*, and much of the tissue fluid flows directly back into the general circulation. Some tissue fluid is drained off into open ended tubes; known as *lymphatic vessels*, which carry it to the lymph nodes and larger lymphatic vessels before it is carried through the general circulation. There are two reasons for this bypass. First, some of the strain is removed from the veins which are not nearly so muscular as the arteries. Secondly, impurities may be removed as the fluid, which is now called *lymph*, passes through the lymph nodes.

It is easy to see that serum, tissue fluid, and lymph are all very similar in nature since they are derived from blood and ultimately return to the general circulation.

Veins, which carry the blood to the heart, are formed from the venules. Small cuplike valves are found within the veins. They help to keep the blood moving forward. They sometimes become weakened and distended, resulting in varicose veins, Figure 31-3.

The Spleen

The spleen is a small organ found in the upper left quadrant of the abdomen. It produces some of the white blood cells and destroys worn-out

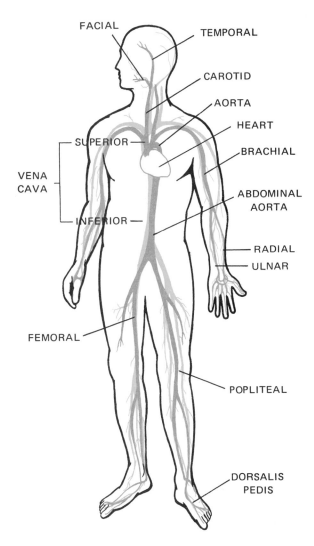

FIGURE 31-2. General plan of circulation (arteries in dark color, veins in light color)

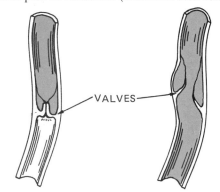

NORMAL VEIN   WEAKENED AND DISTENDED
WITH VALVES   VALVE CAUSING VARICOSITY
FIGURE 31-3. Varicose veins

red blood cells. The spleen always has large quantities of blood passing through it, and so it acts as a type of blood bank.

The Blood

If the blood vessels are the network of highways carrying nutrients and wastes, the blood may be thought of as the trucks and cars traveling along the highway. A person generally has 4 to 6 liters (quarts) of blood depending on size, sex, age, and general health. Both the quality and quantity of blood are indicative of health. Blood consists of a liquid portion and cells.

LIQUID. The liquid portion is called *plasma*, which is the carrier of water, nutrients, and waste products. It carries *fibrinogen*, which helps blood to clot. It also carries *gamma globulin*, a substance that is used to prevent or relieve the symptoms of some of the communicable diseases, such as measles. It transports another protein called *albumin*. *Serum* is plasma from which the fibrinogen, gamma globulin, albumin, and other materials have been removed.

CELLS. There are three kinds of blood cells. They are:

- Red blood cells *(erythrocytes)* that are produced in bone and carry oxygen to the cells and carbon dioxide away from them.
- White blood cells *(leukocytes)*, some of which are produced in the bone and some of which are produced in the lymph nodes and spleen. These cells protect the body by surrounding and destroying germs and other foreign materials.
- Platelets *(thrombocytes)* which are produced in the bone and are important in blood clotting.

COMMON CONDITIONS

Disease conditions of any part of the cardiovascular system will have an effect on the total system. Long standing diseases of the blood vessels will generally result in heart disease.

Peripheral Vascular Diseases

The blood vessels that serve the outer parts of the body, particularly those of the hands and feet, are referred to as *peripheral*—or toward the outer part—blood vessels. Diseases of these vessels affect parts of the body through which they pass and the health of these vessels also influence the heart function.

Those peripheral vascular diseases which affect the arteries diminish the flow of blood to the extremities. Those which affect the venous system result in pooling of the blood in dependent parts. Tissues through which the narrowed arteries pass may not be getting the nourishment they need. Areas affected are the extremities: namely the arms, legs, and brain. Signs and symptoms are associated with a decrease in circulation: coldness, tingling, loss of sensitivity, headaches, dizziness, and memory lapses.

Treatment is aimed at increasing local circulation, preventing injuries (which heal poorly), and lowering the blood pressure. Because injuries heal poorly, special attention must be given to prevent injury to the arms and legs and to prevent pressure areas. Warmth is best supplied by increasing the room temperature and using lightweight blankets and well-fitting, warm socks. Hot water bottles are dangerous because these patients may not realize they are being burned. Positioning and specific prescribed exercises can promote arterial flow and venous return.

Sometimes an oscillating (rocking) bed is employed to improve the circulatory flow. The oscillating bed rocks in cycles up and down, raising the patient's feet six inches above his head and then lowering them twelve to fifteen inches. The steady motion provides both passive exercise for the patient and some circulatory stimulation.

Nothing should be permitted which would hamper the patient's circulation and any new tissue breakdown should be promptly reported. For this reason, circular garters, crossing the legs, and exposure to cold are generally forbidden for peripheral vascular patients. These patients are usually not allowed to smoke either.

Atherosclerosis is a common form of vascular disease. Roughened areas known as *atheromas*, which are deposits of fatty materials, narrow the vessels. The vessels of the heart, brain, and those leading to the legs from the body are often affected.

The atheromas grow gradually larger until they eventually block blood flow to the parts and organs served by the affected vessels. Sometimes clots which have formed over the irregular areas in the vessel walls break off and travel as *emboli* to block distant vessels.

The occlusion of vessels can lead to narrowing and then to angina pectoris, coronary heart attack or strokes.

The exciting cause of this vascular disease is unknown but exercise, proper diet, reduction of stress, control of smoking and obesity are important in limiting the ultimate development of this condition and its serious complications.

Hypertension

Hypertension is another name for high blood pressure. It may follow illnesses which affect organs such as the blood vessels, kidneys, and liver, or it may have no known origin.

The increased pressure damages blood vessels and can cause them to rupture. High blood pressure promotes the development of atherosclerosis which further narrows the vessels, increasing the blood pressure even more and increasing the stress on the heart. Drugs which lower the blood pressure may be prescribed. Diets which are low in sodium are helpful to some patients and smoking is discouraged. Sometimes an operation called *sympathectomy* is needed to help the blood vessels to relax. Moderation in activity and food and avoidance of emotional stress are important. Medication, exercises, and the techniques of biofeedback have helped patients to lower their blood pressure, reducing the need for medication.

Angina Pectoris

Angina pectoris is known as cardiac "pain of effort." Figure 31-4 illustrates one method of diagnosis. In an angina attack the coronary blood vessels which nourish the heart are unable to meet the circulatory need. This may be sudden as the vessel constricts or can develop more gradually due to narrowing of the vessels because of atherosclerosis. Exertion, heavy eating, and emotional stress may bring on an attack by creating a demand for more blood flow than the heart can accomodate. Persons with angina

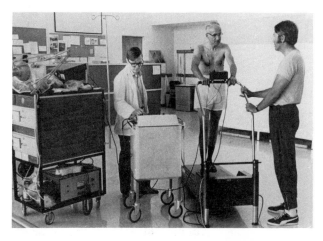

FIGURE 31-4.   The treadmill is a common test to diagnose angina.

pectoris learn to recognize those situations which bring on an attack and often take drugs which will help the muscles in the walls of the coronary arteries to relax. Coronary artery bypass surgery is commonly performed to increase the circulation to the heart muscle. Diet and exercise, carefully monitored, can improve the patient's condition, before occlusion of the vessel results in death of the heart muscle.

HEART CONDITIONS

The term "heart attack" refers to a period in which the heart suddenly cannot function properly, Figure 31-5. There are different kinds of heart attacks, and they differ in their severity and prognosis (expected outcome). Remember that the heart is muscle tissue and may become tired just as any muscle may tire. The cells of the heart require nourishment and oxygen just as all other cells.

Coronary (Heart) Attack

A coronary heart attack occurs when the coronary arteries which nourish the heart are either blocked by becoming narrow or by a blood clot which forms at the site of blockage and is called a *thrombus*. A clot may also be formed somewhere else in the body and then travel to the heart to become lodged in a coronary artery. This moving blood clot is called an *embolus*. When a coronary heart attack occurs, patients experience indigestion or crushing chest pain. The pain frequently radiates up the neck and down the left arm. The patient may feel nauseated, his pulse and breathing can become irregular, and he can begin to perspire and feel very anxious. Immediate treatment has saved many people.

Treatment is directed toward relieving the pain, reducing heart activity, and altering the clotting ability of the blood. Other names for a coronary heart attack are myocardial infarction, coronary occlusion, and coronary thrombosis.

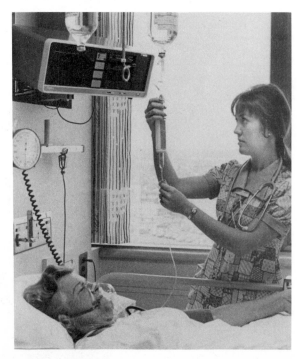

FIGURE 31-5. Professional care is needed during the acute phase of a heart attack. Note the heart monitor (EKG) in upper left of photo, and the oxygen being given by mask. Blood pressure cuff may be left in place, but not inflated, when frequent readings must be taken.

Congestive Heart Failure

The heart, like any other muscle, will tire if it has to work against increasing pressure. When narrowed blood vessels due to atherosclerosis increase the resistance to blood flow and when there is severe damage to major organs like the liver and spleen, it is more difficult to maintain the circulation. The heart must pump harder to maintain the internal flow of blood. At first the heart enlarges *(hypertrophies)* and makes up for *(compensates)* the additional workload. Eventually, however, it reaches a point where it can no longer compensate, and failure follows (cardiac decompensation); also called congestive heart failure.

The heart is unable to pump the blood rapidly enough through the vessels and so more fluid enters the tissue and body spaces than would normally. Swelling (edema) occurs. Frequently the lungs also fill with fluid, making breathing difficult and skin color dusky. The heart rate is irregular and ineffective, so the pulse should be determined apically. Drugs are ordered to help the heart beat more strongly and regularly and to increase the output of fluids (diuresis) by the kidneys. A diet of low sodium is likely to be prescribed and fluids restricted. Careful I & O and daily weighing may also be ordered to insure that the edema is being controlled. Oxygen and the orthopneic or high-Fowler's position will probably be ordered to relieve the associated dyspnea.

CARDIAC CARE PATIENTS. The patient suffering with a heart attack will require someone to care for his basic needs. When a cardiac patient is on complete bedrest, you must provide for any activity that increases the stress on the heart. Bathing, feeding, and assisting in the moving and positioning of the patient may all become part of your responsibility. During the acute stage heart attack patients require professional care. Many hospitals have provided intensive medical care units for these patients.

Cerebral Vascular Accident

A "stroke" is caused by the rupturing of arteries in the brain or blockage of these arteries by clots. Medical names for a stroke include *cerebral vascular accident* (CVA) and apoplexy. Symptoms vary but frequently include loss of consciousness, weakness or paralysis of one side of the body (hemiparesis/hemiparalysis), and difficulties in swallowing and speech. Patients recover in varying degrees, depending on the cause and extent of brain damage, Figure 31-6. Convalescence is long, and the nursing care is demanding.

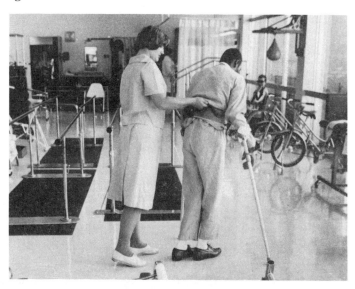

FIGURE 31-6. Following a stroke, extensive rehabilitation may be needed.

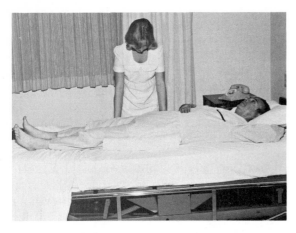

A. The patient's weak hand is tucked under the pillow with fingers open. Rolled sheet or bath blanket is used to maintain position of leg.

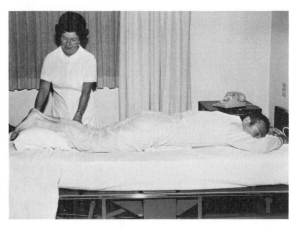

B. When it is not possible for the patient's toes to hang over the end of the mattress, a large pillow can be used to support the feet so that the toes do not touch the mattress.

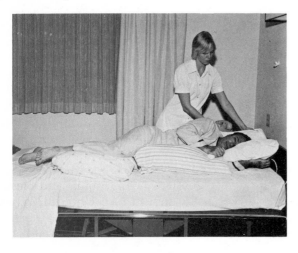

C. In this side-lying position, a pillow is used to support the weak arm. Another pillow is used to support the weak leg and foot.

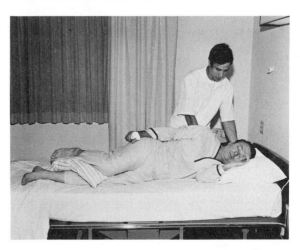

D. Here is one more side-lying position. The weak arm is placed on a pillow right behind the patient. Notice the rolled towel under the hand.

FIGURE 31-7. Four positions of the patient following a CVA. Note: The protective siderails, which would normally be up, have been omitted in each of the photos for clarity.

Vital signs and close observation may be part of your assignment in the initial phases, because keeping a constant and clear airway is essential. Report levels of consciousness and any signs of respiratory distress immediately to your team leader. Frequent changes of position and keeping the body in proper alignment are important throughout, Figure 31-7. Find out what type of movement each body part should receive, since range of motion exercises are often ordered by the physician. When patients are able to eat, allow them to assist themselves as much as possible. Until this happens feeding the stroke patient requires time and an abundant amount of your patience.

Recovery from a stroke is often a very frustrating experience for the patient and requires extreme patience on the part of the care-givers. In your approach to the patient remember two things: (1) the patient has more than enough frustration for the two of you, so be extremely careful not to let yours show—the last thing the patient needs is your silent reinforcement of his helplessness, and (2) it is well known that the degree and speed of recovery is directly related, in most cases, to the patience and encouragement of the caregivers with whom the patient has close contact.

BLOOD ABNORMALITIES

Anemia

Anemia is the result of a decrease in the quantity or quality of red blood cells. There are several causes, such as poor diet, low production of new red blood cells, and blood loss as in hemorrhage. The anemic person has little energy and is usually pale. Dizziness, digestive problems, and dyspnea may be present when anemia is severe. Treatment is aimed at improving the quantity and quality of the blood and eliminating the basic cause of the disease. Whole blood transfusions are sometimes necessary.

Nursing care includes providing for rest, adequate diet, and special mouth care (see Unit 18). Vital signs are checked frequently. Any signs of bleeding should be promptly reported.

Leukemia

Leukemia is sometimes called cancer of the blood. In this condition there is a great production of abnormal white blood cells, and the number and quality of red blood cells and platelets decrease. The cause of the many forms of leukemia is not known. This disease may strike young or old. Treatments, and their effectiveness, are continually improving.

Patients with leukemia are very susceptible to infection, and the least trauma causes bleeding. Treatment is aimed at easing symptoms, maintaining normal blood levels, and slowing the production of the abnormal white blood cells. Drugs, X-ray therapy, blood transfusions, and antibiotics may be ordered.

The nursing care of patients with leukemia is similar to that given to anemic patients. Patients are allowed to be up and care for themselves as long as possible. Handling must be very gentle to avoid injury and bleeding, Figure 31-8. Special care is given to the mouth (see Unit 18). When respiratory difficulties develop, special positioning and oxygen may be required.

Summary

The heart and blood vessels make up the closed circulatory system. The circulatory system is the transportation system of the body carrying products for and of metabolism. Diseases can affect the heart or blood vessels with a related effect on many parts of the body, especially the respiratory tract. Because heart disease is so prevalent the health assistant will probably provide care for many cardiovascular patients.

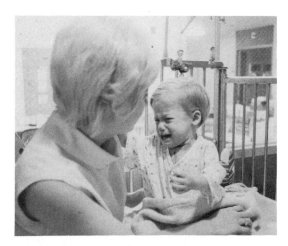

FIGURE 31-8. The leukemic child needs very special nursing care.

SUGGESTED ACTIVITIES

1. Examine a model of a torso or heart and locate its structures.

2. Using charts, trace the pathway of a drop of blood to the brain, right arm, and left foot.

3. Under supervision, give care to patients with blood and cardiovascular conditions.

4. Under supervision, assist with the care of a patient who has suffered a stroke.

VOCABULARY   Learn the meaning and correct spelling of the following words.

albumin	CVA	lymphatic vessels
anemia	diuresis	myocardial infarction
angina pectoris	edema	oxygenation
aorta	embolus	plasma
arteriole	erythrocyte	prognosis
artery	femoral artery	pulmonary artery
arteriosclerosis	fibrinogen	septum
atherosclerosis	gamma globulin	serum
atrium	hemiparalysis	sympathectomy
capillary	hemiplegia	thrombocyte
cardiac cycle	hypertension	thrombus
cardiac decompensation	hypertrophy	vein
congestive heart failure	leukemia	ventricle
coronary occlusion	leukocyte	venule
coronary thrombosis	lymph	

UNIT REVIEW

A. Clinical Situations. Briefly describe how a health care assistant should react to the following situations.

1. Your patient, who has angina pectoris, is having an argument with a visitor.

2. You started to give a tray to your patient with congestive failure and found a salt shaker on the tray.

3. Your CVA patient showed signs of respiratory distress.

B. Completion. Complete the following sentences.

1. The heart is divided into four chambers. They are: _____, _____, _____, and _____.

2. a. The pulmonary artery carries blood to the _____.
   b. The aorta carries blood to the _____.

3. The circulatory system consists of: _____.

4. a. Cells that protect the body by surrounding and destroying germs are the _____.

   b. Red blood cells carry _____ to the cells and _____ away from the cells.

5. Exercise makes the heart beat _____ (faster, slower).

6. a. The heart cannot pump hard enough in the condition called _____.

   b. Because the heart cannot pump hard enough, too much _____ enters the tissues and causes them to _____.

7. Heart attack patients are often put on complete bedrest. This means that you

_____.

8. Adequate _____ of the blood is a goal in the treatment of patients with peripheral vascular disease.

9. Cerebral vascular accident is more commonly called _____.

10. Nursing care of the anemic patient includes providing for _____, _____, and _____.

11. Leukemia is also called cancer of the _____.

12. As leukemia progresses, the patient experiences _____.

Unit 32 The Musculoskeletal System

OBJECTIVES

As a result of this unit, you will be able to:

- Name the bones of the body and their location.
- Name the various parts of the musculoskeletal system.
- List the terms used to describe body movement.
- Demonstrate techniques in caring for orthopedic patients.
- Carry out range of motion exercises.

The muscles and bones give shape and protection to our bodies. *Skeletal muscles* stretch over joints. When these muscles are stimulated by nerves, they shorten (contract), pulling two bones closer together in body movement. Remember that many blood cells are also produced within the living bone tissue. When muscles, bones, or joints have been injured, a long period of rest and inactivity may be required for the part to heal. During this period, it is important that all other moving parts receive sufficient exercise.

STRUCTURE AND FUNCTION

Bones

It will be helpful for you to learn the names and general location of each bone in the body; there are 206. It isn't really as difficult as it may seem. When you look at the skeleton in Figure 32-1, you can immediately see that if a line is drawn down the center there are the same number and kinds of bones on each side. Already, the possible number of bones to learn has been cut in half. Further examination shows us that there are 12 ribs on each side—you have just learned the name of 24 bones.

Many structures within the body take their name from the name of the closest bone. Remember, the femoral artery runs very close to the femur, which is the thigh bone. The radial artery that you use to take the pulse is found beside the radius, which is one of the lower arm bones.

Bones are not all alike, as can be seen by examining Figures 32-2 and 32-3. Some are long, some short, some flat, and some irregular. They meet one another to form *joints*.

Joints

Joints are points of possible movement. Several kinds of body movements are made possible because not all joints are formed in the same way, Figure 32-4. The elbow and knee joints work similarly to a door hinge in that they may move in only one direction. The arm-shoulder joint and thigh-pelvic joints are able to move in a complete circle like a ball and socket. Figure 33-4 illustrates the hinge joint and the ball-and-socket joint. The bones of the wrists, ankles, and spinal column have a more limited, gliding type of motion. Without movable joints walking, bending, lifting, and sitting would not be possible.

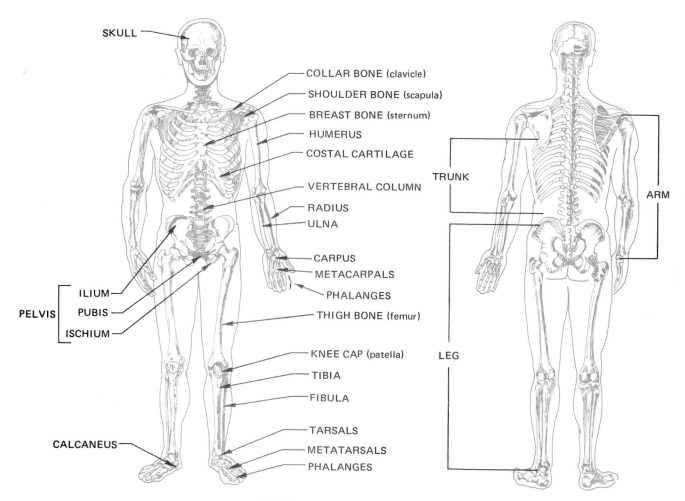

SKULL

COLLAR BONE (clavicle)

SHOULDER BONE (scapula)

BREAST BONE (sternum)

HUMERUS

COSTAL CARTILAGE

VERTEBRAL COLUMN

RADIUS

ULNA

CARPUS

METACARPALS

PHALANGES

THIGH BONE (femur)

KNEE CAP (patella)

TIBIA

FIBULA

TARSALS

METATARSALS

PHALANGES

TRUNK

ARM

LEG

PELVIS

ILIUM

PUBIS

ISCHIUM

CALCANEUS

FIGURE 32-1.   The human skeleton

Joints are held together by bands of fibrous tissue called *ligaments*. Ligaments do not prevent the joint from moving, but they do keep the bones of the joints in the proper relationships.

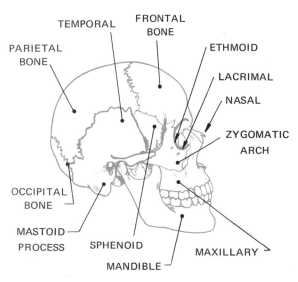

PARIETAL
BONE

TEMPORAL

FRONTAL
BONE

ETHMOID

LACRIMAL

NASAL

ZYGOMATIC
ARCH

OCCIPITAL
BONE

MASTOID
PROCESS

SPHENOID

MANDIBLE

MAXILLARY

FIGURE 32-2.   Bones of the skull

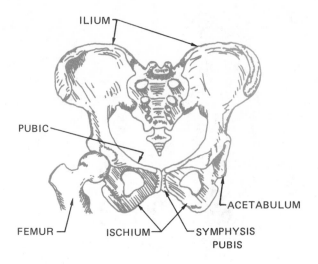

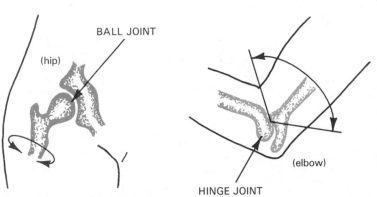

FIGURE 32-4.   Two types of joints

Muscles

There are more than 500 muscles in the body that work in groups. Skeletal muscles are attached to bones and are called *voluntary* because when we wish to pick up something we can make our muscles contract and perform the necessary movements. Other muscles, called *involuntary* or *visceral muscles*, form the walls of organs. These muscles operate without our conscious control. If we had to direct muscles of our intestines to contract each time food is digested or our blood vessels to contract each time slightly higher blood pressure is needed, there would not be time for any other activity. The control of these internal muscles is accomplished by an automatic center in the brain, and the appropriate messages are sent to these muscles by special nerves.

Muscles receive their names in three ways: their location, shape, or action. You can easily locate the major muscle groups responsible for an activity if you remember that:

- Muscles can only shorten: *contract*, and lengthen: *relax*, Figure 32-5. Contraction occurs when nerves bring the message (stimulus) to the muscle cells. Muscles relax when there is no stimulus.
- Muscles have two points of attachment to the bone. As they stretch from one point *(origin)* to the other *(insertion)*, they cross over one or more joints.
- As muscles contract, they shorten, pulling their points of origin and insertion closer together. Bending the forearm at the elbow takes place when the biceps muscle on the anterior arm, extending from the shoul-

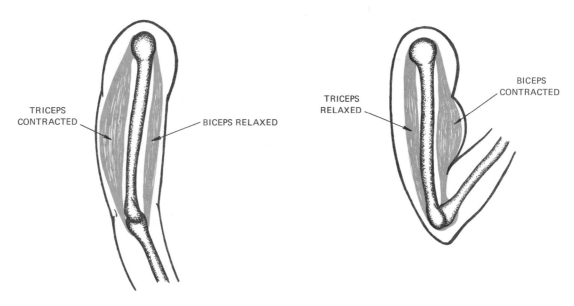

FIGURE 32-5. Coordination of muscles

der to below the elbow, contracts. At the same time, the triceps muscle, which is attached to the posterior shoulder and to the arm below the elbow, relaxes. To straighten the arm at the elbow, the triceps contracts while the biceps relaxes.

Special Terms of Movement

Special terms are used to describe movements. You will hear and see these terms written as you care not only for patients with definite *orthopedic* conditions, but also as you care for patients with any long-term illness.

- *Flexion:* decreasing the angle between two bones, Figure 32-6.
- *Extension:* increasing the angle between two bones, Figure 32-7.
- *Rotation:* circular motion in a ball-and-socket joint, Figure 32-8A.
- *Abduction:* moving away from midline, Figure 32-8B.
- *Adduction:* moving toward midline, Figure 32-8C.

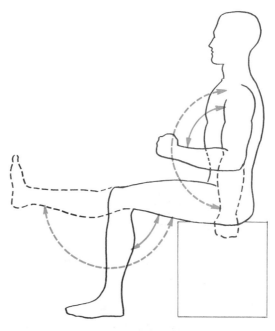

FIGURE 32-6. Flexion

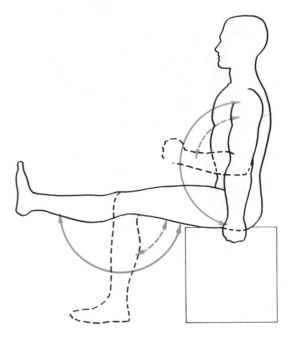

FIGURE 32-7.   Extension

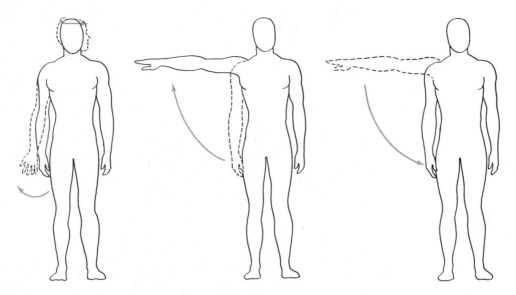

FIGURE 32-8.   Rotation (left) abduction (center) and adduction (right)

COMMON CONDITIONS

Bursitis

Small sacs of fluid are found around joints; they help to reduce friction in the joint and are called *bursae*. At times the bursae become inflamed, and the joint becomes very painful. Treatment of *bursitis* includes applications of heat to promote healing and immobilization so that the joint cannot move. At times the severity of the inflammation warrants the removal of excess fluid from the joint by aspiration with a needle.

Arthritis

This is an inflammatory condition which affects the joints. The exact cause of arthritis is unknown, but many factors are thought to contribute

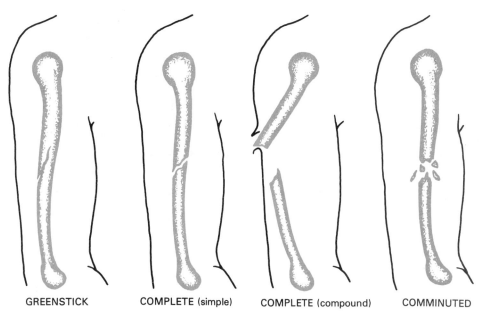

GREENSTICK   COMPLETE (simple)   COMPLETE (compound)   COMMINUTED

FIGURE 32-9. Types of fractures

to its development. These range from infection to metabolic disturbances. Types of arthritis attack all age groups, and crippling is common. Treatment is aimed at reducing deformity, relieving pain, and giving supportive care. A combination of specific exercises and rest periods is prescribed.

Fractures

Any break in a bone is called a fracture. When a bone is fractured, muscles, nerves, and other structures near the site are also injured. Falls are common causes of fractures in elderly people because as we grow older our bones become more brittle. That is partly why fractures of the hip (femur) are common in the elderly.

Children have much more flexibility to their bones since growing is not complete. Their bones tend to bend like young tree limbs, breaking on one side only. This kind of fracture is called *greenstick*.

When the ends of the bone at the fracture site are separated, the fracture is *complete*. When the bones remain within the skin, it is a simple fracture. If the bones protrude (stick out of) the skin, the fracture is *compound*. Sometimes bones are splintered in the trauma, and pieces of bones become embedded in the surrounding tissue. Splintered fractures are known as *comminuted* fractures. Figure 32-9 illustrates the various fractures.

Fractures of any kind are treated by keeping the part that is injured immobilized in proper position until healing takes place. Injured bones take from several weeks to several months to heal. Pins, screws, and bone plates may be used to hold bone pieces together, Figure 32-10. Casts and various forms of traction are used to immobilize the part, Figure 32-11. Sometimes special beds and attachments are used that make nursing care easier. The patient may be placed on a Stryker turning frame or the Circle® bed, Figure 32-12.

Be sure you know exactly how to operate these beds and how to secure the patient safely before attempting to turn the patient.

CARE OF PATIENTS WITH CASTS. Cast material is wet when it is applied and may take up to 48 hours to dry completely. During the drying period, the cast expands and gives off heat. Special care for the newly casted patient includes:

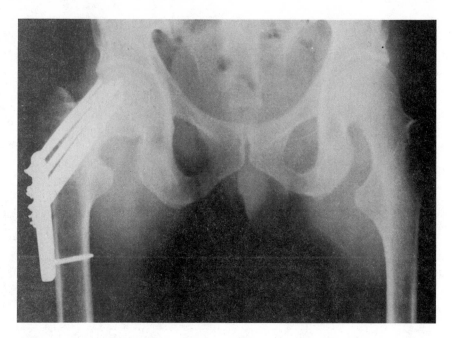

FIGURE 32-10.   Fractured bones are held in place with plates, pins, and screws.

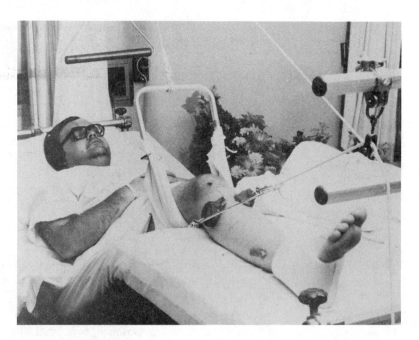

FIGURE 32-11.   Traction can be used to immobilize the bones until healing is complete. *(Photo courtesy of Endo Laboratories, Subsidiary of the Dupont Company)*

- Supporting the cast and body with pillows in good alignment and keeping the cast uncovered, Figure 32-13.
- Turning the patient frequently to permit air circulation to all parts of the cast. Maintain support. Use palm of hand, not fingers, to support the wet cast.
- Close observation of extremities for signs of decreased circulation, Figure 32-14. Report coldness, cyanosis, or numbness immediately.
- Close observation of skin areas around the cast edges for signs of irritation. Pad rough edges carefully.

After the cast has completely dried, remember to turn the patient to the noncasted area. This is particularly important in moving patients with

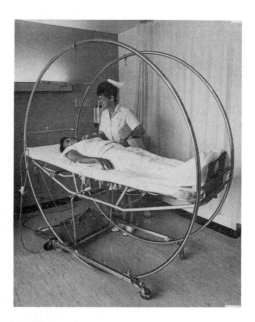

FIGURE 32-12.   Make sure you know exactly how the Circle® bed operates before attempting to provide care.

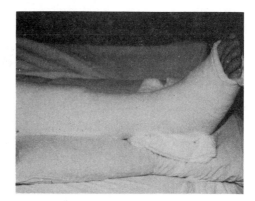

FIGURE 32-13.   Keep the cast uncovered and support in good alignment until dry.

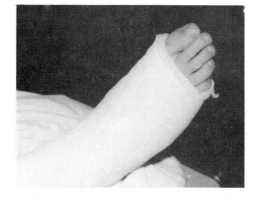

FIGURE 32-14.   Carefully and frequently check skin areas around the edges of the cast for signs of irritation.

body casts *(spica)* because turning to the casted side may result in cracking the cast. Always support the cast. An overhead bar known as a trapeze will greatly assist the patient in helping herself, Figure 32-15. Edges of casts may be padded or taped to prevent pressure areas. Wax paper or plastic secured

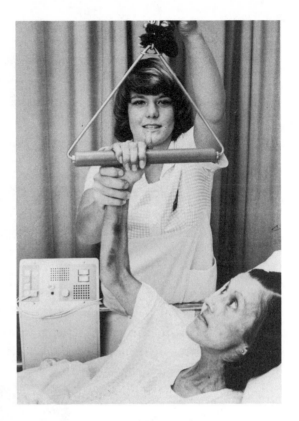

FIGURE 32-15. The overhead bar greatly assists in patient care.

to the cast edges that are near the genitals and buttocks will help to prevent soiling during voiding and defecation.

CARE OF PATIENTS IN TRACTION. Traction is designed to pull two body areas slightly apart to relieve pressure, to help spasmodic (tightly contracted) muscles relax, or to keep the areas in proper position until healing can occur. Traction is applied by attaching weights to a part of the body above or below the area to be treated. The patient's body serves as countertraction by pulling the other side of the area in the opposite direction. Sometimes tongs or pins are placed into bones to hold the traction in place. Belts, halters, or tapes may be applied to the patient's skin to hold the traction. Traction may be applied continuously or intermittently.

- Do not disturb the weights or permit them to swing, drop, or rest on any surface.
- Keep the patient in good alignment and see that his body is properly acting as counterraction. For example, feet pressed against the foot of the bed will decrease the amount of countertraction.
- Check under belts for areas of pressure or irritation.
- Make sure straps of halters and belts are smooth, straight, and properly secured.

Not all patients remain in traction continually. If *pelvic;* Figure 32-16, or *cervical;* Figure 32-17, traction is to be discontinued, the following steps should be taken:

- Slowly raise the weights to the bed. Avoid abrupt or jerking movements. If two sets of weights are being used, raise them at the same time and rate.
- Release the weights from the connection with the halter or belt and place them on the floor.
- To apply traction, reverse the procedure.

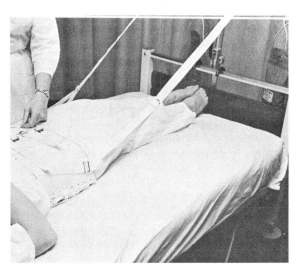

FIGURE 32-16. Pelvic traction

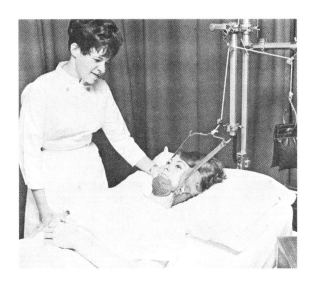

FIGURE 32-17. Cervical traction

• Remember never to jerk or drop the weights quickly or lower them unevenly.

BALANCED TRACTION. Patients in a type of traction which uses several weights and lines to provide a balanced traction tend to look rather strange. However, the same basic principles of traction apply. Usually there is one primary line of traction while the extra ropes and weights provide support.

First locate the primary pull. Figure 32-18 indicates the primary line A. Line B pulls on the Thomas splint which supports the thigh. Line C is connected to the Pearson attachment which supports the calf of the leg. Line D is attached to the foot plate which prevents footdrop and allows the patient to exercise his foot. A trapeze over the bed allows the patient to raise himself with assistance for back care, linen changes, and use of the bedpan.

Bedmaking for orthopedic patients varies according to the type of traction. Two half sheets are often used in place of a large sheet for the bottom, and the top linen is arranged according to the patient's special needs.

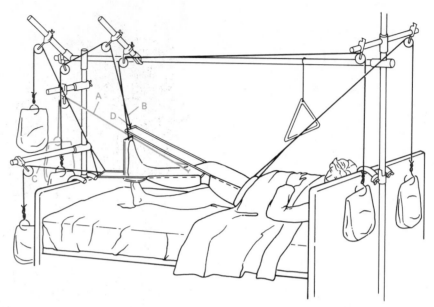

FIGURE 32-18.   Balanced traction—Line **A** is attached to a pin through the tibia. It supplies primary traction to the fractured femur. Patient's body exerts counter traction. Line **B** supports thigh position of Thomas splint. Line **C** supports lower leg portion of Thomas splint. Line **D** supports foot pedal which maintains position of foot and prevents foot drop.

Ruptured or Slipped Disc

There are 31 bones known as *vertebrae* in the spinal column. Between most of these bones, small discs or pads of *cartilage* with soft centers are found. These discs help to cushion the back bones. The anterior of the vertebrae support the head and body while the posterior portions form a tunnel which houses the delicate spinal cord and nerves. It is possible for a disc to slip out of place or for the soft center to rupture. In either case, pressure is placed on the spinal nerves, Figure 32-19. The patient may experience pain, numbness, and tingling or paralysis, depending on which disc is injured.

Treatment is directed toward relieving the pressure. Traction alone may be sufficient, but surgery, with or without casting, may be necessary.

POSTOPERATIVE CARE FOR PATIENTS WITH RUPTURED DISCS. Ruptured disc patients may require special nursing care after surgery. If bone has been grafted into the spinal column, called spinal fusion, care must be taken to treat the patient as if there is a fresh fracture. The spinal column must be kept straight until healing takes place. The patient's position is changed by rolling him like a log. The bed remains flat.

Special orthopedic sheets and linens make bed changing easier when caring for disc patients. Drawsheets may be used instead of large sheets so that one section can be changed at a time.

CHYMOPAPAIN THERAPY. The new technique of enzyme injection is being used in some instances instead of laminectomy or fusion. The major side effect is the possibility of an anaphylactic reaction (severe hypersensitivity reaction). Since this occurs rather rapidly upon injection, the health care assistant would probably not witness it as the patient would be out of the unit.

The enzyme chymopapain, which dissolves the herniated material, is injected into the ruptured disc area while the patient is in the operating room. When the patient returns from surgery, he or she is given routine post-operative followup.

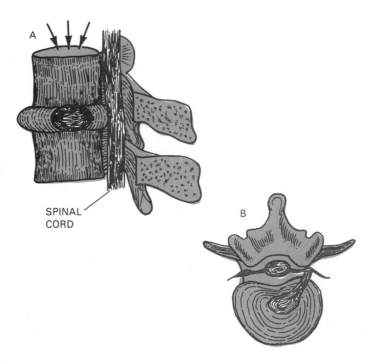

A. Uneven pressure causes the disc to bulge, putting pressure on the nerve root.

B. A herniated disc puts pressure on the nerve root as it oozes backward.

FIGURE 32-19.

Types of Joint Motions	
Extension	Straightening the angle of a joint
Flexion	Bending the angle of a joint
Hyperextension	Straightening the angle beyond 180°
Abduction	Moving away from body center
Adduction	Moving toward body center
Rotation: lateral	Rolling away from center of body
medial	Rolling toward center of body
Eversion	Pointing sole of foot outward
Inversion	Pointing sole of foot inward
Pronation	Palms down
Suppination	Palms up
Plantar flexion	Toes pointed down
Dorsi flexion	Toes pointed up
Opposition	Touching thumb to fingertips
Radial deviation	Turning wrist toward thumb-side
Ulnar deviation	Turning wrist toward little finger side.

FIGURE 32-20. Range of motion exercises

RANGE OF MOTION EXERCISES

Range of motion exercises are usually carried out following the bath and before the bed is made, but may be carried out at other times as well. These exercises aid patients in remaining mobile, stimulate circulation, and help avoid deformities. Patients are encouraged to perform as many of these exercises as their condition permits.

The nurse will instruct you as to the type or limitation of range of motion (ROM) exercises to be performed, Figure 32-20. *Be sure to ask before attempting to carry them out.* Each exercise is usually performed three times, but never exercise a joint to the point of pain. If pain or discomfort develops, stop the exercise and report the fact to the nurse. Always be gentle in handling the patient. Support the part above and below the joint being exercised. Special corrective exercises are performed by the physical therapist.

Procedure

PERFORMING RANGE OF MOTION EXERCISES (FOLLOWING BATH PROCEDURE)

Note: Repeat each action three times. Wash hands prior to performing procedure.

1. Identify the patient and explain what you plan to do and how the patient can assist you.
2. Position patient on back close to you.
3. Adjust the bath blanket to keep patient covered as much as possible.
4. Turn head gently from side to side (rotation), Figure 32-21A.
5. Bend head toward right shoulder and then left (lateral flexion) Note: While rotation (step 4) and flexion (step 5) are very similar movements, the first resembles a "shaking the head" one, while the latter is a shoulder to shoulder move.
6. Bring chin toward chest (flexion), Figure 32-21B.
7. Place pillow under shoulders and gently support head in a backward tilt (hyperextension). Return to straight position (extension). Adjust pillow under head and shoulders.

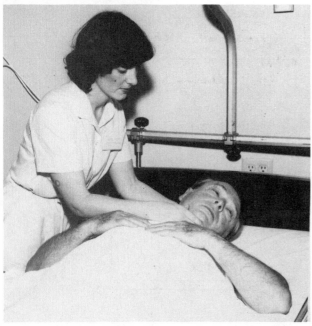

A. Neck rotation. Neck is rotated to the left and right.

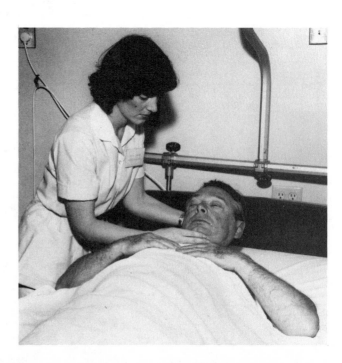

B. Neck flexion, followed by neck extension

FIGURE 32-21.

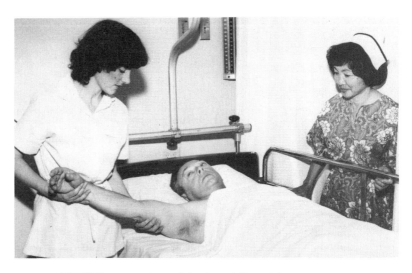

FIGURE 32-22. Arm abduction, followed by adduction

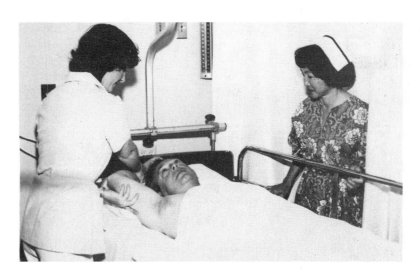

FIGURE 32-23. Shoulder rotation

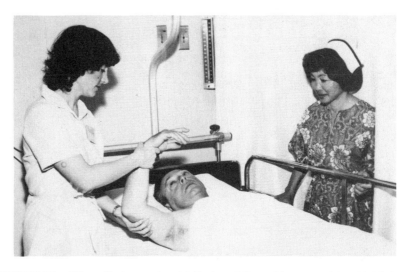

FIGURE 32-24. Elbow flexion and wrist flexion, followed by extension of both joints

8. Supporting the elbow and wrist, exercise shoulder joint nearest you as follows:
   a. Bring entire arm out at right angle to body (abduction), Figure 32-22.
   b. Return to position parallel to body (adduction).
9. With shoulder in abduction, flex elbow and raise entire arm over head (shoulder flexion), Figure 32-23.
10. With arm parallel to body (palm up—suppination), flex and extend elbow, Figure 32-24.
11. Flex and extend wrist and each finger joint, Figure 32-25A and B.
12. Move each finger in turn away from the middle finger (abduction), Figure 32-26 and toward the middle finger (adduction).
13. Touch the thumb to each fingertip (opposition).
14. Turn hand palm down (pronation), then palm up (suppination).
15. Point hand in suppination toward thumb side (radial deviation) then toward little finger side (ulnar deviation).

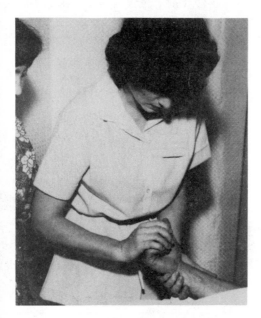
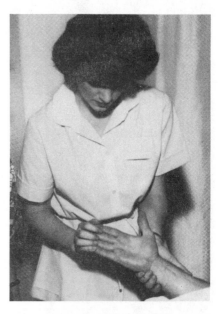

A. Finger flexion   B. Finger extension

FIGURE 32-25.

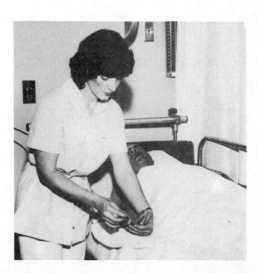

FIGURE 32-26.   Finger abduction followed by finger adduction and rotation

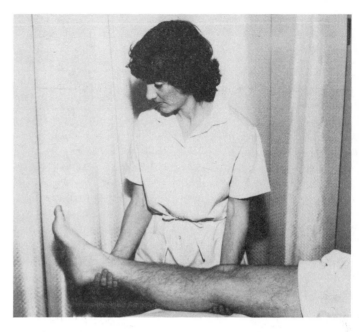

FIGURE 32-27. Leg abduction is followed by leg adduction

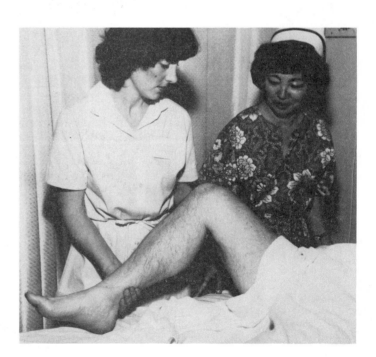

FIGURE 32-28. Knee flexion, which is followed by knee extension

16. Cover the patient's upper extremities and body. Expose only the leg being exercised. Face the foot on the bed.
17. Supporting knee and ankle, move entire leg away from body center (abduction) and toward body (adduction), Figure 32-27.
18. Turn to face bed. Supporting knee in bent position (flexion), raise knee toward pelvis (hip flexion), Figure 32-28. Straighten knee (extension) as you lower leg to bed (hyperextension). Then roll hip in a circular fashion (rotation), Figure 32-29.
19. Grasp toes and support ankle. Bring toes toward knee (dorsi flexion), Figure 32-30, and then point toes toward the foot of the bed (plantar flexion), Figure 32-31.

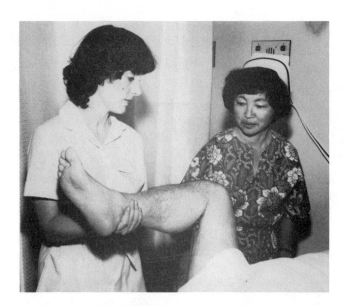

FIGURE 32-29.   Hip rotation

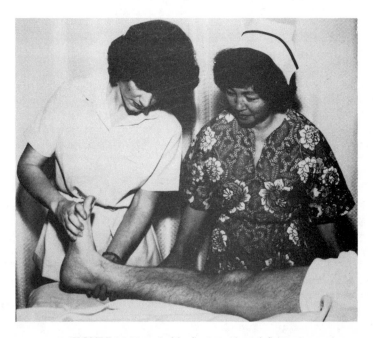

FIGURE 32-30.   Ankle flexion (dorsal flexion)

20. Turn to face foot of bed. Gently turn foot inward (inversion), **Figure 32-32,** and outward (eversion), Figure 32-33.
21. Place fingers over toes, bending toes (flexion) and **straightening toes** (extension).
22. Move each toe away from second toe (abduction), **Figure 32-34, and** then toward second toe (adduction).
23. Cover leg with bath blanket. Raise siderail and move to the **opposite** side of the bed.
24. Move patient close to you and repeat steps 7–21.
25. Complete procedure for making the occupied bed. (See Unit 15.)
26. Wash hands.
27. Report completion of task.

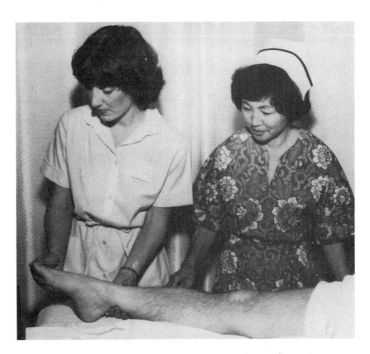

FIGURE 32-31.   Ankle extension (plantar flexion)

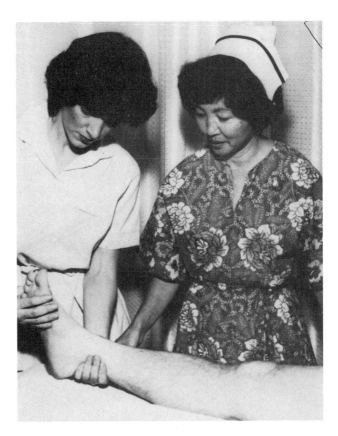

FIGURE 32-32.   Inversion

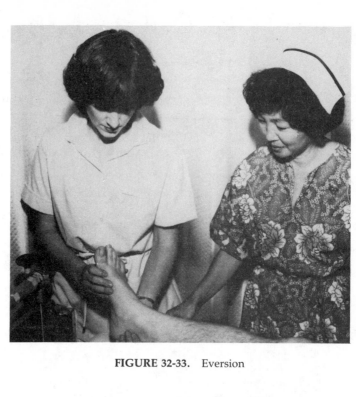

FIGURE 32-33.   Eversion

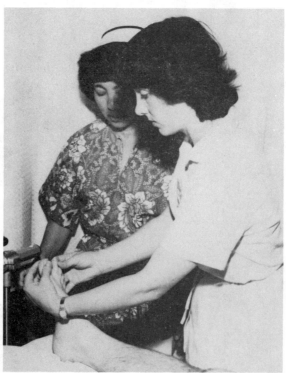

FIGURE 32-34.   Toe abduction

Summary

Healing of bones, muscles, and joints requires long periods of immobilization. Attention must be given to providing exercise for all other joints. Special nursing care to patients in casts and traction insures proper alignment, prevents pressure areas, and avoids skin breakdown. Range of motion exercises help maintain mobility and promote good general circulation.

SUGGESTED ACTIVITIES

1. Examine a skeleton to become familiar with the names and locations of the bones.

2. In small groups of students, try to determine the general location of muscle groups that cause basic body movements. Practice flexion and extension of the elbow and knee joints and abduction and adduction of the shoulder and hip.

3. Under supervision, give care to patients with casts and in traction.

VOCABULARY

Learn the meaning and correct spelling of the following words.

abduction	extension	pronation
adduction	flexion	radial deviation
arthritis	greenstick fracture	range of motion
aspiration	immobilization	rotation
bursae	involuntary muscle	simple fracture
bursitis	joint	skeletal muscle
cartilage	ligament	spica cast
cervical	orthopedic	suppination
comminuted fracture	pelvic	ulnar deviation
complete fracture	plantar flexion	vertebrae
compound fracture	point of insertion	visceral muscle
dorsiflexion	point of origin	voluntary muscle

UNIT REVIEW

A. Clinical Situations. Briefly describe how a health care assistant should react to the following situations.

1. The toes of your patient in a leg cast felt cold or looked bluish.

2. You found that your patient in pelvic traction had the feet pressed against the foot of the bed.

3. Your patient complained of discomfort during range of motion exercises.

B. Completion. Complete the following sentences.

1. When stimulated by nerves, muscles _____.
2. When muscles contract, they pull their points of _____ and _____ closer together.
3. Body movements take place at _____.
4. Two kinds of joint movement are _____ and _____.
5. Joints are held together by _____.
6. We have no control over _____ muscles.
7. Signs of decreased circulation in the extremities include _____, _____, and _____.
8. The cast should be _____ (covered, uncovered) while drying.
9. During range of motion activities, each exercise should be done _____ times.

Unit 33 The Endocrine System

OBJECTIVES

As a result of this unit, you will be able to:

- Define the general function of the endocrine glands.
- Name and locate the glands in the endocrine system.
- Describe the function of each gland.
- Perform a urine test for sugar and acetone.

STRUCTURE AND FUNCTION

Ductless glands found in widely separated areas of the body are called endocrine glands, Figure 33-1. These glands produce an internal secretion called *hormones*, which enter the bloodstream directly and so are quickly carried to all parts of the body. The hormones regulate and control body activities and growth. There are seven endocrine glands, some of which are in pairs. Some endocrine glands secrete several hormones. Some of them also produce an external secretion. In addition to the glands discussed in this unit, there are glandular cells scattered throughout the body which secrete minute amounts of regulatory hormones.

Pituitary Gland

This gland has two portions called lobes, each of which secretes more than one hormone. It is surrounded by bone and located at the base of the brain. The hormones secreted by this gland control growth, urine production, the contractions of involuntary muscles, and influence the activity of all the other glands. Because it controls other glands, the pituitary is called the master gland.

Pineal Body

This is a small gland also located in the skull beneath the brain. Very little is known about this gland. It is thought to be somehow related to sexual growth since it tends to disappear with maturity.

Adrenal Glands

There are two adrenal glands, each located on one of the two kidneys. Each gland has two distinct portions which secrete separate hormones. Two of these hormones, *adrenalin* and *cortisone*, are widely used in medicine. In general, the adrenal hormones control the release of energy to meet emergencies, and water and salt usage by the body. They also have a relationship to the development of male characteristics.

Gonads

The term gonads refers to the male and female sex glands. The female gonads are the two *ovaries* located within the pelvis on either side of

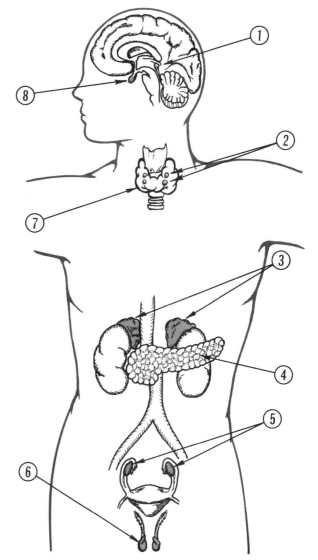

1. PINEAL BODY
2. PARATHYROID GLANDS
3. ADRENAL GLANDS
4. ISLETS OF LANGERHANS (pancreas)
5. OVARIES (female)
6. TESTES (male)
7. THYROID GLAND
8. PITUITARY GLAND

FIGURE 33-1. The endocrine glands.

the uterus. When stimulated by the pituitary gland, they produce two hormones, *estrogen* and *progesterone.* These hormones are responsible for the development of female characteristics such as the development of the breasts, the appearance of pubic and axillary hair, the onset and regulation of menstruation, and pregnancy.

The male gonads, the two *testes,* are located outside of the body in a pouch called the scrotum. They produce the hormone *testosterone* which is responsible for secondary male characteristics. These characteristics include muscular development and deepening voice as well as hair growth.

The male and female gonads also produce the special cells *ovum* and *sperm* which unite to form a new person.

Thyroid Gland

This gland has two lobes and is found in the neck, anterior to the larynx. *Thyroxin* is the main hormone secreted by this gland. It helps to regulate the rate of metabolism, which is the production of heat and energy by the cells. In order for the thyroid gland to produce thyroxin, sufficient iodine must be present.

Parathyroids

There are some tiny glands embedded in the thyroid gland in the neck. The hormone they manufacture is called parathormone, which controls the functioning of two minerals, calcium and phosphorus, by the body. Although they are small, a disorder of these glands results in muscular spasms or tetany, and even death.

Islets of Langerhans

The islets of Langerhans are small groups of cells found within the pancreas. These cells produce the hormone *insulin*. Insulin must be present in order for the cells to utilize sugar.

COMMON ABNORMAL CONDITIONS

Disorders of the Thyroid

When there is not enough iodine in the diet, the thyroid *hypertrophies* (enlarges) and the condition is known as *simple goiter*. The use of iodized salt has largely controlled this problem. *Hypothyroidism*, which involves decreased production of *thyroxin*, has been successfully treated with thyroid extract.

Hyperthyroidism, or overactivity of the thyroid gland, is a condition which results in nervousness, rapid pulse, and weight loss. These patients tend to be restless and irritable and very sensitive to heat; their appetite is increased. Your attitude, when in contact with these patients, must be one of understanding and patience. The room should be kept quiet and cool. The patient's nutritional needs should be met with foods that are liked.

THYROID TESTS. Tests are usually performed to determine thyroid function. One such test, a blood test, is known as *PBI*, which stands for protein-bound iodine, and requires little advance preparation. You may see this test ordered for your patient.

Another thyroid test, the basal matabolism rate, *BMR*, may be ordered. This test measures the amount of oxygen used by the cells when a person is at complete rest. It is done in the morning before breakfast after a restful night. Certain preparations must be made before the test. If your patient is to have a BMR, do not awaken for AM care, withhold breakfast and fluids and, if necessary, provide a bedpan rather then allow patient to get up. It is most important to maintain a quiet, restful environment.

THYROIDECTOMY. It may be necessary to treat hyperthyroidism with surgery. Following surgery the patient is placed in a semi-Fowler's position with neck and shoulders well supported. You may be assigned to assist in the postoperative care. Remember at all times to support the back of the neck. Hyperextension of the neck may damage the operative site. Oxygen may be ordered for the patient. In addition to routine postoperative care, note and report the following:

- Any signs of bleeding—this may drain toward the back of the neck. The pillows behind the patient as well as the dressings should be checked.
- Signs of respiratory distress.
- Inability of the patient to speak. Initial hoarseness is common, but any increase should be reported.
- Greatly elevated temperature and pulse, pronounced apprehension, or irritability.
- Numbness, tingling, or muscular spasm of the extremities.

Diabetes Mellitus

When the islets of Langerhans do not produce enough insulin, sugar cannot be used, and so it accumulates in the blood and is excreted by the kidneys in the urine. This condition is called *diabetes mellitus,* and the people with the condition are known as *diabetics.* Acetone and ketone bodies also build up in the urine of diabetics. This is because the patient's body uses fats for energy, since sugar is not being used efficiently. By testing for sugar; known as *glucose,* and acetone, the physician can determine the level of these substances in the blood.

Treatment of diabetes mellitus consists of balancing the diet by controlling the available sugar, exercise; which controls the rate at which sugar will be used, and insulin, Figure 33-2A, B, and C. Patients are taught to give themselves exact amounts of insulin based on the amount of sugar being excreted in the urine.

Injuries to diabetic patients do not heal easily, and care must be taken to prevent trauma, especially to the extremities. Cutting the toenails of the

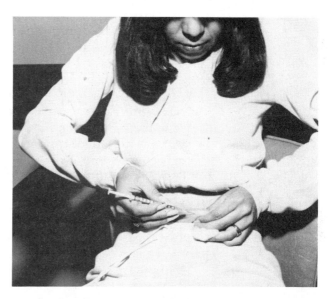

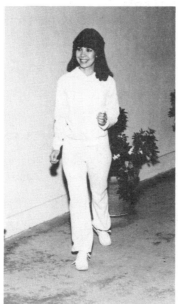
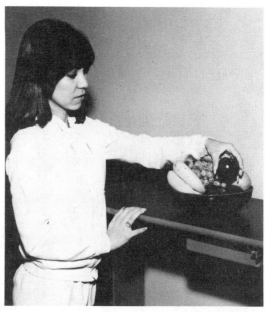

FIGURE 33-2.   The life style of the diabetic must be balanced in three areas: A) insulin intake, B) exercise, and C) diet.

diabetic patient requires a doctor's order and should be done by a licensed person. Your special responsibilities in the care of the diabatic patient in the hospital concern diet and urine testing.

DIET. Make sure you serve the patient the proper tray. You must have permission for additional nourishments. A record of the food consumed should be made on the patient's chart. If the patient does not eat his meal, report this to your team leader.

URINE TESTING. You may be asked to perform two tests on urine, one for sugar or glucose (Clinitest® or Tes-Tape®) and one for acetone (Acetest®). Dipstick methods are recommended for quantitative glucose in stable diabetes. All urine to be tested should be freshly voided. It is well to have patients empty their bladder about one hour before the test is to be done. Collect the specimen for testing immediately before the test is to be done. If the patient cannot void, be sure to report this to the nurse.

As a precaution, test the initial sample of urine just in case a fresh, second specimen cannot be obtained. The second specimen is preferred since this urine has recently accumulated while the first sample may have been in the bladder for an unspecified period of time.

Procedure

TESTING URINE FOR SUGAR: CLINITEST

1. Wash hands. Identify the patient and explain what you plan to do. Follow procedure for obtaining a routine urine specimen.
2. Wash hands again and assemble the following equipment on a tray:
   - Freshly voided urine in specimen container
   - Test tube and rack
   - Medicine dropper
   - Clinitest tablet and color chart
   - Container of fresh water
3. Read manufacturer's directions carefully.
4. Place clean, dry test tube in rack.
5. Place five drops of urine in test tube with a clean medicine dropper. Hold medicine dropper upright so that urine does *not* touch the sides of the test tube.
6. Rinse medicine dropper in cold, running water.
7. Add 10 drops of fresh water to test tube with dropper. Note: If you miscount the drops, empty the tube, wash it and dry it, and start again.

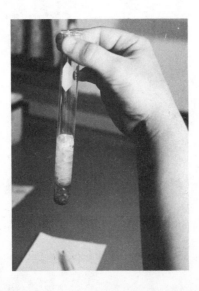

FIGURE 33-3. After the reaction has stopped, wait 15 seconds and then gently shake the test tube. *(From Simmers, Diversified Health Occupations, 1983, Delmar Publishers Inc.)*

8. Remove Clinitest tablet from wrapper. *Do not touch tablet.* Drop it into the test tube. If a bottle of tablets is used, drop one tablet into the inside lid of the bottle. Then drop the tablet into the test tube from the cover. Re-cover the bottle immediately.

9. Watch the reaction carefully. Note: **Do not handle the tube during the reaction,** since burns can occur if the test tube is handled at the bottom, where the reaction is occurring. Fifteen seconds after the reaction has stopped, shake the test tube gently, holding it at the top, Figure 33-3. (Time the 15-second interval with the second hand of your watch.) Compare the resulting color of the solution with the Clinitest color chart. Match up the color on the chart that most closely resembles the color of the solution in the test tube, Figure 33-4.

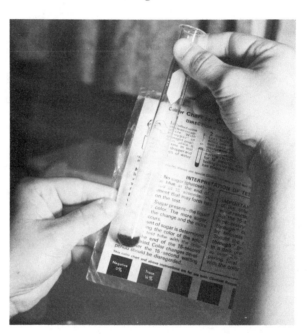

FIGURE 33-4.   Compare the color of the test tube solution with the color chart. *(From Simmers*, Diversified Health Occupations, *1983, Delmar Publishers Inc.)*

10. Record the results noted and report them. Include the patient's name, date, time, and type of test on the chart.
11. Clean and replace equipment according to hospital policy. Invert the test in the rack so it will dry thoroughly.
12. Wash hands.

Procedure

TESTING URINE FOR SUGAR: TES-TAPE

1. Wash hands. Check testing area for Tes-tape strips.
2. Identify patient and explain what you plan to do.
3. Screen unit and obtain a fresh, fractional urine specimen following the procedure for fractional urine collection.
4. Take sample to test area.
5. Wash your hands.
6. Withdraw approximately one and one-half inches of Tes-tape from the container. Touch only the tip closest to your fingers.
7. Dip approximately one-quarter inch of the Tes-tape strip into the urine sample. Withdraw, holding tip downward above container.
8. Time reaction for 60 seconds.
9. Check darkest area of wet strip against Tes-tape color chart (on back of

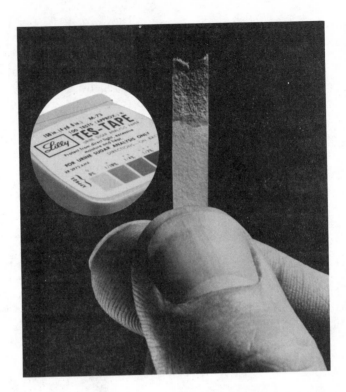

FIGURE 33-5. The color of the Tes-Tape, which has been dipped in the specimen, is compared with a color chart. *(Photos courtesy of Eli Lilly and Company)*

Tes-tape container). Read the figures above the color match. This is the value to record and report.

10. Discard tape and urine sample.
11. Clean equipment and return it to its proper place. Be sure to measure urine if patient is on I & O.
12. Wash hands. Report findings to the nurse and record on appropriate record form.

Procedure

TESTING URINE FOR ACETONE: ACETEST

1. Wash hands. Identify the patient and explain what you plan to do. Follow procedure for obtaining a routine urine specimen.
2. Wash hands again and assemble the following equipment on a tray:
   - Freshly voided urine specimen in container
   - Acetest tablet and color chart
   - White paper
   - Fresh water
   - Medicine dropper
3. Pour one tablet from the Acetest bottle into the bottle cap. Carefully drop the tablet from the cap onto the white paper, Figure 33-6. Note: **Do not touch the tablet,** as it is a chemical that can burn or injure the skin. Replace the cap on the bottle immediately.
4. Place one drop of urine on Acetest tablet with a clean, dry medicine dropper.
5. Wait 30 seconds. (Time interval with second hand on your watch.)
6. Compare the resulting color of the tablet with the color chart, matching it to the color on the chart that it most resembles.
7. Record the results of the test, noting the patient's name, date, time, type of test, and results. Report the results.
8. Discard tablet, paper, and urine.

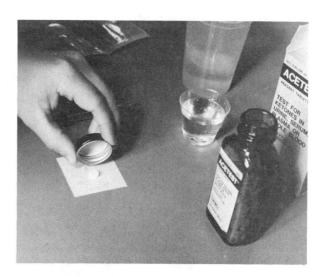

FIGURE 33-6. Place one Acetest tablet on a piece of white paper. Do not touch the tablet. *(From Simmers,* Diversified Health Occupations, *1983, Delmar Publishers Inc.)*

9. Clean and replace equipment according to policy.
10. Wash hands.

Procedure

TESTING URINE FOR ACETONE: KETOSTIX STRIP TEST

1. Wash hands. Identify patient and explain what you plan to do. Follow procedure for obtaining a routine urine specimen.
2. Wash hands again and assemble the following equipment:
   - Ketostix reagent strips
   - Sample of freshly voided urine in container
3. Dip one end of the Ketostix strip (the end with the reagent areas) into the urine.
4. Remove and hold strip horizontally.
5. Fifteen seconds later, compare the strip with the color chart on the bottle label, matching it as closely as possible to one of the colors on the chart. (See Figure 33-7, page 368.)
6. Record the results of the test, noting the patient's name, room number, date, time, type of test, and results.
7. Dispose of urine specimen unless orders have been given to save it.
8. Clean and replace equipment according to hospital policy.
9. Report the results.
10. Wash hands.

Summary

The endocrine glands produce small amounts of powerful chemicals called hormones. They regulate and control body functions. Hyperthyroidism and diabetes mellitus, conditions caused by malfunction of endocrine glands, are fairly common.

The responsibilities in caring for patients with endocrine disease includes urine testing. Urine testing gives an indication of the presence of sugar or acetone. Endocrine glands act together with the nervous system to exert control over body activities.

SUGGESTED ACTIVITIES

1. Examine a torso or wall chart and locate the endocrine glands.

2. Test a specimen of your own urine for sugar and acetone.

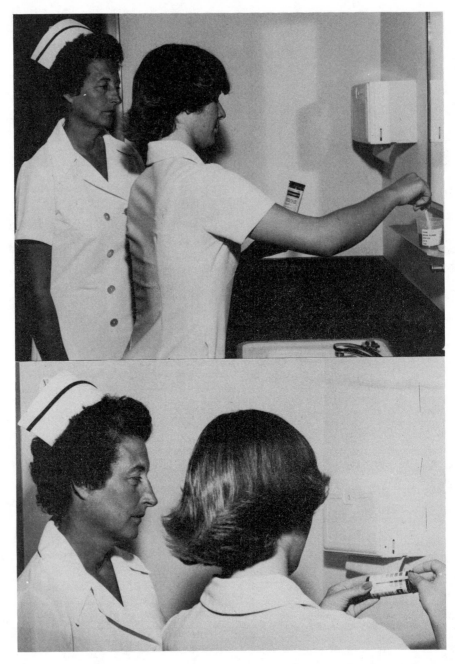

FIGURE 33-7.   Testing urine for the presence of ketones.

3. Test a specimen of prepared urine containing glucose for sugar.

4. Under supervision, give care to patients with conditions of the endocrine system.

VOCABULARY   Learn the meaning and correct spelling of the following words.

adrenalin	hyperthyroidism	PBI
BMR	hypertrophy	progesterone
cortisone	hypothyroidism	simple goiter
diabetes mellitus	insulin	sperm
endocrine gland	iodine	testes
estrogen	lobe	testosterone
glucose	ovary	tetany
hormone	ovum	thyroxin

UNIT REVIEW

A. Clinical Situations. Briefly describe how a health care assistant should react to the following situations.

1. You miscounted the drops of urine during a Clinitest procedure.

2. Your young diabetic patient refuses to eat his dinner.

3. Your postoperative thyroidectomy patient has increasing difficulty speaking.

4. Your postoperative thyroidectomy patient has moved down in the bed so that the neck is hyperextended.

B. Completion. Complete the following sentences.

1. The general function of the endocrine glands is to _____.
2. Following a thyroidectomy, it is especially important to support _____.
3. Three things that must be balanced in the treatment of the diabetic patient are _____, _____ and _____.
4. The hormone produced by the parathyroid gland controls the body's use of phosphorus and _____.
5. Name the endocrine glands and give their locations:

Gland	Location
_____	_____
_____	_____
_____	_____
_____	_____
_____	_____
_____	_____
_____	_____

6. Complete the following chart:

TEST	AMOUNT OF URINE USED	AMOUNT OF WATER USED	TIME WAITED	HOW RESULTS ARE CHECKED
Clinitest				
Acetest				

Unit 34 The Nervous System

OBJECTIVES

As a result of this unit, you will be able to:

- Locate the parts of the central nervous system.
- Name the common conditions of the central nervous system.
- Describe the function of the autonomic nervous system.
- Describe some of the functions of the assistant in caring for patients with neurological conditions.

STRUCTURE AND FUNCTION

The nervous system controls and coordinates all voluntary and involuntary body activities, even the production of hormones. Special parts of the nervous system are concerned with maintaining normal day-to-day functions while other parts act during emergency situations and others control voluntary activities. Neurological conditions require highly specialized nursing care. You will assist with the less technical aspects of that care.

Neurons

Cells of the nervous system are called *neurons,* Figure 34-1. They are specialized to conduct electric-like impulses. The neuron has extensions called *axons* and *dendrites*. Impulses enter the neuron only through the dendrites and leave only through the axon.

Although neurons do not actually touch each other, the axon of one neuron lies close to the dendrites of many other neurons. In this way impulses may follow many different routes. The space between the axon of one cell and the dendrites of others is called a *synapse*.

Nerves

Some axons and dendrites are very long and others are short. Axons and dendrites of many neurons are found in bundles, and are held together by connective tissue. These bundles resemble telephone cables and are called *nerves*. The cell bodies of the axons and dendrites in these nerves may be found at far distances from the ends of the nerves.

Sensory nerves, made up of dendrites, carry sensations to the brain and spinal cord from the various body parts. Feeling is lost when these nerve impulses are interrupted *(anesthesia)*. Motor nerves carry impulses from the brain and spinal cord to muscles that cause body activity. Paralysis, or loss of function occurs when these nerves are damaged.

For easier study, the nervous system can be divided into two parts. Remember, though, that the nervous system is one interwoven system, a complex of millions of neurons.

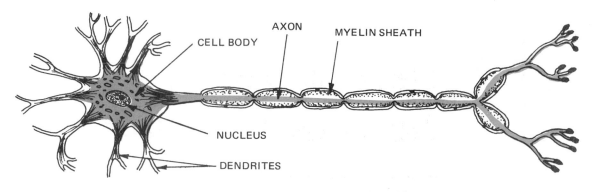

FIGURE 34-1. The neuron

THE CENTRAL NERVOUS SYSTEM

The term *central nervous system* or CNS, refers to the brain and spinal cord. These vital tissues are surrounded by bone and membrane called *meninges* and cushioned by *cerebrospinal fluid* for protection. The brain and spinal cord are a continuous structure found within the skull and spinal canal. The spinal cord itself is about 17 inches long, ending just above the small of the back. Nerves extend from the brain and spinal cord.

The Brain

The brain is a large, soft mass of nerve tissue contained within the cranium; also called the encephalon. It consists of gray and white matter. Gray matter is composed principally of nerve-cell bodies and white matter of nerve-cell processes which form connections between various parts of the brain.

CEREBRUM. The largest portion of the brain is called the *cerebrum*. The outer portion is formed in folds known as convolutions and separated into lobes which take their name from the skull bones that surround them. The outer

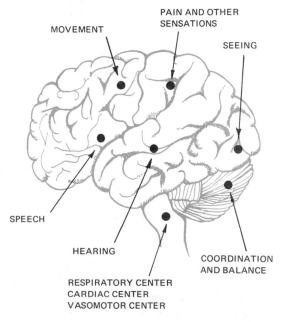

FIGURE 34-2. Functional areas of the brain

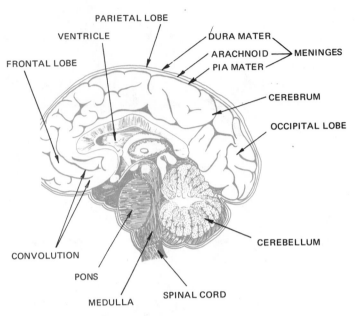

FIGURE 34-3. Cross section of the brain

portion, the cerebral cortex, is composed of cell bodies and appears gray. The inner portion is composed of axons and dendrites and so appears white. All mental activities: thinking, voluntary movements, interpreting sensations, and emotions are carried out by cerebral cells, Figure 34-2. Certain activities are centered in each lobe. In general, the right side of the cerebrum controls the left side of the body and vice versa.

CEREBELLUM. Beneath the occipital lobe of the cerebrum, Figure 34-3, is the smaller *cerebellum*. It, too, has an outer layer of gray cell bodies. This portion of the brain coordinates muscular activities and balance.

THE BRAIN STEM. The *pons* and *medulla* are in the brain stem. They are composed mainly of axons and dendrites. These fibers serve as connecting pathways between the control centers in the cerebrum and cerebellum and the spinal cord.

Control centers for involuntary movements of such vital organs as the heart, blood vessels, lungs, stomach, and intestines are found within the brain stem.

The Spinal Cord

The spinal cord extends from the medulla to the second lumbar vertebra in the spinal canal, which is just above the small of the back, a distance of about 17 inches. The cell bodies of the spinal cord are found on the inner part of the cord. Nerves entering and leaving the spinal cord carry impulses to and from the control centers. Certain *reflex* activities performed without conscious thought are controlled within the cord. Pulling your hand away from something hot is an example of this type of reflex activities.

THE MENINGES. Three membranes surround both the brain and spinal cord. The outermost, the *dura mater*, is tough. The middle layer, the *arachnoid mater*, is loosely structured and filled with cerebrospinal fluid. The innermost layer, the *pia mater*, is very delicate and clings closely to the surface of the brain and spinal cord.

CEREBROSPINAL FLUID. Ventricles are cavities within the cerebrum which are lined with highly vascular tissue. These tissues produce *cerebrospinal fluid*. The fluid flows to other ventricles which are connected to the central canal of the spinal cord and the space between the arachnoid mater and pia mater. The fluid is continually being produced in the ventricles and then returned to the general circulation. In normal amounts and freely circulating, the cerebrospinal fluid bathes the central nervous system as tissue fluid and cushions it.

Tests on the cerebrospinal fluid give information about pressure within the system. Other tests measure the presence of blood, proteins and infectious materials. Each abnormal finding or value provides clues to the condition of the central nervous tissues. For example, blood in the cerebrospinal fluid indicates bleeding into the system such as occurs in stroke patients, and lowered sugar or increased white blood cells are indicative of bacterial infections.

SPECIAL RELATIONSHIPS: THE AUTONOMIC NERVOUS SYSTEM (ANS)

The autonomic, or peripheral, nervous system is concerned with involuntary body activities. It is made up of special nervous pathways that begin in the central nervous system and reach out through cranial and spinal nerves to the glands, smooth muscle walls of organs, and to the heart. It is made up of two parts called the *sympathetic* and *parasympathetic* systems. The center of control is in the brain stem. Nerve fibers which carry impulses to control the usual functions of moderate heartbeat, digestion, elimination, respiration, and glandular activity are called parasympathetic.

In times of stress or danger, the heart beats faster, the lungs work harder, and certain glands increase their production. Blood pressure is increased as the body prepares for action. These activities are brought about by stimulation of the sympathetic nerve fibers.

Sensory Receptors

The ends of the dendrites carrying sensations to the central nervous system are found throughout the body. Some end in joints and bring information about body positions to the brain. Others in the skin carry sensations of pain, heat, pressure, and cold, Figure 34-4.

The sense of smell originates with stimulation of dendrites in the lining of the nose. The sense of taste is due to stimulation of dendrites found in the tongue. Sensory dendrites also receive stimulation through two very

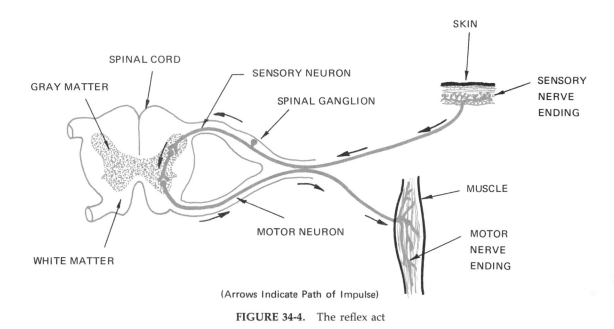

(Arrows Indicate Path of Impulse)

FIGURE 34-4.   The reflex act

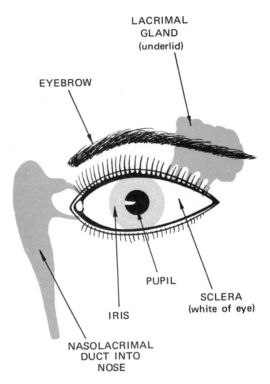

FIGURE 34-5. External view of the eye

special end organs, the eye and the ear. All of these structures are called sensory receptors because they carry information about the outside world to the brain. The brain interprets and uses the information.

THE EYE. The eye, Figure 34-5, is a hollow ball filled with a semiliquid called vitreous humor. The wall of the eye is made up of three layers. A tough white fibrous outer coat known as the *sclera* has a transparent portion in the front called the *cornea*. Beneath the sclera is a vascular layer called the *choroid*. Its job is to nourish the eye. The innermost lining, the *retina*, is made up of dendrites highly sensitive to light. These dendrites join together and leave the eye as the *optic nerve*. The two nerves cross beneath the brain and carry their impulses to the occipital lobe of the cerebrum to let us know what we see.

Light enters the eye through the cornea. The amount of light entering the eye is controlled by the colored portion of the eye, the iris, found behind the cornea. Fluid between the cornea and *iris* helps to bend the light rays and bring them to focus on the retina. The opening in the iris is called the *pupil*. The pupil appears black because there is no light behind it. Directly behind the iris is the *lens*. Small muscles pull on either side of the lens to change its shape. The changing shape of the lens makes it possible for us to adjust the range of our vision from far to near or from near to far. Figure 34-6 shows a cross-section of the eye.

The eye is held within the bony socket by muscles which can change its position. A mucous membrane, the *conjunctiva*, lines the eyelids and covers the eye. The eyelids, eyelashes, and tears combine to protect the delicate eye. Tears are manufactured by the *lacrimal gland* which is found beneath the lateral side of the upper lid. Tears wash across the eye, keeping it moist, and drain into the nasal cavity.

THE EAR. Just as the eye is sensitive to light, the ear is sensitive to sound, Figure 34-7. The ear has three parts, the outer, the middle, and the inner ear. The outer ear consists of the visible external structure known as the *pinna*, and a canal which directs sound waves to the middle ear.

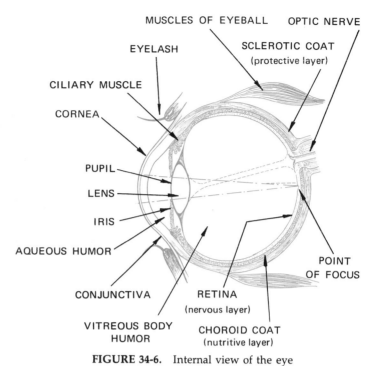

FIGURE 34-6. Internal view of the eye

Fig. 33-6 Internal view of the eye

At the end of the canal is the eardrum or *tympanic membrane*. Sound waves cause the eardrum to vibrate. Three tiny bones called *ossicles* form a chain across the middle ear from the tympanic membrane to an opening in the inner ear. These bones, known as the *incus,* or anvil; *stapes,* or stirrup; and *malleus,* or hammer, carry the sound waves across the middle ear and, by pushing against the opening of the inner ear, they start fluid moving in the inner ear. A small tube, called the *eustachian* tube, leads from the nasopharynx into the middle ear. Air carried through this tube helps to keep pressure equal on both sides of the eardrum.

The inner ear is a very complex structure having two main parts. One looks somewhat like a coiled snail shell and is called the *cochlea.* Within the

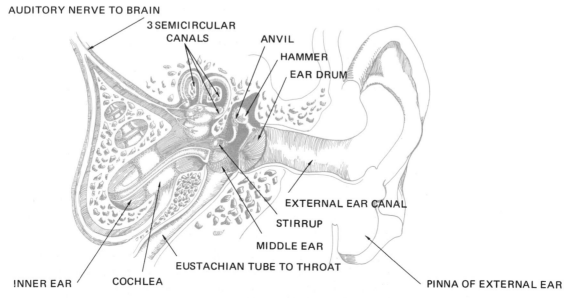

FIGURE 34-7. Internal view of the ear

cochlea are the tiny dendrites of the hearing or *auditory* nerve. Fluid covers the dendrites, and when the fluid is set in motion by the vibrating of the middle ear bones, it stimulates the dendrites with sound sensations. The auditory nerve, one from each ear, carries the sensations to the temporal lobe of the cerebrum to let us know what we are hearing. Also found in the inner ear are three *semicircular canals* that also contain liquid and nerve endings. Stimulation of these nerve endings sends impulses to the brain about the position of the head. This helps us keep our balance.

COMMON CONDITIONS

Head Injuries

Any head injury can cause damage to the delicate brain, Figure 34-8. Bleeding from damaged blood vessels and swelling puts pressure on the brain cells. This *intracranial* pressure (pressure within the skull) is capable of altering the ability of one or both irises to respond to light. In a normal eye the pupil should become smaller when a flashlight is directed at each eye, so the equality of the pupils and their ability to react to light is an important observation when a head injury occurs.

Intracranial pressure can also result in headache, vomiting, loss of consciousness and sensation, paralysis, and *convulsions,* which are uncontrolled muscular contractions that are often violent. Right now it is important to realize that almost any condition which causes increased intracranial pressure will give rise to these signs and symptoms. For example, toxins and high temperatures may also cause convulsions.

With regard to head injuries though, how long all or part of the symptoms remain depends upon the extent and cause of damage to the brain cells. The assistant should remember also that paralysis is not always accompanied by sensory loss. It is important to keep a careful check on vital signs of any patient with a head injury. A special record (head chart) may be kept for recording all observations.

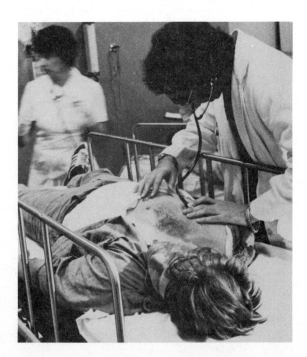

FIGURE 34-8. Auto accidents often result in severe head injuries which require immediate attention.

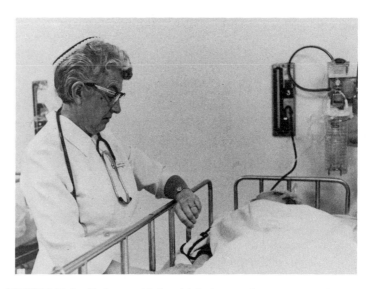

FIGURE 34-9.   Patients with head injuries require expert nursing care.

Patients acutely ill with head injuries or increased intracranial pressure require the most skilled of nursing care, Figure 34-9. Level of consciousness and orientation, reaction to pain and stimuli, and vital signs must be regularly and frequently monitored, Figure 34-10. The nurse will handle this responsibility. If, as you are assisting in the care, you should note any change in the patient's response or behavior, it must immediately be brought to the nurse's attention. Such changes that might be very significant include incontinence, uncontrolled body movements, disorientation, deepening or lessening in the level of consciousness, dizziness, vomiting, or alterations in speech, Figure 34-11.

Once improved, the patient may be moved from critical to an intermediary care unit, then to a long-term care facility for a potentially prolonged period of convalescence. The nursing measures first established in the critical care unit must be maintained throughout this extended period, however.

Loss of sensation and decreased mobility makes these patients more prone to pressure sores, infection, and contractures. You must continue special skin care, range of motion exercises, and positioning faithfully. Early signs of infection should be immediately reported. Elimination must be

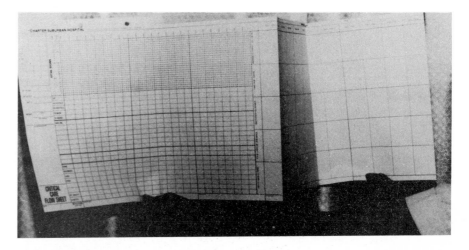

FIGURE 34-10.   The head chart is a detailed record of the patient care and response during a critical period of illness.

Note changes in levels of consciousness/orientation
Pupilary reflex response
  equality
  response to light
Response to stimuli
  verbal
  pain
Vital signs
Behavior/Speech
Motor instability

FIGURE 34-11.   Summary of some important observations pertaining to head injury patients

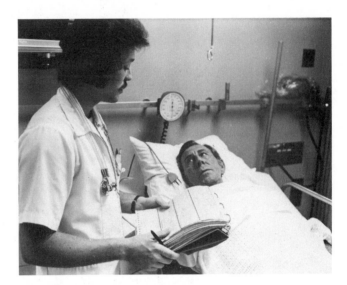

FIGURE 34-12.   Be alert to mood changes and provide the necessary emotional support.

watched since loss of muscle tone and inactivity may lead to constipation and impaction. Drainage tubes such as indwelling catheters must receive careful attention.

Patients recovering from these illnesses often experience anxiety and depression. Be alert to any indication of mood decline and plan extra time to provide essential emotional support, Figure 34-12.

Epilepsy

Epilepsy is one of the oldest known diseases. It involves recurrent, transient attacks of disturbed brain function. It is characterized by various forms of convulsions, called seizures. Convulsions range from momentary loss of consciousness to violent random or uncoordinated movements. The cause and cure are often unknown, but drugs which control the seizures are widely used and permit the epileptic—seizure syndrome—patient to live a normal, productive life.

CARE DURING CONVULSIONS. The main nursing focus during a convulsion is to (1) prevent injury and (2) to maintain an airway. A mouth gag, made of tongue blades padded with a sponge and taped, is inserted between the back teeth to prevent the patient from biting his tongue. Never force the mouth open because teeth may be loosened, and do not leave the person alone. Clothing should be loosened, and any object the patient may hit should be moved away. No attempt should be made to move the patient or restrain his movements, however. Place a pillow under the head, turn head to one side so that saliva may drain out, and if necessary, open an airway by lifting the shoulders and allowing the head to fall back. Careful

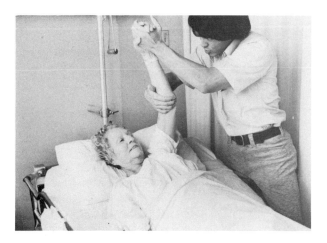

FIGURE 34-13. It is particularly important to carry out range of motion exercises when patients are paralyzed.

observation of the patient should be made during and following the convulsion. Breathing should be carefully monitored. Ring for assistance if possible.

Spinal Cord Injuries

Injuries to the spinal cord result in loss of function and sensation below the level of the injury, Figure 34-13. These patients are particularly prone to contractures and pressure areas. Special terms have been given to the conditions resulting from such injury:

- Quadriplegia: both arms and legs are paralyzed (paralyzed from the neck area down)
- Paraplegia: lower part of the body is paralyzed
- Hemiplegia: one side of the body is paralyzed, Figure 34-14

RESPONSIBILITIES OF THE HEALTH CARE ASSISTANT. The loss of sensory and motor functions often makes self-care difficult and depressing. In response, your approach must be consistently calm and patient. The patient's expressions of irritability, fear, and depression as well as clumsy attempts at self-care must be accepted in a matter-of-fact manner. Remember that the patient's ability to think is not necessarily impaired. His frustration is even greater because he can no longer will his actions.

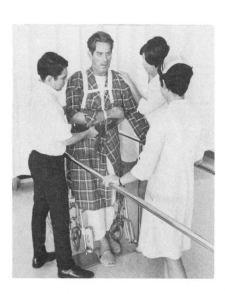

FIGURE 34-14. This patient is recovering from a head injury that resulted in right hemiplegia.

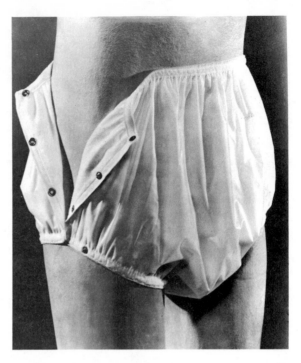

FIGURE 34-15.   Adult incontinence pants

Incontinence causes the patient embarrassment and discomfort and makes adequate skin care more difficult. Suppositories may be used to stimulate and control daily bowel movement. A catheter can be inserted into the urinary bladder to drain the urine. Special pads within plastic incontinent pants may also be used, Figure 34-15.

Skin breaks down more easily because the lack of nervous stimulation decreases circulation to the part. Since pressure and pain cannot be felt, pressure sores and contractures can become serious problems. The skin must be kept clean and dry and inspected frequently. Regular turning and proper positioning are necessary if contractures are to be prevented.

Success has been achieved in bladder and bowel retraining, but it requires consistent professional supervision.

Meningitis

Meningitis is an inflammation of the meninges usually caused by microorganisms. Headache, nausea, and stiffness of the neck are commonly associated symptoms. This condition is treated with antibiotics, and if communicable, strict isolation precautions are taken. Convulsions, chills, and elevations in temperature should be promptly reported.

CEREBROSPINAL PUNCTURES. Punctures are done to verify the existence of meningitis, as well as to diagnose cord injury. The physician inserts a long, sterile needle between the lumbar vertebrae into the fluid-filled space between the arachnoid and pia mater. The pressure of the cerebrospinal fluid is measured, and a sample withdrawn and placed in a sterile test tube.

There are special positions in which the patient can be placed in preparation for the spinal puncture: (1) The patient is placed on the side facing away from the doctor; knees are drawn up on the abdomen as far as possible, Figure 34-16. The head is bent down on the chest and the arms are flexed comfortably. (2) An alternate position is one in which the patient is seated on the edge of the bed with the shoulders hunched forward, Figure 34-17. He may also lean on the over-the-bed table. Be sure to offer ample

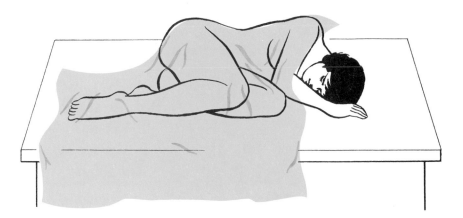

FIGURE 34-16. One position of the patient for a cerebrospinal puncture

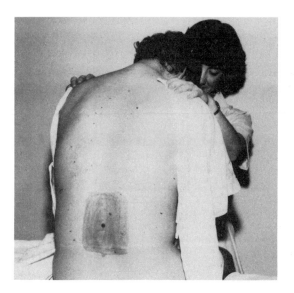

FIGURE 34-17. Alternate position for cerebrospinal puncture or anesthesia

support. It is important that the patient not move during the procedure. Patients are usually kept flat in bed for 8 hours following the puncture to reduce the possibility of headache. Do not elevate the head of the bed or provide patient with a pillow during this time.

Cataracts

When the normally clear lens of the eye becomes cloudy, vision is impaired and the condition is called a cataract. *Cataracts* are sometimes present at birth. Removal or replacement of the lens permits light rays to enter the eye, and sight is restored. Since the lens is necessary for adjusting vision to different distances, glasses must be worn to compensate for the loss when the lens is removed. Following any eye surgery, stress on the suture line through coughing, sneezing, and abrupt movements must be avoided. Orders regarding postoperative activity are usually detailed and must be followed carefully.

Otitis Media

Infections of the nose and throat can move along the eustachian tube to the middle ear, causing inflammation of the middle ear which is known as *otitis media*. Fluid and pus forms within the middle ear and may result in *fusion* (locking) of the middle ear bones. Increased pressure may cause rupturing of the eardrum. Both conditions decrease the ability to transmit sound waves. Antibotics are usually given, and sometimes a surgical opening (myringotomy) is made in the eardrum to drain the pus. Tubes may be inserted.

Summary

Our complex nervous system enables us to know our environment and react to it. Diseases of the nervous system interfere with these functions. The health assistant assists the professional nurse in the care of patients with neurological conditions.

Patients with head injuries may demonstrate loss of either sensory or motor control and often some degree of both. Although the professional nurse is responsible for neurologic assessment and intervention, the alert health care assistant can be very valuable. Observations of changes in levels of consciousness, response and behavior must be accurately and promptly reported.

Diseases and injuries of the nervous system often require a long recovery period. During the convalescent period, the health care assistant plays a vital role. Patience, empathy and skill are needed in full measure to assist these patients in their recovery period.

SUGGESTED ACTIVITIES

1. Examine a wall chart or torso and locate the parts of the central nervous system.

2. Under supervision, give care to patients with neurological conditions.

3. Practice neurological checks with your classmates.

VOCABULARY

Learn the meaning and correct spelling of the following words.

anesthesia	eustachian tube	paraplegia
arachnoid mater	hemiplegia	parasympathetic
auditory	intracranial	pia mater
autonomic nervous system	iris	pinna
cataract	lacrimal gland	pons
central nervous system	lens	pupil
cerebellum	medulla	quadriplegia
cerebrospinal fluid	meninges	reflex
cerebrum	meningitis	retina
choroid	motor nerve	sclera
cochlea	nerve	semicircular canals
conjunctiva	neuron	sensory nerve
convulsion	optic nerve	sensory receptor
cornea	ossicles	sympathetic
dura mater	otitis media	synapse
epilepsy	paralysis	tympanic membrane

UNIT REVIEW

A. Clinical Situations. Briefly describe how a health care assistant should react to the following situations.

1. You found a patient convulsing.

2. You noticed a change in the level of consciousness of your head-injured patient.

3. You were asked to position the patient for a lumbar puncture.

4. You were asked to state two special nursing care measures required for a paraplegic.

B. Completion. Complete the following sentences.
1. The spinal cord and brain form the _____ system.
2. The nerve cell is called (a, an) _____.
3. Dendrites carry _____ toward the central nervous system. If they are damaged, the patient cannot _____.
4. Impulses leave the cell body by way of the _____.
5. Meningitis is inflammation of the _____ membranes which cover the brain and spinal cord.
6. The autonomic portion of the nervous system has two parts: _____ and _____.
7. The _____ fibers prepare the body for emergencies.
8. Dendrites in the retina are sensitive to _____.
9. Dendrites in the cochlea are sensitive to _____.
10. General care for neurological patients includes _____, _____, _____, _____.
11. Describe the two positions of the patient during a cerebrospinal puncture:
12. The main nursing care during a convulsion should be to _____ and _____.

Unit 35 The Gastrointestinal System

OBJECTIVES

As a result of this unit, you will be able to:

- Locate the organs of the gastrointestinal system.
- Name the common conditions of the gastrointestinal system.
- Demonstrate the procedure for giving enemas and Harris flushes.
- Name the various types of enemas.

STRUCTURE AND FUNCTION

The gastrointestinal system is also called the GI or digestive tract. It extends from the mouth to the *anus* and is lined with mucous membrane, Figure 35-1. The organs along the length of this system change food into simple forms able to pass through the walls of the small intestine and into the circulatory system. The circulatory system then carries the nutrients to the body cells.

Proteins are changed to amino acids; carbohydrates to simple sugars like glucose; and fats to fatty acids and glycerol. The changes are brought about by mechanical action and chemicals called *enzymes*. The nondigestible portions of what we eat are moved along the intestines, and are finally excreted from the body as feces. Many organs contribute to the digestive process, and many disease conditions affect them.

The Mouth

Food is chewed by the teeth so that it can be swallowed and digested easily, Figure 35-2. Together, the teeth and tongue mix the food with *saliva*, which contains the first enzymes that food encounters. Several quarts of liquid saliva are produced daily by the salivary glands.

During our lives we have two natural sets of teeth. There are 20 teeth in the first set (deciduous). They begin to appear at about 6 months of age and are gradually replaced by 32 permanent adult teeth.

The Stomach

After the food has been chewed and swallowed it passes through the pharynx and esophagus to the stomach. The stomach is a hollow, muscular organ where food is mixed with and acted upon by *gastric* or stomach enzymes. Food is held within the stomach by muscles at either end while it is thoroughly mixed with the digestive enzymes.

The narrow, tapered, lower end of the stomach is called the *pylorus*. The muscle guarding this exit point is called the *pyloric sphincter*. Sometimes in babies the muscle is so tight (pyloric stenosis) that milk cannot get through and the muscle must be cut surgically. In addition to enzymes, the cells of the stomach lining produce *hydrochloric acid* (HCl), which helps to digest protein.

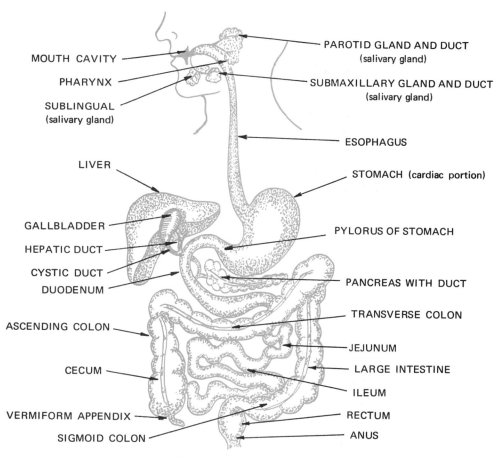

FIGURE 35-1. The digestive system

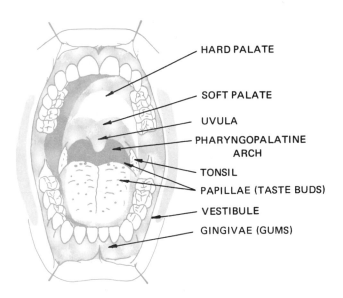

FIGURE 35-2. The mouth

The Intestines

When food leaves the stomach, it is in a semiliquid form called *chyme*. Chyme enters the small intestine where any undigested nutrients are broken down by intestinal and pancreatic enzymes and *bile* from the liver.

The small intestine is about 20 feet long and coils within the peritoneum. There are three main portions: the duodenum, the jejunum, and

ORGAN	IMPORTANT ENZYMES	FOOD ACTED UPON
Salivary glands	{ Ptyalin	Starches
Stomach	{ Pepsin { Lipase { Renin	Proteins Fats Milk protein
Pancreas	{ Steapsin { Amylopsin { Trypsin	Fats Starches Proteins
Small intestine	{ Lactase { Sucrase { Maltase { Erepsin	Lactose (sugar) Sucrose (sugar) Maltose (sugar) Protein

FIGURE 35-3. Enzymes and digestion

the ileum. The duodenum is about 12 inches long and has an opening in the back to receive the bile and pancreatic enzymes. Materials are moved through the intestines by waves of rhythmic contractions of the involuntary muscles in the intestinal wall, called *peristalsis*. Most of the nutrients and food the body needs is absorbed into the bloodstream through the walls of the small intestine. Figure 35-3 gives the digestive enzymes, their sources, and the foods they act on.

The small intestine is separated from the large intestine by the ileocecal valve. The large intestine is also called the *colon*. Names have been given to different portions of the large intestine: cecum, ascending colon, tranverse colon, descending colon, sigmoid colon, *rectum*, and anus.

No digestive enzymes are secreted in the colon, but an alkaline fluid normal to the colon aids in the completion of digestion. The colon is also the place where the more complex carbohydrates are acted upon by bacteria. Much of the remaining water is absorbed through the walls of the large intestine, changing wastes to a more solid form. In this way the large intestine helps to maintain the water balance of the body. Peristalsis moves waste through the large intestine until it reaches the rectum. When a certain amount has been collected in the rectum, it is eliminated as feces through the anus.

The Liver and Gallbladder

The liver is a large gland located just beneath the right side of the diaphragm. It helps to control the amount of proteins and sugar in the blood by changing and storing excess amounts. Two proteins, prothrombin and fibrinogen, which are necessary for blood clotting, are produced by the liver. The liver also manufactures bile, which is used for the digestion of fats. Bile is stored in the *gallbladder*, a small saclike organ found on the underside of the liver. When needed, bile is sent from the gallbladder to the duodenum. Bile gives feces their brown color.

The Pancreas

This glandular organ extends from behind the stomach into the curve of the duodenum. It manufactures pancreatic juice which is sent into the duodenum to aid in the digestion of foods. Remember, too, that special cells in the pancreas produce insulin.

COMMON CONDITIONS

Malignancy

Malignancies known as cancers of the gastrointestinal tract are very common. The symptoms they cause depend on their location. *Obstruction*, which is blocking of the passageway, is sometimes the first major indication of a long-growing tumor. Other things like indigestion, constipation, and changes in the shape of stool are signs and symptoms that might be overlooked.

Malignancies of the intestinal tract are usually treated surgically by removing the affected part. It may be necessary to make an artificial opening in the abdomen, a *colostomy*, so that feces may continue to be eliminated.

Ulcerations

Ulcers can occur anywhere along the digestive tract, but common places are the stomach; *gastric ulcers*, the duodenum; *duodenal ulcers*, and the colon; *ulcerative colitis*, whose cause is unknown. Excess production of HCl in the stomach contributes to the development of ulcers in that region.

In colitis, malnutrition and dehydration are brought about by loss of fluids in frequent, watery, offensive stools with mucus and pus. Drugs may be ordered to slow down peristalsis and reduce patient anxiety. A high-protein, high-calorie, low-residue diet is recommended. A low-residue diet is one in which the foods are almost completely digested, so there is little waste.

Patients with ulcers of the upper tract have periodic, burning pain about 2 hours after eating. Most patients improve when they are placed on a bland diet in which no foods are served that can cause distress. Medications are given to neutralize the hydrochloric acid, to coat the stomach, and to decrease anxiety. Often the first diet is a modified Sippy diet. This diet consists of half milk and half cream in small quantities every hour. The Sippy diet is gradually increased to include small amounts of soft-cooked eggs and creamed foods. If you are assigned to assist in providing a Sippy diet, make sure servings are on time. If the half-and-half is kept at the bedside, check to be sure it is being taken on time and is kept sufficiently cool.

Despite medical treatment, it is sometimes necessary to remove part of the stomach (*gastrectomy* or *gastric resection*). Following surgery, the patient is placed on NPO. Special mouth care is, therefore, essential. Usually a nasogastric tube (NG tube), Figure 35-4, which is inserted through the patient's nose and extends into his stomach, is attached to a drainage bottle. Miller-Abbot and Canter tubes are inserted into the intestinal tract. Be careful not to disturb this tube and do not allow anything to block the drainage. If the drainage becomes blocked, report it to your supervisor at once. The type and amount of drainage are noted and recorded.

Hernias

Hernias result from the *protrusion* of a structure, such as the intestines, through a weakened area in a normally-restraining wall. Frequent sites of herniation are the groin area (inguinal hernia), near the umbilicus (umbilical hernia), through a poorly healed incision (incisional hernia) and through the diaphragm (hiatal hernia). The danger of each of these abnormal protrusions is that some of the protruding tissue can become trapped in the weakened area and the circulation becomes limited so that the tissue is in danger of dying. This is called an incarcerated hernia.

Gallbladder Conditions

Inflammation of the gallbladder, known as *cholecystitis*, and the formation of stones in the gallbladder, or *cholelithiasis*, are fairly common. When the flow of bile is obstructed, symptoms of indigestion, pain, and *jaundice*—yellowing of the skin—are present. It may be necessary to remove the diseased gallbladder and stones. This operation is called a *cholecystectomy*.

After surgery the patient is most comfortable in a semi-Fowler's po-

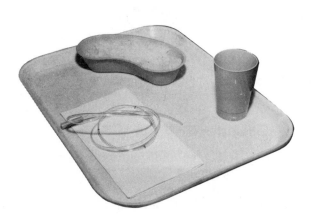

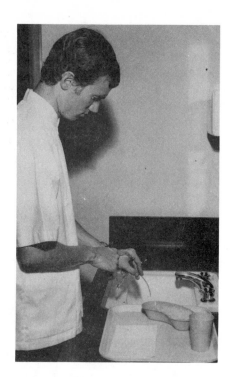

A. Tray setup includes tubing, water, and ice

B. Tubing must be iced before insertion.

FIGURE 35-4.   Preparing for nasogastric tube insertion

sition. Drains are often placed in the operative areas, and large amounts of yellowish-green drainage may be expected. Care must be taken not to disturb the drains.

If you notice fresh blood on the dressing, increased jaundice, or dark urine, report it immediately to your team leader.

SPECIAL DIAGNOSTIC TESTS

Gastrointestinal Series

When disease of the GI tract is suspected, a GI series is ordered. In this test a liquid called barium is either swallowed (upper GI series) or given as an enema (lower GI series). Then X-rays are taken. The entire GI tract must be emptied before the X-rays. No food is permitted for 8 hours, and enemas are given before the series until only the clear liquid returns.

Gallbladder Series

A GB series is an X-ray examination similar to the GI series except that the dye tablets are swallowed. Orders for preparing patients for this test vary. Cleansing enemas are frequently ordered and a special diet may be required beforehand.

ENEMAS

An enema is a means of injecting fluid into the rectum in order to remove feces and flatus (gas) from the colon and rectum. A soap solution, a salt solution, or tap water are the fluids usually ordered. These solutions create a feeling of urgency in the patient's bowel and are expelled a short time after they are given. *Urgency* is a term used to describe the need to empty the bowel.

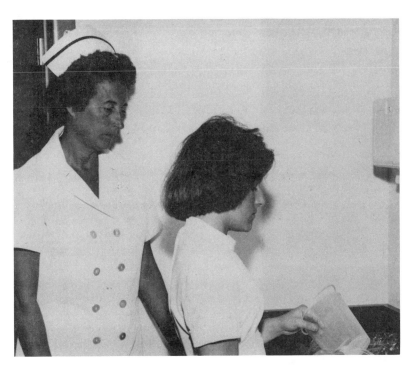

FIGURE 35-5.   Preparing to administer a soapsuds enema using a disposable unit

Sometimes a small amount of oil is given and temporarily retained by the patient to soften the feces. This is called an *oil-retention enema*. A retention enema of this type is followed by a cleansing enema (non-retention enema) in about half an hour.

Disposable enema units contain a special solution which draws fluid from the body to stimulate peristalsis. The amount of solution administered is usually 4 ounces. These units have proved most successful for patients who are unable to hold the large amount of fluid which is necessary when a soap or saline solution is being used.

In addition, they are less tiring to the patient. Oil-retention enemas may come in disposable sets as well. Disposable equipment for administering a soapsuds enema is also available, Figure 35-5. Administration is simple and time is saved in preparing and cleaning the equipment.

When possible, the enema should be given before the patient's bath or before breakfast. It should not be given within an hour following mealtime. Remember that you must have a doctor's order.

Procedure

GIVING AN OIL-RETENTION ENEMA

Note: This type of enema is frequently followed by a soapsuds enema.
1. Wash hands and assemble the following equipment:
   • Prepackaged oil for retention enema
   • Bedpan and cover
   • Bed protector
   • Toilet tissue
   • Bath blanket
   • Towel, soap, and basin with water
2. Identify patient and explain what you plan to do. Instruct patient that it will be necessary to hold the solution at least 20 minutes.
3. Place chair at foot of bed, cover with towel, place bedpan on it.
4. Cover patient with bath blanket and fan-fold linen to foot of bed.
5. Place bed protector under buttocks.
6. Help patient assume the Sims' position.
7. Open the prepackaged oil-retention enema.

8. Expose the patient's anus. Remove cap from enema and insert the pre-lubricated tip into anus as the patient takes a deep breath.
9. Squeeze container until all the solution has entered the rectum.
10. Remove container and place in package box to be discarded.
11. Encourage patient to remain on the side.
12. Check patient every five minutes until fluid has been retained for 20 minutes.
13. Position patient on bed pan or assist to bathroom.
14. If patient is on the bed pan, raise head of bed to comfortable height.
15. Place toilet tissue and signal cord within easy reach of patient. If patient is in bathroom, stay nearby.
16. Dispose of expendable material per hospital policy.
17. Remove bedpan or assist patient to return to bed. Observe contents of bedpan or toilet. Cover pan and dispose of, or flush toilet.
18. Give the patient soap, water and towel to wash and dry his hands.
19. Replace top bedding and remove bath blanket and bed protector. Dispose of according to hospital policy.
20. Wash hands and chart:
    - Date and time
    - Procedure: oil-retention enema
    - Returns
    - Patient reaction to procedure

Procedure
GIVING A SOAPSUDS ENEMA

1. Wash hands. Obtain disposable enema equipment consisting of a plastic container, tubing, clamp, and lubricant which is commercially available.
    a. Connect tubing to solution container.
    b. Adjust clamp on tubing and snap shut.
    c. Fill container with warm water (105 degrees F) to the 1000 ml line.
    d. Open packet of liquid soap and put the soap in the water.
    e. Using the tip of the tubing, mix the solution gently so that no suds form.
    f. Run small amount of solution through tube to get rid of air and warm the tube.
    If disposable equipment is not available, you will need:
    - A funnel
    - Tubing and clamp
    - Connecting tube
    - Rectal tube
    - Graduate pitcher with warm soapy water, 105°F
2. Take the following equipment to bedside:
    - Disposable enema unit/or prepared one
    - Pack of lubricant
    - Toilet tissue
    - Bedpan and cover
    - Towel, soap, and basin with water
    - Bath blanket
    - Bed Protector (Chux)
3. Identify the patient and tell what you plan to do, Figure 35-6.
4. Place chair at foot of bed and cover with towel. Place the bedpan on it.
5. Cover the patient with a bath blanket and fanfold linen to foot of bed.
6. Place bed protector under buttocks.
7. Help patient to turn on left side and flex knees (Sims' position).

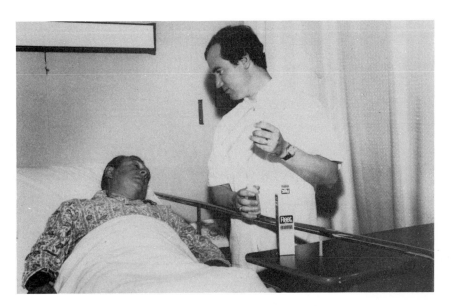

FIGURE 35-6. The health care assistant explains that the patient will only have to hold a small amount of fluid.

8. Place container of solution on chair so tubing will reach patient. Lubricate tip.
9. Adjust bath blanket to expose anal area.
10. Expose anus by raising upper buttock.
11. Never force the tube. If tube cannot be inserted easily, get help. There may be a mass of feces blocking the bowel. This is known as an *impaction*.
12. Open the clamp and raise container so that the fluid flows in slowly. Ask the patient to take deep breaths to relax the abdomen. If the patient complains of cramping, clamp tube and wait. Then open the tubing to continue fluid flow.
13. When enough solution has been given, clamp the tubing.
14. Tell the patient to hold his breath while upper buttock is raised and tube is gently withdrawn.
15. Wrap tubing in paper towel. Put it in the disposable container.
16. Place patient on bedpan or assist to bathroom.
17. Raise head of bed to comfortable height if patient is on bedpan.
18. Place toilet tissue and signal cord within reach of patient. If patient is in bathroom, stay nearby.
19. Take tray to utility room. Rinse enema equipment thoroughly in cool water and then wash in warm soapy water. Return it to bedside or discard according to hospital policy.
20. Remove bedpan or assist patient to return to bed and observe contents. Cover bedpan. Remove bed protector.
21. Give the patient soap, water, and a towel to wash his hands.
22. Replace top bedding and remove bath blanket. Air the room. Leave room in order.
23. Clean and replace all other equipment used according to hospital policy. Wash hands.
24. Chart:
    - Date and time
    - Procedure, enema (type, amount, and temperature of solution)
    - Return (color, consistency, unusual materials, flatus)
    - Patient reaction to the procedure

Procedure

GIVING A ROTATING ENEMA

Note: The procedure for the rotating enema varies only slightly from the regular soapsuds enema. The same equipment is used, and about 1000 ml of fluid is allowed to flow into the rectum.

1. Follow steps 1 through 8 for the soapsuds enema.
2. Raise foot of bed about 30 degrees, Figure 35-7.

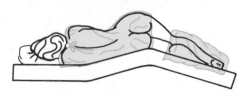

A. PATIENT ON LEFT SIDE

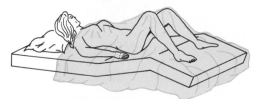

B. PATIENT ON BACK

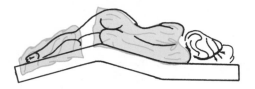

FIGURE 35-7.   Positions for rotating enema

3. Insert lubricated tip into the rectum from 2 to 4 inches.
4. Allow about 300 ml of fluid to flow slowly into the rectum.
5. Help patient to turn on back while holding tube in place.
6. Administer about 300 ml more of the solution.
7. Holding tube in place, move solution can under patient's legs to other side of bed.
8. Assist patient to turn on right side and administer the remaining solution.
9. Follow steps 13 through 24 for the soapsuds enema.

The Harris Flush

The Harris flush is used to relieve abdominal distention caused by gas. In this procedure a small amount of fluid is injected into the rectum and then allowed to return by lowering the irrigation can. The Harris flush is also called a return-flow enema.

Procedure

GIVING A HARRIS FLUSH (RETURN-FLOW ENEMA)

1. Wash hands and assemble the following equipment on a tray:
   • Irrigating can
   • Enema tubing and clamp
   • Lubricant
   • Covering for tray
   • Bed protector
   • Toilet tissue
   • Solution: 500 ml tap water at 105 degrees F

2. Pour the solution into the irrigating can and cover. Carry tray to bedside.
3. Identify the patient and tell what you plan to do.
4. Screen, drape, and place patient in Sims' position if possible, as for enema.
5. Put lubricant on a square of tissue. Lubricate end of enema tubing.
6. Allow a small amount of fluid to run through the tubing to remove air.
7. Insert tube into rectum about 4 inches.
8. Handle the Harris flush in the following way to bring about peristalsis:
   a. Open clamp, raise irrigating can to a height of 12 to 18 inches above the patient's hips and allow about 200 ml of fluid to run into the rectum.
   b. Lower irrigating can about 12 inches below the level of the bed and allow fluid to flow out of rectum into can.
9. Continue procedure until some gas is expelled. When all fluid has been returned, clamp tube and remove.
10. Straighten bedclothes and make the patient comfortable.
11. Return tray to utility room. Clean equipment as for regular enema. Wash hands.
12. Chart:
   • Date and time
   • Procedure, Harris flush (temperature of solution, amount of flatus expelled, reaction of patient)

Other Gas-expelling Methods

The rectal tube is used to reduce the amount of flatus (gas) which is in the bowel since flatus distends the intestines, causing pain and stress on incisions. The disposable tube is used once in a twenty-four hour period for no more than 20 minutes each time. Relief is sometimes dramatic as soon as the tube is inserted. Be sure to check the amount of abdominal distension and to question the patient about the degree of relief.

Procedure
INSERTING A RECTAL TUBE AND FLATUS BAG

1. Wash hands and gather the following equipment:
   • Disposable rectal tube and flatus bag
   • Lubricant
   • Tissue
   • Tape
   • Paper towel
2. Identify the patient and explain what you plan to do.
3. Screen unit for privacy.
4. Lower head of bed to horizontal position.
5. Assist the patient to assume the left Sims' position (see procedure, Unit 26).
6. Expose only the patient's buttocks by drawing the bedding upward in one hand.
7. Lubricate tip of rectal tube.
8. Separate buttocks, exposing anus and ask patient to bear down gently.
9. Insert lubricated tip of rectal tube 2–4 inches.
10. Secure rectal tube in place with small piece of adhesive.
11. Adjust bedding and make patient comfortable. Leave unit tidy.
12. Wash hands.
13. Return to unit in 20 minutes and wash hands.
14. Identify patient and screen unit.
15. Gently remove rectal tube and place on paper towel.

16. Assist patient to assume a comfortable position and adjust bedding. Leave unit tidy.
17. Dispose of wrapped rectal tube and bag according to hospital policy.
18. Wash hands and report and record:
    • Procedure including time of insertion and removal
    • Degree of relief
    • Any observations you have made

RECTAL SUPPOSITORIES

Suppositories are given to stimulate bowel evacuation or to instill medications. Medicinal suppositories must be inserted by the nurse. You may be asked to insert suppositories that soften the stool and promote elimination, if you have been trained in this advance procedure and if your facility allows it. Instruction are detailed in Unit 39.

CARE OF THE PATIENT WITH A COLOSTOMY

Sometimes disease of the bowel makes it necessary to remove part of the bowel or at least temporarily rest that organ. To make this possible, a section of the bowel is brought to the surface of the abdomen and an opening is made. The procedure is called a *colostomy* and the new opening is called an *ostomy* or stoma.

There are different surgical techniques which may be employed. For example, part of the bowel may be removed and the remaining end be brought through the wall. When there is the potential to reunite the bowel in the future, both segments may be brought to the surface (this is called a double-barrelled colostomy).

Since the normal sphincter control has been lost, there may be problems of leakage, odor control, and irritation of the surrounding area. It is very important to keep the area clean and dry. To collect the drainage, a disposable colostomy bag covers the stoma and is held in place with a belt. Irrigation of the fresh colostomy is done by the nurse. If this procedure is to be permanent, patients are taught to carry out this procedure for themselves. You may be assigned to assist the nurse in the routine care of an established colostomy. This, again, is an advanced procedure which is covered in detail in Unit 39. It can be done only by those who are trained, and provided the rules of your hospital allow you to either assist or to perform the care.

The following advanced procedures are included in Unit 39:

• Inserting Rectal Suppositories
• Giving Routine Stoma Care (Colostomy)
• Routine Care of an Ileostomy (patient in bed)
• Routine Care of an Ileostomy (patient in bathroom)

These procedures are to be carried out only after adequate practice and supervision and only in accord with specific hospital policy.

Summary

The digestive tract breaks food into simple substances that can be used by the body cells to carry on their work. Because of the complexity of the many organs that contribute to the digestive process, disease of these organs is fairly common. Enemas are frequently ordered before tests and most kinds of surgery. Other procedures you may perform for patients include the insertion of rectal tubes to relieve flatus and other irrigations.

Great care must be exercised when performing the procedures. The comfort and privacy of the patient should be protected at all times.

SUGGESTED ACTIVITIES

1. Examine a wall chart or torso and locate the organs of digestion.

2. Under supervision, give care to patients with conditions of the gastrointestinal tract.

3. Under direct supervision, administer various types of enemas; insert rectal tubes to relieve flatus.

VOCABULARY   Learn the meaning and correct spelling of the following words.

anus	gastrectomy	modified Sippy diet
bile	gastric	obstruction
cholecystectomy	gastric resection	peristalsis
cholecystitis	gastric ulcers	proctoscopy
cholelithiasis	gavage	pyloric sphincter
chyme	hernia	pylorus
colon	herniorrhaphy	rectum
colostomy	hydrochloric acid (HCl)	saliva
duodenal ulcers	impaction	strangulated hernia
enzymes	jaundice	suppository
flatus	lavage	ulcerative colitis
gallbladder	masticate	urgency

UNIT REVIEW   **A. Clinical Situations.** Briefly describe how a health care assistant should react to the following situations.

1. You have an order to give a soapsuds enema and the patient has just finished breakfast.

2. You wished to encourage a patient to relax the anal sphincter so the rectal tube could be inserted.

3. The patient complains of cramping while you are giving an enema.

B. Completion. Complete the following sentences.

1. Digestion is the process by which _____ are made into simple forms.
2. There are _____ teeth in the deciduous set.
3. There are _____ teeth in the permanent set.
4. A cholecystectomy is performed to remove the _____.
5. Two functions of the pancreas are _____ and _____.
6. Two functions of the liver are _____ and _____.
7. Diets prescribed for gastric ulcers include _____ and _____.
8. Enemas are usually given to promote _____.
9. A Harris flush is given to relieve _____.
10. Another name for a Harris flush is _____.

Unit 36 The Urinary System

OBJECTIVES

As a result of this unit, you will be able to:

- Name and locate the parts of the urinary system.
- Describe the function of the urinary system.
- List the conditions of the urinary system.
- Name and describe the special tests given for urinary conditions.

STRUCTURE AND FUNCTION

The urinary system is also referred to as the excretory system. As the name implies, the organs of this system produce urine—liquid waste—which is excreted from the body. The urinary system also helps to control the vital water and salt balance of the body. Inability to secrete urine by the kidneys is known as *suppression*. Inability to excrete urine that has been produced is called *retention*. The organs of this system include: the *kidneys*, *ureters*, *urinary bladder*, and *urethra*.

The Kidneys

The two bean-shaped kidneys are located behind the peritoneum and are held in place by capsules of fat. The outer portion of the kidney is called the *cortex*, and it is in this area that the urine is produced. The middle area, known as the *medulla*, is a series of tubes which drain the urine toward the *pelvis* of the kidney.

URINE PRODUCTION. The renal arteries carry blood to each kidney. Their many branches pass through the medulla to the cortex, Figure 36-1. In the cortex the blood vessels branch to form balls of capillaries called *glomeruli*, of which there are approximately one million in each kidney. Each glomerulus is surrounded by a blind tube, the end of which resembles a cup: called Bowman's capsule. The tube twists and coils within the cortex, dips down into the medulla, and eventually drains what is now called the urine through the structures of the medulla into the pelvis of the kidney and then into the ureter. Waste products in large amounts of water are passed from the glomerulus to Bowman's capsule.

All of the water needed to pass the waste products cannot be permanently lost from the body. Much of it is reabsorbed back into the bloodstream as the branches of the glomerulus encircle the twisted tubule in the cortex. The blood vessels then merge to leave the kidney as the renal vein. Hormones also influence how much urine is produced.

Waste products excreted in urine include *urea, creatinine, uric acid*, and various salts. The average urine output is 1,500 to 2,000 ml every 24 hours.

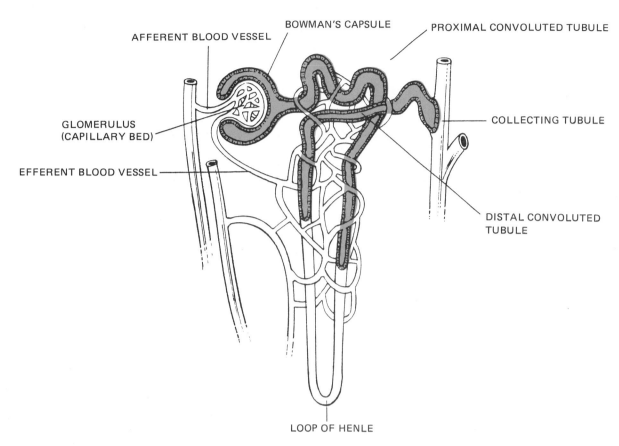

AFFERENT BLOOD VESSEL

BOWMAN'S CAPSULE

PROXIMAL CONVOLUTED TUBULE

GLOMERULUS
(CAPILLARY BED)

COLLECTING TUBULE

EFFERENT BLOOD VESSEL

DISTAL CONVOLUTED
TUBULE

LOOP OF HENLE

FIGURE 36-1.   The nephron is the functional unit of the kidney which produces urine. One million of these units are found in the cortex. *(From Fong, Ferris, and Skelly,* Body Structures and Functions, *1984, Delmar Publishers Inc.)*

Ureters

The two ureters extend from the pelvises of the kidneys to the urinary bladder, Figure 36-2. The ureters are approximately 10 to 12 inches long and 1/4 inch wide. They simply act as passageways for the urine.

Urinary Bladder

The urinary bladder, found within the pelvic cavity, is a reservoir for urine until it is expelled from the body. The muscular walls of the bladder are able to contract and force the urine out. The urge to urinate (*micturate* or *void*) occurs when there is 200 to 300 ml of urine in the bladder. The bladder is capable of holding much more urine than this amount.

Urethra

The urethra in the female is about 1-1/2 inches long. In the male it is about 8 inches. The opening to the outside is called the *external urinary meatus*. The meatus is guarded by a round sphincter muscle which relaxes to release the urine.

COMMON CONDITIONS

Cystitis

Cystitis, or inflammation of the urinary bladder, is fairly common, particularly in women because of the shortness of the urethra. Frequency of urination, *hematuria*, which is blood in the urine, and *dysuria*, or painful voiding, are symptoms of cystitis.

Treatment is aimed at relieving the symptoms and eliminating the cause. Medicated sitz baths, rest, and vaginal douches are ordered.

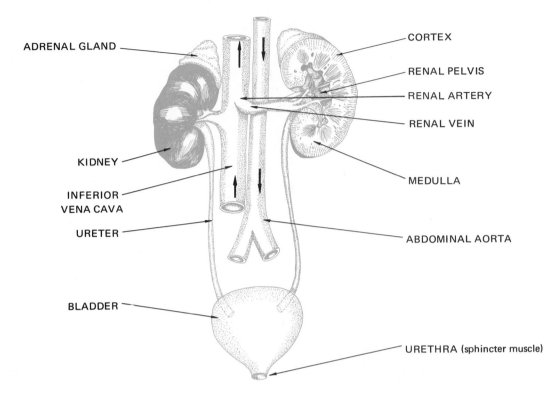

FIGURE 36-2. The urinary system

Nephritis

Inflammation of the kidney is called *nephritis*. It may follow an attack of a communicable disease or may result from general arteriosclerosis. In either case, the destruction of kidney cells results in decreased urine production. The course of the disease may be acute (rapid) or chronic (slow). Decreased kidney function causes hypertension and edema. Treatment includes absolute bedrest, a low-sodium diet, and, at times, restricted fluid. Frequent checks on vital signs and accurate I & O are part of your responsibility.

If both kidneys are involved, there is eventual death unless the diseased kidneys are replaced with a healthy kidney (kidney transplant) or the waste products can be removed from the blood by a hemodialysis machine—commonly called an artificial kidney.

Smaller dialysis units are now successfully being used by patients at home.

Renal Calculi

Just as stones sometimes form in the gallbladder, stones may also form in the kidney and along the urinary tract. Kidney stones; known as *renal calculi*, can cause obstruction when they become lodged in the ureters. The resulting pain *(renal colic)* is sudden and intense. Many renal calculi are passed in the urine, Figure 36-3. Forcing fluids encourages increased output. All urine must be strained through gauze and inspected for stones before discarding it, Figure 36-4.

When it is impossible for the patient to pass the stones, surgery may be necessary. This type of surgery can take one of two forms, minor, or major. In the minor form, sometimes it is possible for the doctor to pass an instrument into the bladder through the urethra. The instrument is called a *cystoscope* and the procedure a *cystoscopy*. With the cystoscope, the doctor is able to see inside the bladder and locate stones. The stones may then be crushed so they may be flushed out in the urine.

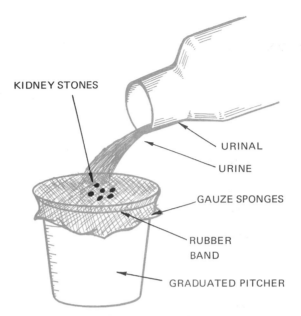

FIGURE 36-3.   Straining urine for kidney stones

At other times, the stones may be reached and removed only through a surgical incision. When a surgical incision is made, the patient usually returns from surgery with two drainage tubes in place: one in the urinary bladder and the other inserted in the ureter or kidney. The nurse will see that the proper drainage is established. You must check frequently to be sure the drainage is not blocked by kinks in the tubes or by the patient's

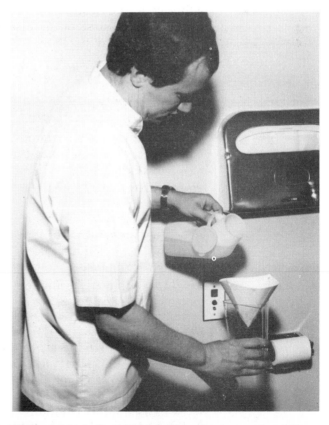

FIGURE 36-4.   The urine is strained through filter paper to retrieve kidney stones that are excreted from the bladder.

body lying on the tubes. The amount and type of drainage from each area should be carefully noted.

Hydronephrosis

Urine is constantly being produced even if it cannot be excreted. Obstruction of the flow of urine may be caused by renal calculi, kinking of the ureters, and tumors. The increasing pressure of urine causes pressure on the kidney cells which results in their destruction. The condition is known as *hydronephrosis*. Symptoms may be acute or occur so gradually as to go unnoticed. The condition is treated by draining the urine above the blockage to relieve pressure and then to correct the cause.

SPECIAL TESTS

Urinalysis

One of the most common means of learning about the condition of the kidneys is to examine the urine. You learned how to collect a specimen for routine urinalysis in Unit 24.

Cystoscopy

Cystoscopy is a test performed during surgery which enables the doctor to look inside the bladder. An instrument called a cystoscope is inserted through the urethra. Following this examination, frequency is to be expected, but heavy bleeding or a complaint of sharp, intense pain should be reported at once.

Pyelograms

Pyelograms are X-ray examinations of the urinary tract similar to the GB and GI series. The dye may be given intravenously: *intravenous pyelogram* or IVP, or inserted during cystoscopy: *retrograde*, that is, through the urethra. Preparation of the patient usually includes cleansing enemas. Satisfactory results of the X-ray examination are largely based on proper patient preparation.

RESPONSIBILITIES OF THE HEALTH CARE ASSISTANT

Careful measurement of intake and output is required for all patients with urinary problems. Signs of bleeding, chills, temperature elevation, increased edema, and pain are all significant and should be reported promptly. Orders regarding positioning, drainage, and activity after urological (urinary) surgery vary. Be sure you understand the orders for each individual patient before you assist in their nursing care.

Urinary Drainage

Urine is usually drained from the bladder through a catheter into a container. Most catheters are attached to a closed drainage system, but some facilities still employ open drainage systems, Figure 36-5. French catheters, Figure 36-6A, are hollow tubes, usually made of soft rubber or plastic. Some catheters have a balloon surrounding the neck which is inflated to keep the catheter in place. This type is called the Foley (retention or indwelling) catheter, Figure 36-6B. The insertion of a catheter is a sterile procedure and is performed by the nurse or physician.

Once the Foley catheter is inserted, the urinary meatus must be kept clean and free of secretions. The area around the meatus is washed daily with a solution approved by your hospital. This care is called indwelling

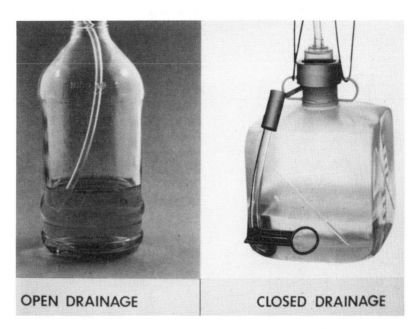

FIGURE 36-5. Although some facilities employ open drainage, the closed system ensures greater safety for the patient. *(Photo courtesy of Burroughs Wellcome Co.)*

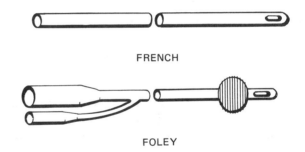

FIGURE 36-6. Two types of catheters used to drain urine

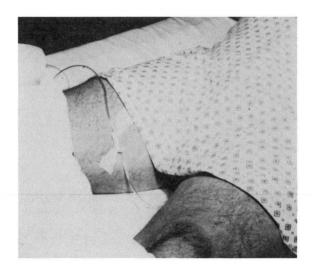

FIGURE 36-7. Urinary drainage

catheter care. Report any signs of irritation or urinary discomfort.

Indwelling catheter care may be performed during the routine morning care, as part of perineal care, or as a separate procedure. It must be done on a regular basis to be effective.

Procedure

GIVING DAILY INDWELLING CATHETER CARE

1. Wash your hands and collect the following equipment:
   - Disposable gloves
   - Bed protector
   - Bath blanket
   - Plastic bag for disposables
   - Daily catheter care kit
   - Antiseptic solution
   - Sterile applicators
   - Tape
2. Identify patient and explain what you plan to do. Screen unit.
3. Raise bed to working height and lower siderail closest to you. Be sure opposite siderail is up and secure. Position patient on his or her back, legs separated and knees bent, if permitted.
4. Cover patient with bath blanket and fanfold bedding to foot of bed.
5. Position bath blanket so that only genitals will be exposed (Unit 26).
6. Ask patient to raise his hips and place bed protector underneath.
7. Arrange catheter care kit, plastic bag on overbed table. Open kit.
8. Put on gloves and draw drape back.
9. **For the male patient:**
   a. Gently grasp penis and draw foreskin back.
   b. Using an applicator dipped in antiseptic solution, for each stroke, cleanse the glans from meatus toward shaft for approximately 4 inches.
   c. Do not return the applicator to the solution after use.
   d. Put it into disposable plastic bag.
   e. Use a new, freshly-dipped applicator for each stroke.
   For the female patient:
   a. Separate the labia.
   b. Using an applicator, freshly dipped in antiseptic, stroke from front to back.
   c. Discard each used applicator after one stroke and dispose in plastic bag.
10. Remove gloves and discard in plastic bag.
11. Check catheter to be sure it is taped properly. Retape and adjust for slack, if needed.
12. Check to be sure tubing is coiled on bed and hangs straight down into drainage container. Check level of urine in container. End of tubing should not be below urine level. Empty bag and measure if necessary.
13. Replace bedding and remove bath blanket.
14. Fold bath blanket and leave in bedside stand for reuse.
15. Help patient to assume a comfortable position, call bell within easy reach.
16. Lower bed and raise and secure siderail. Leave unit tidy.
17. Dispose of equipment per hospital policy.
18. Wash hands and report completion of task. Record:
    - Procedure: Catheter care
    - Antiseptic solution used
    - Any observations you have made

Condom Drainage

When male patients require long periods of urinary drainage, external drainage is preferred because of the reduced risk of infection. A condom (sheath) to which tubing has been connected is applied to the penis and changed by the male assistant daily during morning care.

You have definite responsibilities when patients have urinary drainage:

- Make sure tubes are in good position and unblocked.
- Measure output carefully. Note color and anything else unusual.
- Keep the end of the drainage tubing above the urine in the bag.
- Do not permit the drainage bag to touch the floor. Connect it to the bed frame. Always keep the bag below the patient's hip level.

• Keep the drainage tubes smoothly coiled in the bed so that there is a direct drop to the drainage bag.

Procedure
REPLACING A URINARY CONDOM

1. Wash hands and assemble the following equipment:
   - Basin of warm water
   - Wash cloth
   - Towel
   - Bed protector/Bath blanket
   - Gloves
   - Plastic bag
   - Tincture of Benzoin
   - Condom with drainage tip
   - Paper towels
2. Identify patient and explain what you plan to do.
3. Screen unit and elevate bed to comfortable working height. Arrange equipment on overbed table.
4. Lower siderail on the side on which you are working.
5. Cover patient with bath blanket and fanfold bedding to foot of bed. Place bed protector under patient hips.
6. Adjust bath blanket to expose genitals only. (See Unit 26.)
7. Put on gloves.
8. Remove present sheath by rolling toward tip on penis. Place in plastic bag if disposable. Place on paper towels to be washed and dried if reusable.
9. Wash and dry penis carefully. Observe for signs of irritation.
10. Check to see if condom has "ready stick" surfaces. If not, a thin spray coat of tincture of benzoin may be applied to the penis. Do not spray on head of penis.
11. Apply fresh condom and drainage tip to penis by rolling it toward base of penis. If the patient is uncircumcised, be sure that the foreskin remains in good position.
12. Reconnect drainage system.
13. Remove gloves.
14. Adjust bedding and remove bath blanket. Fold bath blanket and leave in bedside stand.
15. Lower bed and raise side rail. Make patient comfortable, call bell at hand. Leave unit tidy.
16. Clean and replace equipment and disposables according to hospital policy.
17. Wash hands.
18. Report completion of task to the nurse. Record:
    - Procedure: urinary condom replaced
    - Any observations you have made.

Procedure
DISCONNECTING THE CATHETER

Note: It is preferable never to disconnect the drainage setup, but at times it is necessary. If sterile caps and plugs are available, they should be used. If not, the disconnected ends must be protected with sterile gauze sponges.

1. Wash hands.
2. Identify patient and tell him what you plan to do.
3. Clamp the catheter.
4. Disinfect the area to be disconnected.
5. Disconnect the catheter and drainage tubing. Do not put them down or allow them to touch anything.
6. Insert a sterile plug in the end of the catheter. Place a sterile cap over the exposed end of the drainage tube.
7. Secure the drainage tube to the bed in such a way that it will not touch the floor. Wash hands.

Note: Reverse the procedure to reconnect the catheter. If you find an unprotected disconnected tube in the bed or on the floor, *do not reconnect it. Report it at once.*

Procedure

EMPTYING A URINARY DRAINAGE UNIT

1. Wash hands.
2. Identify patient and tell him what you plan to do.
3. If drainage bag has an opening in the bottom, place a graduate under it and allow the urine to drain.
4. If there is no opening, the tube must be removed before emptying. Protect the end of the drainage tube with a sterile cap or a sterile gauze sponge, Figure 36-8.
5. Empty urine and measure it.
6. Remove protective cover from the end of the tube and reinsert it in the bag. Be careful not to hit the sides of the bag.
7. Wash hands.

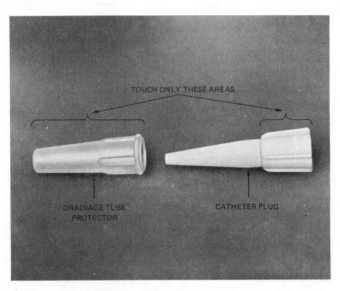
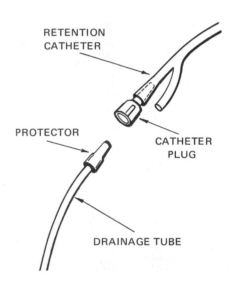

FIGURE 36-8. Left: sterile catheter plug and protector Right: plug and protector in place

---

Summary

Maintaining adequate urinary drainage is one of the most important aspects of the nursing care of urological patients. Making sure that the drainage equipment is kept free of contamination is of equal importance. The health assistant must know how to disconnect the catheter from the drainage setup and how to empty drainage safely. The urinary tract is considered a sterile area. Very special sterile techniques must be employed when the doctor or nurse introduces catheters into this area.

SUGGESTED ACTIVITIES

1. Examine a wall chart or torso and locate the organs of the urinary system.
2. Under supervision, give care to patients with urological conditions.
3. Under direct supervision, practice:
   a. Emptying and measuring drainage
   b. Ambulating patients with urinary drainage

VOCABULARY Learn the meaning and correct spelling of the following words.

catheter (Foley, French)   hydronephrosis   retention
cortex   intravenous pyelogram (IVP)   retrograde pyelogram
creatinine   kidneys   suppression
cystitis   medulla (of kidney)   urea
cystoscopy   micturate   ureter
dysuria   nephritis   urethra
external urinary meatus   pelvis (of kidney)   uric acid
glomeruli   renal calculi   urinalysis
hematuria   renal colic   urinary bladder

UNIT REVIEW **A. Clinical Situations.** Briefly describe how a health care assistant should react to the following situations.

1. Your patient has an indwelling catheter. Explain your daily care.

2. Your patient has a condom drainage. Review your responsibilities.

3. Your patient is on intake and output. Explain how to measure the drainage when the patient has an indwelling catheter.

B. Completion. Complete the following sentences.

1. Urine is produced in the _____.
2. The tube leading from the urinary bladder to the outside of the body is the _____.
3. The tubes leading from the kidneys to the urinary bladder are _____.
4. Patients with urinary conditions should have their _____ and _____ measured.
5. Catheters are small, hollow _____.
6. Foley catheters differ from other catheters in that they have an inflatable _____.
7. If the drainage tube must be removed when you empty the drainage bag, you must protect it from _____.
8. The drainage bag must never be _____ (higher, lower) than the level of the patient's bladder.
9. The end of the drainage tube should never be _____ (above, below) the level of the urine in the drainage bag.
10. The drainage bag should be attached to the _____.

Unit 37 The Reproductive System

OBJECTIVES

As a result of this unit, you will be able to:

- Name and locate the organs of the reproductive system in the male and female.
- Describe the functions of the male and female reproductive systems.
- Name and describe the common diseases of the reproductive system.
- Prepare and give a nonsterile vaginal douche.

Both the male and female organs of reproduction have dual functions. They produce the hormones responsible for masculine and feminine characteristics and the living cells—sperm and ovum—which unite to form a baby. The female also houses the new baby until birth. The female breasts, known as mammary glands, produce milk after delivery to nourish the newborn. In the male the urethra is a common passageway for both urine and sperm. Conditions affecting the urethra in the male may result in both urinary and reproductive problems.

Disease conditions of the reproductive organs and surgery have tremendous psychological effects on patients. Communicable diseases that are transmitted through direct sexual contact are called *sexually-transmitted disease*; STD, or venereal diseases (VD). The most common venereal diseases are herpes II, gonorrhea, and syphilis. These are not, however, the only diseases transmitted in this way.

THE MALE REPRODUCTIVE ORGANS: STRUCTURE AND FUNCTION

The male organs include the *penis* and the two *testes* found in the *scrotum*, Figure 37-1. The testes produce sperm and masculine hormones, mainly testosterone. Leading from each testis is a tube. The first part of the tube (epididymis) is coiled on top of the testis. The next part (the vas deferens) passes with the nerves and blood vessels into the pelvis. The vas deferens passes behind the urinary bladder to the seminal vesicle, a pouch which stores the sperm. A small tube (ejaculatory duct) leads from the seminal vesicles, entering the urethra just below the bladder. Urine and seminal fluid, which is composed of sperm and other secretion, do not mix.

Surrounding the urethra just below the bladder is the *prostate gland*. It secretes a fluid which increases the ability of the sperm to move in the seminal fluid. Enlargement of the prostate gland may prevent urine from passing through the urethra. This is a fairly common occurrence in older men.

The penis is composed of special tissue that can become filled with blood, making the organ enlarge and become stiffened so that it may enter the *vagina* to deposit seminal fluid. Loose-fitting skin covers the penis (the prepuce or foreskin). The section of foreskin which covers the penis tip (glans) is often removed by a surgical procedure called circumcision shortly after birth.

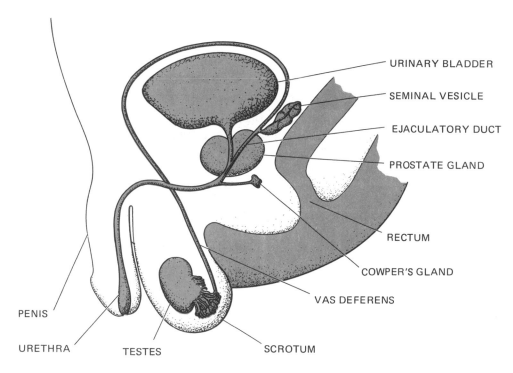

FIGURE 37-1. The male reproductive organs

Prostate Conditions

Tumors of the prostate gland are common. As men grow older, the prostate gland tends to enlarge even without tumor formation. This kind of enlargement is called *benign hypertrophy*. An enlarged prostate, for whatever the reason, puts pressure on the urethra, causing urinary retention.

Various surgical approaches are used to remove all or part of the prostate gland *(prostatectomy)* to relieve the retention. Sometimes only enough of the gland is removed from inside the urethra to permit urine to pass. This operation is called a *transurethral prostatectomy* or (TURP). At other times the entire gland is removed through surgical incisions in the perineum; called a *perineal prostatectomy* or through an incision right over the bladder; known as a *suprapubic prostatectomy*.

A Foley or indwelling catheter is always in place following prostate surgery. In addition, a suprapubic drain through the surgical incision or a perineal drain may be present. Be careful the tubes do not become kinked, stressed or dislodged when positioning the patient.

You must carefully note the amount and color of the drainage from all areas. Any sudden increase in bright redness or the appearance of clots that seem to block the tube must be reported at once. If dressings become wet with urinary drainage, report it to your team leader who will reinforce them. At times it will be necessary to irrigate (wash out) the drainage tubes. This is a sterile procedure that will be carried out by the nurse or the doctor.

Male patients are very apt to be disturbed by the necessity of prostate surgery. You must be patient, calm, and understanding of their fears and of their frustrations. Men often fear that they will not be able to have sexual intercourse after a prostatectomy. Be sure to refer these questions to your team leader so that he or she may provide the patient with accurate information.

THE FEMALE REPRODUCTIVE ORGANS: STRUCTURE AND FUNCTION

The female internal organs include the *ovaries*, fallopian tubes *(oviducts)*, *uterus*, and *vagina*, Figure 37-2. The external genitals include the *vulva*,

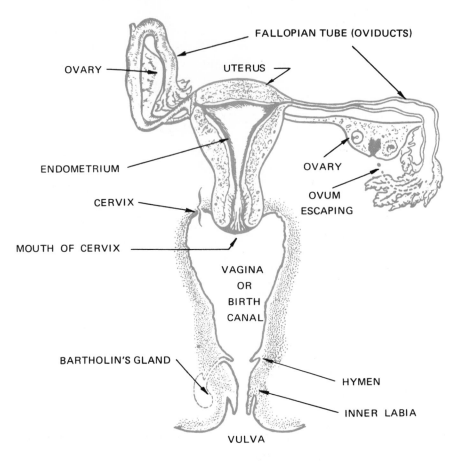

FIGURE 37-2.   The internal female reproductive organs

which is made up of two liplike structures, the *labia majora* and *labia minora*. When the labia are separated, other external structures may be seen: the clitoris, the urinary meatus and the vaginal opening, Figure 37-3.

Ovaries and Oviducts

The ovaries are two small glands, found on either side of the uterus, at the ends of the oviducts in the pelvis. They produce two female hor-

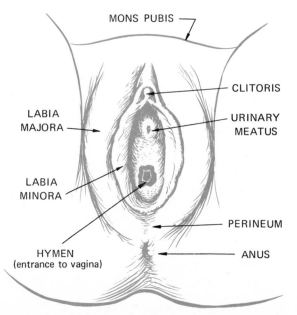

FIGURE 37-3.   The external female reproductive organs

mones—estrogen and progesterone—and the living ova. The ova are contained in many little sacs called follicles. About once each month a follicle matures and releases an ovum which makes its way into one of the 4-inch oviducts. This process is called *ovulation*. The cells of the follicles that are left produce progesterone which causes changes within the uterus, readying it for the possibility of receiving a fertilized ovum.

Uterus

The uterus is a hollow, pear-shaped organ. Its walls are made up of involuntary muscles and it is lined with special tissue called endometrium. The uterus has three main parts: the *fundus*, the body, and the cervix. The body and the fundus can stretch enough to hold a baby, the placental sac, and the afterbirth. The cervix extends into the vagina and, during labor, it opens up to allow the baby to be delivered.

Vagina

The vagina is found between the urinary bladder and rectum. Its muscular walls are capable of much stretching, and it is lined with mucous membrane. Two glands known as Bartholin's glands are found on either side of the external vaginal opening.

Menstruation and Ovulation

Menstruation is the loss of an unneeded part of the endometrium. It occurs for approximately 3 to 5 days each month.

At the end of each menstrual period, an ovum begins to mature in a follicle in one of the ovaries. As the follicle and its ovum grow, it produces the hormone estrogen, which causes the endometrium to develop new blood vessels and tissues. Ovulation takes place about 12 to 14 days after the first day of the last menstrual period. When ovulation occurs, the follicle secretes progesterone, a hormone which causes the endometrium to become somewhat soft and sticky in preparation for pregnancy.

Sperm are capable of moving by means of a flagellum so that they can travel from the vagina, through the uterus, to the oviduct. If the ovum unites with a sperm in the oviduct, it begins to divide into many cells and journeys to the uterus where it grows and develops into a baby. If the ovum does not meet a sperm as it passes through the oviduct, it is expelled from the body. It is too small, however, to be seen.

If pregnancy does not occur after ovulation, the production of progesterone is slowed down about 12 days later. Shortly thereafter the unneeded, newly built-up portion of the endometrium is shed as menstrual flow. The processes of ovulation and menstruation are known as the menstrual cycle. It occurs from puberty (sexual maturity) to the menopause (about 50 years of age). Terms used in discussing menstruation include *dysmenorrhea*, painful menstruation; *amenorrhea*, without menstruation; and *menorrhagia*, excessive bleeding.

The Breasts

The breasts are two glands located on the anterior chest wall. They develop at puberty, but they do not produce milk until pregnancy occurs. Ducts from the glandular cells drain into a central duct which opens into the nipple. Surrounding the nipple is tissue that is slightly darker in color called the areola.

SEXUALLY TRANSMITTED DISEASES (STD)

Sexually-transmitted diseases or venereal diseases affect both men and women. Although they can be cured, there is no immunity to repeated infections.

Gonorrhea

Gonorrhea is caused by a microorganism. It causes inflammation of the reproductive system, and usually there is a greenish-yellow discharge. The male experiences the discharge and painful urination usually within 2–5 days after exposure. The female may not experience discomfort until the infection has spread. She may then develop pelvic inflammatory disease (PID). If untreated with antibiotics, sterility, which is the inability to produce children, may result from the formation of scars which close the reproductive tubes of both sexes. It is important that both sex partners be treated since the infection can reoccur. When a pregnant woman has gonorrhea, her baby's eyes may be permanently damaged if they are contaminated by the disease during birth. As a preventative measure, the baby's eyes are treated with silver nitrate drops shortly after birth.

Syphilis

Syphilis also is caused by a microorganism. If untreated, this disease passes through three stages. The first stage after contact is the development of a sore *(chancre)*, within 90 days of contact, which heals without treatment. Since it is not painful, it may go entirely unnoticed. During the second stage the patient may have a rash, sore throat, or other mild symptoms suggestive of a viral infection. Again, the signs and symptoms disappear without treatment. The disease may be spread during either the first or second stage. By this time, the microorganisms have gained entrance into vital organs such as the heart, liver, brain, and spinal cord. Signs of the third stage, in which permanent damage is done to vital organs, may not appear for many years.

An additional danger of syphilis in pregnancy is that the microorganism can attack the growing baby, causing it to die or be seriously deformed.

Herpes

Herpes simplex II (genital herpes) is an infectious disease caused by the herpes simplex virus. It is transmitted primarily through direct sexual contact. The person who has herpes may develop red blister-like sores on the reproductive organs. The sores are associated with a burning sensation and usually heal in about two weeks. The fluid in the blisters is infectious.

People with herpes infection may have only one episode or may have repeated attacks.

There seems to be a greater incidence of cancer of the cervix and miscarriages among female sufferers than among women who do not have this condition. There is the danger of seriously infecting the newborn children when the pregnant mother gives birth.

Although there is treatment which reduces the discomfort, there is no cure at the present time.

COMMON FEMALE CONDITIONS

Rectocele and Cystocele

Rectoceles and *cystoceles* are hernias and usually occur at the same time. The conditions are due to a weakening of the muscles in the walls between the vagina and bladder *(cystocele)* and between the vagina and rectum *(rectocele)*. Cystoceles cause urinary incontinence; rectoceles cause constipation and hemorrhoid development.

A surgical procedure called colporrhaphy tightens the vaginal walls. Following surgery, ice packs, heat lamps, sitz baths, and sterile vaginal douches (irrigations) may be ordered. Patients should be checked carefully after any vaginal surgery for signs of excessive bleeding or foul discharge.

Infections

Vaginitis, or inflammation of the vagina is most often caused by a parasite known as trichomonas or a fungus infection caused by Candida albicans.

Trichomonas infections cause large amounts of white vaginal discharge, called *leukorrhea*. This condition is very difficult to control, but vaginal suppositories, douches, and new medications have made very good progress in that direction.

The vaginal discharge in a fungus infection is watery, and inflammation and itching are intense. Douches are not given for this condition, but special drugs and creams are prescribed to combat the infection.

Tumors

Benign and malignant tumors of the uterus and ovaries are frequent. Malignancies of the cervix are very common. The cure rate is very high if treated in time. A simple test, called the *Pap smear*, is used to detect cancer of the cervix. It is painless and can be performed in the doctor's office during the pelvic examination. It is recommended that a Pap smear be done regularly. The most common sign of tumors of the uterus and ovaries is changes in the menstrual flow such as excessive flow, spotting between periods, and amenorrhea.

To diagnose conditions of the uterus, a surgical procedure, called *dilatation and curettage* (D & C), is performed. A D & C is an operation in which the opening of the cervix is made larger, and the uterus is scraped with a surgical instrument, known as a curette. It may be found to be necessary to remove all of the uterus because of tumors, (total hysterectomy) or only that portion that is diseased. *Oophorectomy* and *salpingectomy* (excision of ovaries and oviducts) may also be necessary. In younger women at least a portion of the ovary is left to continue hormone production whenever possible. If a pan hysterectomy is performed, in which the uterus, ovaries, and oviducts are removed, the patient experiences surgically induced menopause. The more uncomfortable symptoms are usually relieved with hormone injections.

Following a hysterectomy, the patient will have a Foley catheter and may have a nasogastric tube to relieve abdominal distention and nausea. Special attention is given to maintaining good circulation because slowing of the blood supply to the pelvis may result in clot formation. Fluids and foods are gradually introduced after the initial nausea subsides. You should be very careful to observe your patient for low back pain, decreased urine output, and increased bleeding. Check both the abdominal incisional area and the vagina for presence and type of drainage.

Breast Surgery

A *simple mastectomy* means removal of the breast tissue only. A *radical mastectomy* includes the breast tissue, underlying muscles, and the glands in the axillary area. A *lumpectomy* removes the abnormal tissue and only a small amount of the breast tissue. Any form of a mastectomy requires a great deal of psychological adjustment for the patient.

Since a large amount of blood can be lost during a mastectomy, transfusions are likely to be ordered. Pressure dressings must be checked frequently for signs of excess bleeding. The bed linen should also be checked since blood may drain to the back of the dressing. Since the circulation to the arm may be lessened, swelling and numbness should be reported immediately. Walking may be difficult since the patient feels unbalanced. Be ready to offer your fullest physical and emotional support.

You should also know that there are many excellent breast forms now available for the mastectomy patient. There are also support groups to aid in the psychologic adjustment.

Procedure

GIVING A NONSTERILE VAGINAL DOUCHE

1. Wash hands. Obtain disposable douche and bring to bedside with the following equipment:
   - Irrigating standard
   - Bed protector (Chux)
   - Rubber gloves
   - Monel cup with cotton balls and disinfectant
   - Toilet tissue
   - Bedpan and cover
   - Bath blanket
   - Paper bag
2. Identify patient and tell what you plan to do.
3. Pour a small amount of the specified disinfecting solution over the cotton balls in the Monel cup.
4. Close clamp on tubing. Leave protector on sterile tip.
5. Measure water in douche container. Temperature should be about 105 degrees F. Add powder or solution as ordered.
6. Assemble the remaining equipment conveniently at bedside and screen unit.
7. Remove the perineal pad from front to back and discard in paper bag.
8. Give bedpan to patient and ask her to void.
9. Drape patient with bath blanket. Fanfold top bedding to foot of bed.
10. Assist the patient into the dorsal recumbent position.
11. Place bed protector beneath the patient's buttocks.
12. Place bedpan under patient.
13. Wash hands. Put on gloves.
14. Cleanse perineum. Use one cotton ball with disinfectant for each stroke. Cleanse from vulva toward anus. Cleanse labia minora first. Expose labia minora with thumb and forefinger and cleanse. Give special attention to folds. Discard cotton balls in emesis basin.
15. Open clamp to expel air. Remove protector from sterile tip.
16. Allow small amount of solution to flow over inner thigh and then over vulva. Do not touch vulva with nozzle.
17. Allow solution to continue to flow and insert nozzle slowly and gently

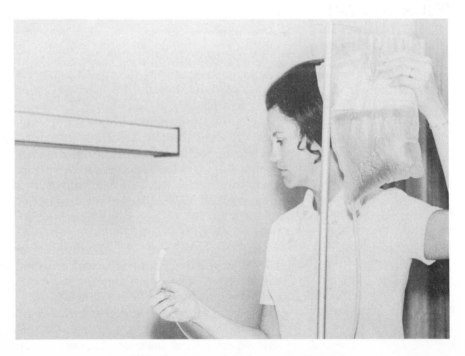

FIGURE 37-4.   Preparing the nonsterile douche

into the vagina with an upward and backward movement for about 3 inches.
18. Rotate nozzle from side to side as solution flows.
19. When all solution has been given, remove nozzle slowly and clamp tubing.
20. Have patient sit up on bedpan to allow all solution to return.
21. Remove douche bag from standard and place on paper towels.
22. Dry perineum with tissue. Discard tissue in bedpan.
23. Cover bedpan and place on chair.
24. Have patient turn on side. Dry buttocks with tissue.
25. Place clean pad over vulva from front to back.
26. Remove bed protector and bath blanket. Replace with top bedding.
27. Make patient comfortable and leave unit in order.
28. Observe contents of bedpan. Note character and amount of discharge if any. Remove gloves.
29. Clean and return equipment according to hospital policy. Wash hands.
30. Chart:
    • Date and time
    • Procedure, vaginal irrigation (type, amount, and temperature of solution)
    • Patient's reaction
    • Your observations regarding douche returns

Perineal Care

Perineal care is a simple procedure that greatly adds to the comfort of many patients. The technique reduces odor and provides an opportunity to closely inspect the patient for abnormalities. Daily attention to the perineum is also given in conjunction with indwelling catheter care.

Procedure
GIVING ROUTINE PERINEAL CARE

1. Wash your hands and assemble the following equipment:
   • Pitchers for warm water (100°) or solution per hospital policy
   • Cotton balls
   • Gloves
   • Bedpan and cover
   • Bed protector
   • Bath blanket
   • Emesis basin lined with paper towels
2. Take equipment to bedside and identify the patient. Explain what you plan to do.
3. Drape the patient with a bath blanket similar to the procedure for vaginal douching.
4. Place bed protector under buttocks.
5. Fill pitcher with warm water or proper solution.
6. Place patient on bedpan. Put gloves on.
7. Position pitcher slightly above the pubis and allow fluid to flow over the vulva into the bedpan.
8. Using cotton balls, wipe area dry. Wipe from top to bottom with each ball and dispose of it in emesis basin. Do not place in bedpan. If a perineal pad is needed, apply at this time.
9. Remove gloves and deposit in emesis basin.
10. Remove bedpan and cover.
11. Remove drape and adjust bedding. Help patient assume a comfortable position.
12. Wrap cotton balls and gloves, if disposable, in paper towels and discard.

13. Empty bedpan—note any discharge. Wash hands.
14. Record time, procedure, including type of solution and any unusual observations.

Summary

A knowledge of the normal male and female reproductive structures is important for the health care assistant who wishes to understand the related nursing care. Disposable equipment available in many hospitals makes nursing care most convenient and safer for the patient. Any surgery to either a man or woman's reproductive organs will have a strong psychological effect on the patient. The health care assistant must remain calm, patient, and understanding.

SUGGESTED ACTIVITIES

1. Examine a wall chart or torso and locate the male and the female reproductive organs.

2. Under supervision, give care to selected patients with conditions of the reproductive organs.

3. Under direct supervision, prepare and give a nonsterile vaginal douche.

4. Under direct supervision give perineal care.

VOCABULARY

Learn the meaning and correct spelling of the following words.

amenorrhea	labia minora	prostate gland
cervix	leukorrhea	rectocele
circumcision	mastectomy	scrotum
cystocele	menorrhagia	sexually transmitted disease (STD)
D & C	menstruation	sterility
dysmenorrhea	ovaries	syphilis
endometrium	oviducts	testes
fundus	ovulation	uterus
gonorrhea	Pap smear	vagina
herpes	penis	vaginitis
hysterectomy	perineum	venereal disease (VD)
labia majora	prostatectomy	vulva

UNIT REVIEW

A. Clinical Situations. Briefly describe how a health care assistant should react to the following situations.

1. A patient expresses concern about being able to perform sexually after a prostatectomy.

2. A patient is to have a lumpectomy and wants to know if the entire breast will be removed.

3. The temperature of the douche solution is 110 degrees.

4. You are to remove a perineal pad.

5. You are asked how to insert the irrigating nozzle during a douche.

B. **Completion.** Complete the following sentences.
1. The testes and ovaries have two functions: _____ and _____.
2. There is need for great _____ adjustment when there is surgery performed on the reproductive organs.
3. During menstruation _____ tissue called _____ is shed.
4. Menstruation usually occurs about once each _____ for _____ days.
5. Venereal diseases are transmitted by sexual intercourse. Two of these sexually transmitted diseases are _____ and _____.
6. Following any pelvic surgery such as a hysterectomy or prostatectomy, you should check carefully for _____.
7. A simple test to detect cancer of the cervix is the _____.
8. Mastectomy is the removal of _____.
9. Hypertrophy of the prostate gland results in urinary _____.
10. When inserting a vaginal douche tip, the fluid should be _____.
11. Perineal care is included as part of daily _____ catheter care.
12. Used cotton balls should not be discarded in the _____.

Section Ten
Self-evaluation

A. Match Column I with Column II.

Column I	Column II
___ 1. Break in a bone	a. flexion
___ 2. Ovaries and testes	b. abduction
___ 3. Simple sugar	c. pallor
___ 4. Bringing the arm toward the midline	d. adduction
___ 5. Chemical messengers	e. crusts
___ 6. Scabs	f. fracture
___ 7. Color less than normal	g. hormones
___ 8. Cerebrovascular accident	h. stroke
___ 9. Carry blood toward the heart	i. gonads
	j. veins
	k. glucose
	l. cyanosis

B. Choose the phrase which best completes each of the following sentences by encircling the proper letter.

10. Patients in pelvic traction require special care. Remember to
    a. allow weights to rest on the floor.
    b. allow the patient's feet to rest on the foot of the bed.
    c. adjust the belt and straps smoothly and snugly.
    d. All of the above.

11. The best position for the patient with respiratory problems is.
    a. lithotomy.
    b. high Fowler's.
    c. prone.
    d. Sims'.

12. You may be asked to weigh the cardiac patient daily because
    a. decreased appetite may cause weight loss.
    b. increased appetite may cause weight gain.
    c. fluid tends to collect in the tissues, increasing weight.
    d. urine output is increased causing weight loss.

13. Remember in caring for patients with arteriosclerosis that
    a. hot water bottles may cause serious burns.
    b. injuries heal well.
    c. circulation is very adequate.
    d. a cool room is most comfortable.

14. The patient who has suffered a CVA usually
    a. is paralyzed.
    b. speaks clearly.
    c. is able to assist in his care.
    d. has a short convalescence.

15. Fractures of children's bones are frequently incomplete. These fractures are called
    a. compound.
    b. simple.
    c. comminuted.
    d. greenstick.

16. A patient with skin lesions must
    a. be washed off with soap and water.
    b. have crusts removed daily.
    c. have frequent back rubs with alcohol.
    d. be handled gently.

17. A bed patient may develop pressure areas if
    a. his position is not changed at least every 2 hours.
    b. his bed is kept dry and clean.
    c. he is bathed frequently.

    d. pressure areas are frequently massaged.

18. When assigned to give an emollient bath, remember
    a. to gently sponge areas not submerged in water.
    b. to have temperature of water 110 degrees F.
    c. to allow the patient to soak only 5 minutes.
    d. to help the patient remain active after the bath.

19. The patient with emphysema has respiratory problems because
    a. he cannot inspire completely.   c. he inspires more deeply than usual.
    b. he cannot expire completely.   d. he expires more deeply than usual.

20. In caring for patients receiving oxygen, remember
    a. no smoking in the area is permitted.
    b. electric call bells may be used.
    c. woolen blankets are used for warmth.
    d. electrical equipment such as suction may be used without discontinuing the oxygen.

21. Following a thyroidectomy, check your patient carefully for
    a. signs of respiratory distress.   c. bleeding.
    b. inability to speak.   d. All of the above.

22. During a convulsion, remember to
    a. force the mouth open and insert a mouth gag.
    b. restrain the patient.
    c. move objects away that the patient may hit.
    d. not turn the head to one side.

23. Your patient has anemia. You should carry out which of the following nursing procedures?
    a. Oxygen by cannula   c. Vital signs
    b. Special mouth care   d. Urine measurement

24. You are assigned to care for a convalescing patient who has suffered a stroke. You will pay particular attention to
    a. skin care.   c. evidence of infection.
    b. development of contractures.   d. All of the above.

25. To protect a newborn baby from gonorrhea, which of the following procedures will be carried out?
    a. Medication is placed in the eyes.
    b. The urine is cultured.
    c. Isolation technique is used for the first twenty-four hours.
    d. Nursing is encouraged to provide the baby with antibodies.

Unit 38 The Obstetrical and Neonatal Patient

OBJECTIVES

As a result of this unit, you will be able to:

- Define terms related to pregnancy.
- Assist in the care of the normal newborn.
- Assist in the care of the normal postpartum patient.

Normally, when a baby, *fetus*, is ready to be born, it is upside down in the mother's uterus with it's head toward the birth canal, Figure 38-1. It is surrounded by a membraneous bag known as an *amniotic sac* or *membrane* and floating in a liquid called *amniotic fluid*.

Nourishment for the fetus is derived from the mother through the *umbilical cord* which is attached to the baby and the *placenta*. The placenta is attached to the wall of the mother's uterus.

After the baby is born and separated from the umbilical cord, the placenta, membranes and remaining cord will be expelled as the *afterbirth*. After a period of time, the mother's *uterus*: or womb, which had greatly stretched to accommodate the pregnancy, will return to its normal size and shape.

PRENATAL CARE

The care of the mother begins in the *prenatal* period when she first learns she is pregnant, Figure 38-2. During this period, she is regularly weighed, her blood pressure is checked and a urine sample is collected. Nursing assistants sometimes help with these procedures. A nurse or physician counsels the patient about any problems that might be occurring.

Anything unusual such as elevated blood pressure, vaginal bleeding or discharge, complaints of dizziness, or swelling of hands and feet should be called to the attention of the professional health worker.

LABOR AND DELIVERY

When the mother reaches her *due date* and begins labor, she will experience contractions of her uterus which prepares the birth canal for passage of the baby. The contractions are irregular at first but become more

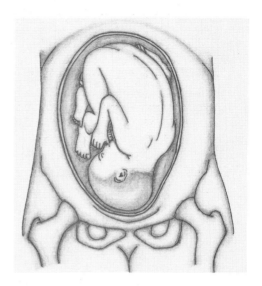

FIGURE 38-1.   The usual position of the fetus at term

Presumptive Signs
   cessation of menses (amenorrhea)
   breast enlargement
   darkening of areola
   fatigue
   morning sickness
   linea nigra (line of pigmentation along midline of abdomen)
Positive Signs
   Hearing the fetal heart beat
   Feeling fetal movement
   Visualization by X-ray or ultrasound

FIGURE 38-2.   Some signs of pregnancy

regular and closer together as labor progresses.

Sometimes the amniotic sac ruptures early in labor and there is a rush of fluid from the vagina. If this doesn't happen the doctor may rupture the membranes once the patient is in the hospital.

In many hospitals, *fetal monitors*, Figure 38-3, which are instruments to check the well-being of the baby during the labor, are attached to the baby's head.

As the labor progresses, the cervix opens up, *dilates*, and thins out, *effaces*, so that the baby may move downward into the birth canal and out of the mother's body. The degree of *dilatation* at any given time is determined by the nurse or doctor who places a gloved finger in the patient's rectum and indirectly measures the cervical opening, called a rectal examination.

The actual delivery usually takes place after the patient is moved to a special delivery room where sterile precautions can be carried out to protect both mother and baby.

In the delivery room, the mother may be given an anesthetic to decrease the discomfort of the delivery. The type of medicine the mother receives during this time will influence the type of *postpartum*, or after delivery care the mother must receive.

It may be necessary to enlarge the vaginal opening at this time by making a cut in the perineum called an *episiotomy*, which is *sutured* together after delivery.

There is a trend to try to encourage the mother and father to participate fully in the birth of their baby, Figure 38-4. Special training, which

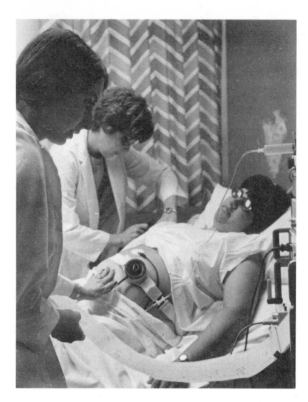

FIGURE 38-3.   A fetal monitor helps measure the condition of the baby as the labor progresses.

begins in the prenatal period, prepares the parents to participate in "natural childbirth" necessitating minimal, if any, pain-controlling medication. One of the most popular of these methods is called the Lamaze method. Further advances have combined the Lamaze method with a refinement developed by Frederick Leboyer.

The Leboyer method of natural childbirth is based on the principle of "birth without violence." With this technique all unnecessary stimuli are limited. Lighting is lowered consistent with safety. No noise or very soft music only is allowed in the delivery area. The cord is not cut or tied until the pulsations cease and the baby is then placed on the mother's abdomen for approximately 3–6 minutes. The mother traces the outline of the baby's eyes with her own while gently stroking its back.

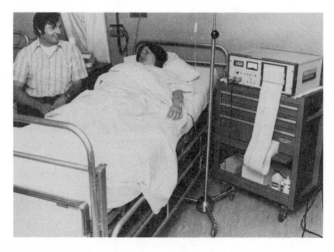

FIGURE 38-4.   The father offers support and frequently acts as coach during labor and delivery.

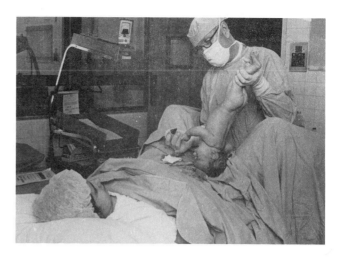

FIGURE 38-5.   Immediately following delivery, the baby is held head down to clear the respiratory tract.

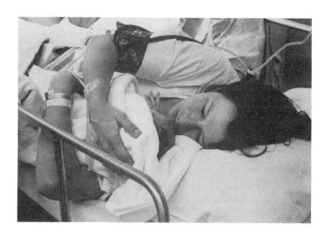

FIGURE 38-6.   The baby is placed in the mother's arms to establish bonding.

Shortly thereafter the baby is placed, with its head carefully supported, in a tub of warm water for another 3–6 minutes. Then the baby is carefully dried and wrapped and returned to the mother for an extended period.

This technique is believed to encourage parental interaction with the baby and birthing process and to encourage bonding between parents and child.

Immediately following the delivery, after the baby's respiratory tract has been cleared, Figure 38-5, the mother is encouraged to hold her newborn, now called a *neonate,* to establish emotional bonding, Figure 38-6. Both mother and child are identified with name tags before being separated. The baby may also be footprinted and have the eyes treated right in the delivery room, Figure 38-7. After several procedures have been completed, Figure 38-8A and B, the baby is then usually taken to the newborn nursery and the mother to her room. In some hospitals, both mother and child are cared for in a single unit. This form of care is called *rooming in.*

POSTPARTUM CARE

You may be assigned to assist with the care of the mother following delivery. This is known as the *postpartum* period.

With other team members, you will assist the mother from the stretcher

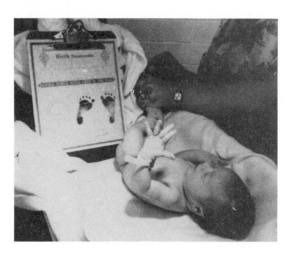

FIGURE 38-7.   Footprinting is done in the delivery room or nursery. Note the name tag on the baby's arm, which matches the mother's identification band.

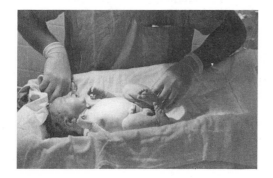

A. The infant is placed head down in a bassinette. Note that the umbilical cord has been clamped and cut.

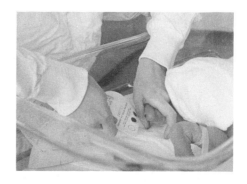

B. The foot is punctured and a drop of blood is checked for a disease called PKU (phenylketonuria).

FIGURE 38-8.

into bed. A protective pad (Chux) may be placed under the patient's buttocks.

Anesthesia

If an anesthetic has been used, follow the procedures for postop care of surgical patients which was covered in Unit 27. Keep the patient flat on her back. In addition, make sure each patient has a fresh gown and the bed linen is kept clean. Check the blood pressure, pulse, and respirations as ordered until stable, Figure 38-9, and then usually every four hours for twenty-four hours. Patients may complain of chilling—an extra blanket may provide comfort.

Drainage

Carefully check the condition of the perineum and the perineal pad for the amount and color of drainage. When removing the pad, always lift it away from the body from front to back. Red vaginal discharge, called *lochia*, is expected but the amount and any clotting should be reported.

The Uterus

The size and firmness of the uterus should be checked and reported. A soft and enlarging uterus indicates excessive bleeding. Massaging the *fundus* stimulates the uterine muscles to contract, firming up the uterus.

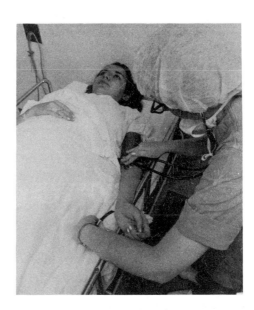

FIGURE 38-9.   Check blood pressure, pulse, and respirations until stable.

The top of the uterus, the fundus, is massaged in a circular fashion while the opposite hand is held against the pubic bone. Be sure that your hospital policy allows assistants to perform this procedure and that you are completely skilled before attempting to do it.

The level of the fundus is measured by placing the fingers lengthwise across the abdomen between the fundus and umbilicus. On the first post-partal day, the level of the fundus is at the umbilicus or may be one to two fingers below.

As the uterus begins to return to its normal size, *involution*, the patient may experience strong uterine contractions or cramps. Cramping may also be associated with breast feeding. This is normal but be sure to report any complaints of pain to your team leader, who can administer medication for relief.

Check carefully for signs of urine retention. The uterus may be unusually high, a swelling may be noted just above the pubis, or the patient may complain of *urgency*, which is the need to void but will only be able to void 200 ml of urine or less. Report signs of possible urine retention immediately to the nurse so the patient's recovery will not be impeded. Also report any inability to void within the first 8 hours postpartum.

Ambulation

After the initial recovery, many of the patients are usually up and about and care is self-directed, Figure 38-10. Unless otherwise indicated, the mother is allowed to be up and will be able to care for most of her personal needs. Remember to check on the new mother periodically, especially when showering, as she may become faint.

TOILETING AND PERINEAL CARE

The nurse will instruct the patient as to how to care for herself after toileting but you should also be aware of the proper procedure.

In some hospitals, the mother is provided with a squeeze-type bottle which is filled with tap water. She is instructed to rinse the genitals and perineum after voiding or defecating. She is then instructed to gently *touch*, not wipe, the perineal area containing the stitches with tissue or special medicated pads, once only from front to back and then dropping the tissue in the toilet.

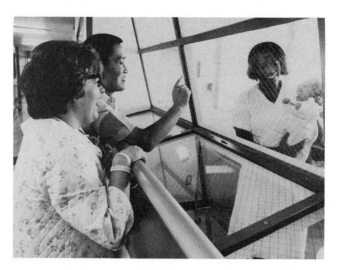

FIGURE 38-10. The mother is often up and about early and a visit to the nursery is a pleasant diversion.

If the perineum is very uncomfortable, specially medicated pads may be used for cleansing but the procedure is always the same—front to back and discard. Relief is also afforded by use of a sitz bath (see Unit 25), anesthetic sprays, and sometimes the use of a *peri light* to encourage drying and healing.

Procedure

USING A PERI LIGHT

CAUTION: Care must be taken so that the patient is protected from burns.
1. Check with your team leader for the length of time the light is to be applied.
2. Wash your hands and assemble the following equipment:
    * Perineal heat light
    * Bath blanket
    * Tape measure
3. Identify the patient and explain what you plan to do.
4. Draw curtains to assure privacy.
5. Place the patient in the lithotomy or dorsal recumbent position and drape in an appropriate manner.
6. Remove perineal pad from front to back—fold soiled side in. Wrap in a paper towel and dispose in proper container. Do not place in toilet. Wash hands.
7. Place the light approximately 18 inches from the perineum. Be careful— a closer placement could result in burns. Use the tape measure to be sure of accuracy.
8. Turn light on so it focuses on the perineum.
9. Leave light on for the prescribed time period (usually 5–10 minutes). Check patient frequently. Discontinue procedure if patient becomes uncomfortable.
10. At the end of the prescribed period, shut light off. Apply a clean perineal pad. Be careful fingers do not touch the inside of the pad. Wash your hands.
11. Remove drape and adjust bedding. Make the patient comfortable.
12. Clean the light per hospital policy and return to storage area.
13. Record the procedure including the time the procedure began, its duration and any unusual observations.

BREAST CARE

The first mothers milk is watery and called *colostrum*. It carries protective *antibodies* to the child and has a mild laxative effect. It usually begins to flow about 12 hours after delivery but milk itself, *lactation*, doesn't begin to flow until the second or third postpartum day.

Keeping the breasts clean is especially important when the mother is planning to breast feed. Hands and breasts should be washed just prior to the arrival of the baby for feeding. During the shower, the mother should wash the breasts first using a circular motion from the nipples outward. Sometimes creams are used to help the nipples remain supple. Breast pads absorb milk leakage and should be frequently changed.

If the mother chooses not to breast feed, the breasts should be supported by a well-fitted brassiere. Medication to suppress the milk production is sometimes ordered.

Mothers and healthy newborns, whose delivery is uncomplicated, do not remain in the hospital very long and are able to go home within one or two days.

NEONATAL CARE

The newborn is admitted to the nursery where those procedures not carried out in the delivery room are completed at this time. The doctor or nurse will examine the baby and make an evaluation of the baby's condition, called status, Figure 38-11.

The vital signs of the baby are determined; measurements and weight are taken. The child is then cleaned and dressed according to hospital policy and placed in a crib or isolette. Since a baby's temperature is not yet stabilized, it is important to keep him as warm as possible while these procedures are being carried out.

Sometimes an admission bath using an antiseptic soap or oil is administered, but procedures for bathing newborns varies from hospital to hospital. In some hospitals, the bath is omitted and the cheesy material known as *vernix caseosa* is allowed to remain on the skin.

If the eyes were not treated with silver nitrate drops in the delivery room and the footprints not taken, these procedures will also be taken care of at this time.

Feeding is not usually started for 12 hours after birth. During these hours, the baby is monitored carefully for successful, independent life, Fig-

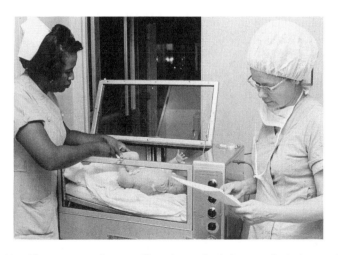

FIGURE 38-11. The nurse or doctor will evaluate the baby on admission to the nursery.

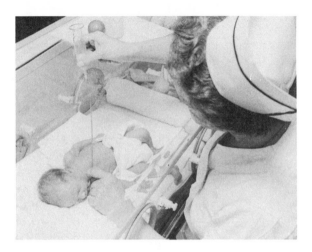

FIGURE 38-12. Babies who are too small or weak to nurse may have to be gavaged.

ure 38-12. After 12 hours, the baby is either taken to breast or started on feedings of glucose and water. Babies whose mothers are unable to feed will be fed in the nursery.

Male babies may be circumcised before discharge. Circumcision removes the excess tissue *(foreskin)* over the tip of the penis.

Procedure

ADMITTING A NEWBORN INFANT

1. Wash your hands and place a paper protector in the scale and open the isolette cover if the baby has been transported in this way.
2. Check identification of infant.
3. Uncover the infant and grasp the ankles, lifting legs and buttocks with one hand while sliding the other under the buttocks to shoulders and neck to support the head, Figure 38-13. Carefully lift the infant out of the isolette or crib and place him gently in the scale tray. Never turn your back or leave the baby for an instant. Keep one hand over the baby at all times. Weigh the baby by adjusting the weights on the balance bar.
4. Return the baby to the isolette or crib, being sure to always support the shoulders, neck and head. Work quickly to prevent undue body heat loss. Newborns have very little temperature control.
5. Measure the baby's head circumference, shoulder width, and length.
6. Take the infant's temperature; usually axillary or rectal, and respira-

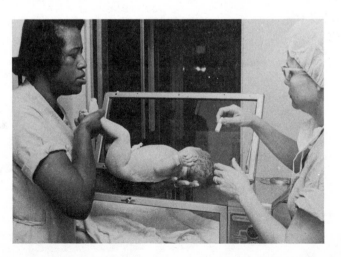

FIGURE 38-13. While grasping the legs securely, the other hand is slipped under the back to support the head and neck. Note the vernix caseosa on the infant's back.

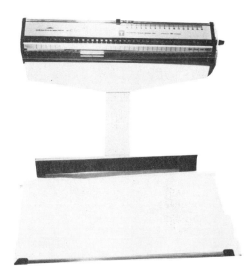

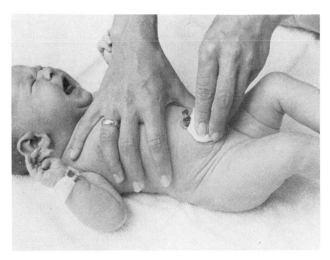

A. The infant scale

B. Carefully clean around the cord with solution prescribed by the hospital.

FIGURE 38-14.

tions per hospital policy. The apical pulse and blood pressure are determined also.

7. Examine the child carefully for any obvious abnormalities such as extra fingers or toes. Note first black-green stool, called *meconium*, urine, condition of cord, cord clamp and the infant's color.

8. The nurse may take the footprints and treat the eyes to prevent infection at this time.

9. If the bath is given, do so at this time. Dress the baby in a diaper and shirt according to hospital policy.

10. Wrap in a lightweight blanket, placing the child with his head lower than his body in the bassinet so that excess mucus can drain freely.

11. Make out the bassinet identification card. Check it carefully with the baby's identification anklet or bracelet.

12. Record the information according to hospital policy.

Procedure
TAKING THE INFANT FOR FEEDING

1. Wash hands and check the identification band and bassinet card.

2. Be sure baby is dry and wrapped for delivery. If diaper is wet or soiled, be sure to wash and dry hands thoroughly after changing.

3. Check the order for breast, glucose and water, or formula.

4. Pick up baby. Get the bottle if needed. Cradle infant in your arms (see Figure 38-15 for proper way to carry infant). In some hospitals, the entire bassinet is used for transportation. If infant is carried, always back through doorways as an added safety precaution.

5. Identify mother and match baby identification with that of mother.

6. Ask mother to position herself on her side for breast feeding and in a comfortable position for bottle feeding (put up side rail if mother is on her side with head of bed elevated).

7. Position baby safely with mother.

8. Baby is returned to the nursery following feeding.

9. Change the diaper and shirt if soiled. Position on right side with head of the bed elevated. Be sure to wash hands before and after handling each baby and after each diaper change.

10. Record type and amount of feeding, defecation and voiding. If breast fed, babies are sometimes weighed before and after feeding period.

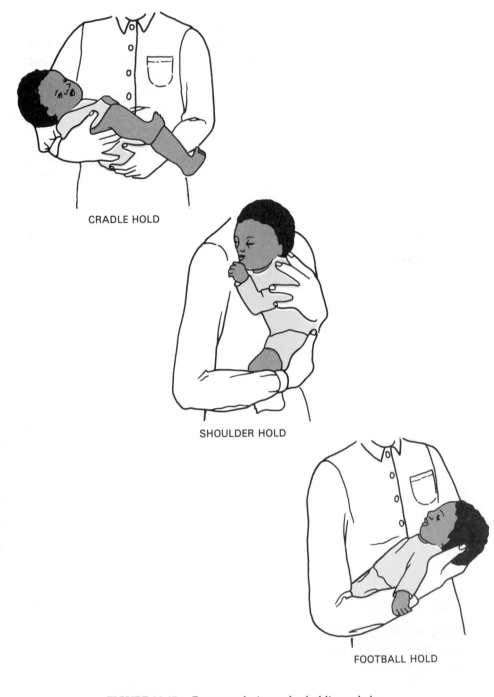

CRADLE HOLD

SHOULDER HOLD

FOOTBALL HOLD

FIGURE 38-15. Proper techniques for holding a baby

Procedure

FEEDING THE INFANT IN THE NURSERY

1. Wash hands, check identification band and bassinet card.
2. Check order for type of feeding.
3. Check for wetness or soiled diaper. Be sure to wash and dry hands before proceeding with feeding.
4. Pick up baby and proper feeding and position yourself comfortably in a chair.
5. Cradle baby in your arms and insert nipple in baby's mouth. A few babies need encouragement to start sucking. Gently stroke the cheek or rotate the nipple in the infant's mouth.

6. After 1/2 to 1 oz has been taken, remove bottle and place in a safe, clean place.
7. Place a protective pad over your shoulder and position baby with its head on the pad. Gently rub the back. This helps gas trapped in the stomach to be expelled. Be sure to support head and neck with opposite hand.
8. After burping, resume feeding. Repeat burping procedure every 1/2 to 1 oz.
9. Change diaper and shirt if necessary. Be sure to wash and dry hands.
10. Position baby on right side with head of crib elevated.
11. Record type and amount of feeding, defecation, and voiding.

Procedure

FOOTPRINTING THE INFANT

1. Wash hands and check identification band, bassinet card, and print card.
2. Expose baby's feet.
3. Apply ink with roller or pad to one foot at a time.
4. Firmly but gently press prepared foot against print card.
5. Clean ink from foot.
6. Repeat procedure with opposite foot.
7. Dress or cover baby.
8. Wash hands and recheck name on print card with baby's identification.

Post Circumcision Care

The circumcision should be checked each time the diaper is changed and should be a routine part of that care. Observe the incision site for bleeding and report anything unusual. The crib identification should note the new circumcision. A note should be included as to the condition of the circumcision on the nursery record and a record of first voiding after circumcision.

Eye Care

This procedure is usually performed by the nurse but if you are assigned this responsibility, consider your hospital policy, then carry it out in the following manner.

Procedure

GIVING EYE CARE TO THE NEWBORN INFANT

1. Wash hands and assemble the necessary equipment.
   • Small, wax container of silver nitrate 1%
   • A sterile needle to pierce the container
   • Sterile distilled water
   • Cotton balls
2. Check identification band and bassinet card.
3. Turn baby's head to the right, shading the eyes, and gently separate the eye lids with thumb and forefinger of one hand by drawing the lower lid down. This is sometimes difficult because babies tend to squeeze their lids together especially when crying. Put no pressure on the eyeball.
4. Pick up the wax vial and puncture with sterile needle.
5. Insert two drops in the conjunctival sac of the right eye—wait two minutes.
6. Flush with sterile water—wipe with cotton ball from nose to outer canthus and discard.
7. Turn infant's head to opposite side and repeat procedure.
8. Dispose of used materials properly according to hospital policy.
9. Wash hands and record procedure.

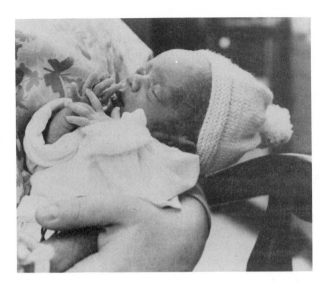

FIGURE 38-16.   Dressed in his own clothes, the baby is ready for discharge.

DISCHARGE

The discharge procedure begins as the baby's identification is matched with the mother's and he is dressed in his own clothing, Figure 38-16. This may be done in the nursery or in the mother's room. Be sure the mother has received and understands any special discharge instructions and equipment or needed formula is ready.

Carrying her baby, the mother is transported by wheelchair to the discharge area. After discharge, notations are made on the discharge record of both mother and child which include condition of each and time of release.

Summary

Care of the obstetrical patient is a very specialized area of medicine. It includes the care given to both mother and child and begins long before the birth of the baby.

The health of the mother is supervised throughout the prenatal period and through the labor and delivery and postpartum periods to discharge. The health care assistant participates in this care under the close direction of the professional staff.

Care of the newborn is also very special and you may function in this area as well. A thorough understanding of your responsibilities and close attention to the details of care helps ensure a successful and safe pregnancy.

Remember, all the procedures presented in this unit require advanced training and supervision before you attempt to perform them. In addition, you may do so only under proper authorization.

VOCABULARY

Learn the meaning and correct spelling of the following words.

amniotic sac	episiotomy	lochia	postpartum
antibodies	fetus	meconium	prenatal
circumcision	foreskin	membranes	rooming in
colostrum	fundus	monitors	umbilical cord
dilatation	Isolette	neonate	urgency
due date	labor	Peri light	vernix caseosa
efface	lactation	placenta	

**SUGGESTED
ACTIVITIES**

1. If possible, observe the care given to the pregnant woman during labor and delivery at your hospital.

2. Write a short statement which summarizes your experiences.

3. Practice, under supervision, the admission of the baby to the normal newborn nursery. Carry out as many procedures as your hospital policy allows.

4. Provide care, under supervision, for the postpartum care of the mother.

5. Demonstrate the proper way to lift and support the newborn.

UNIT REVIEW

A. Brief Answer. Briefly answer the following questions.
   1. Name three functions or characteristics of colostrum.
      a.
      b.
      c.
   2. Four routine observations regarding the newborn that should be made and noted are:
      a.
      b.
      c.
      d.
   3. Four presumptive signs of pregnancy include:
      a.
      b.
      c.
      d.
   4. List the procedures you would carry out when admitting a newborn to the nursery.

B. Clinical Situations. Briefly describe how a health care assistant should react to the following situations.
   1. The young pregnant woman asks what to expect when she visits the prenatal clinic each month.

   2. The young mother is told the form of care in this hospital is "rooming-in" and asks what this means.

   3. The patient has just delivered and returned to her bed. She has had a spinal anesthesia. Your responsibilities include:

C. Completion. Complete the following sentences.
   1. The placenta is known as the _____.
   2. The pregnant woman regularly has her blood pressure, urine, and _____ checked during her prenatal visits.
   3. During the delivery, the perineum may be cut and then sutured together. This procedure is called an _____.

4. The newborn baby is called a _____.
5. When changing or removing the perineal pad, it should always be lifted from the body and removed from _____ to _____.
6. During a perineal heat light treatment, the light should be _____ inches from the perineum.
7. The chemical used in the baby's eyes to prevent gonococcal infection is called _____ _____.
8. The first feeding for the newborn is _____ and water.
9. Circumcision is a surgical procedure which removes _____.
10. After feeding, babies are usually placed on the _____ side with the head of the crib _____.

Unit 39 Special Advanced Procedures

OBJECTIVES

As a result of this unit—and with advanced training—you will be able to:

• Open and handle sterile equipment.
• Perform advanced urine and stool tests.
• Give routine stoma and ileostomy care.

INTRODUCTION

The use of nursing care assistants varies throughout the nation. Basic preparation, experience, specific advanced training in procedural skills, and facility policy all influence the type and scope of assignments that are made to ancillary workers.

Some procedures considered routine for some workers would not be appropriate or permitted in other situations. Even basic procedures such as bed bathing might be restricted to professionals if the situation or patient conditions warrant such precautions.

Under no circumstances must it be assumed that because the following procedures are included in this text that they should be assigned to all health care workers.

Each facility should establish policies and surpervisory practices that are consistent with legal regulations and that ensure competency on the part of the caregiver and safety for the patient.

These procedures are to be carried out only after adequate practice and supervision and only in accord with specific hospital policy. Additional information supporting these advanced procedures may be found in the units indicated.

STERILE TECHNIQUES

Sterile technique is an exacting procedure. *There can be no mistakes.* For this reason, usually only very specially trained people like you are given this responsibility. There will be times that you might be called upon the assist someone as they perform these duties or to perform them yourself. Therefore, you will need to develop an awareness of correct technique and be ready to assist without fear of contamination.

The term *sterile field* refers to an area of sterile equipment and materials. This may be a table covered with a sterilized sheet or a sterile towel placed on an over-bed table. Only the center of the towel is actually used and equipment is kept two inches in from the edges all around as an added precaution.

Never reach or pass anything that is unsterile over a sterile field. Go around or hold the article away from the side. You might drop the unsterile article onto the field or touch the field. In either case, the field would be contaminated and the entire set-up would have to be discarded.

Opening a Sterile Package

Sterile equipment such as gloves, dressings, instruments, swabs and throat sticks are double wrapped in cloth or paper and sealed. Most will have a seal which changes color to indicate that the sterilizing process has been completed. Commercially-prepared products will be sealed. If the color code has not changed or a seal does not look intact, do not consider it sterile. If you have any question, do not take a chance. Touch only the outside of the package. Remember, only sterile surfaces may contact sterile surfaces.

Transfer forceps, which are instruments used to pick up sterile equipment, are sometimes soaked in a disinfectant solution and are used almost like sterile fingers. Your hand touches only the non-sterile handle; the soaked, disinfected tips are used to arrange sterile equipment and supplies.

Sometimes, transfer forceps are double wrapped, and must be opened like any sterile package. Once the package is safely opened, it forms a sterile field. The forceps are lifted by the handle, being careful not to touch the tips to anything not sterile.

Procedure
OPENING A STERILE PACKAGE

Note: Background information is given in Unit 10.
A. *Wrapped in paper*
  1. Wash hands.
  2. Check seal to be sure it is intact.
  3. With two hands, grasp each side of separated end and gently pull apart, Figure 39-1.

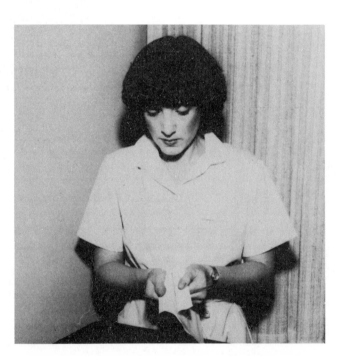

FIGURE 39-1.   Note that the fingers never touch the inner contents of the package as it is opened.

  4. If the article is to be taken by the nurse or doctor, open only enough to expose the end sufficiently to be withdrawn without contamination.
  5. Do not open until the nurse or doctor is ready to use the article.
B. *Double wrapped in cloth*
  1. Wash hands.

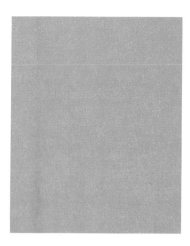

2. Check tape seal to be sure color change indicating sterility has taken place, Figure 39-2A.
3. Place package fold side up on a flat surface.
4. Remove tape.
5. Unfold flap farthest away from you by grasping outer surface only between thumb and forefinger, Figure 39-2B.
6. Open left flap with left hand using same technique, Figure 39-2C.
7. Open right flap with right hand using same technique, Figure 39-2D.
8. Open final flap (nearest to you). Touch only the outside of flap. Be careful not to stand too close. Do not allow uniform to touch flap as it is lifted free, Figure 39-2E. Be sure the flaps are pulled open completely to prevent them from folding back up over the sterile field.

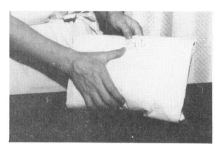

A.

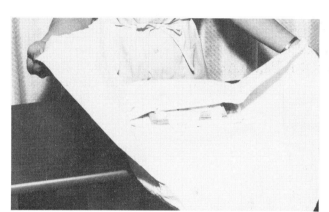

D.

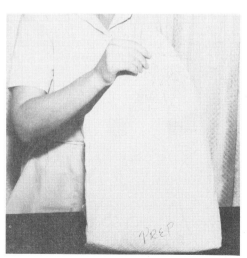

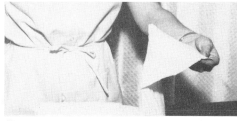

B.

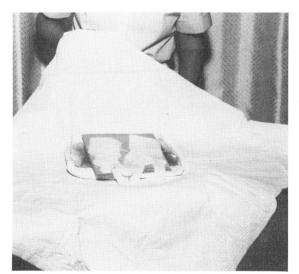

C.

E.

FIGURE 39-2. Technique for opening a sterile package.

Procedure

TRANSFERRING FORCEPS IN SOLUTION

Note: Background information is given in Unit 10.

1. Wash hands.
2. Grasp handle of forceps.
3. Gently raise forceps out of solution. Do not allow forceps to touch sides of container, Figure 39-3A. Area above level of solution must be considered contaminated. If the forceps touch the sides or top of container do not use them.
4. When free of container, hold forceps out parallel to the table so that the solution will drip straight down and not run toward handle, which is contaminated, and then back down to tip, Figure 39-3B. Do not allow solution to drip onto sterile field, or it will be contaminated.
5. Gently touch tips together to remove excess fluid.
6. Use only tips to handle sterile materials.
7. After use, return to container by reversing this procedure.

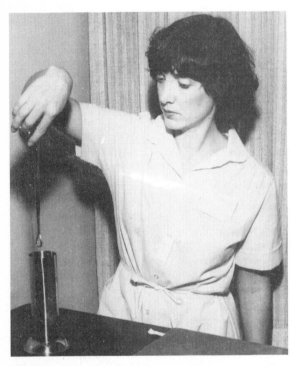

A. Forceps in solution are grasped and held clear of the container.

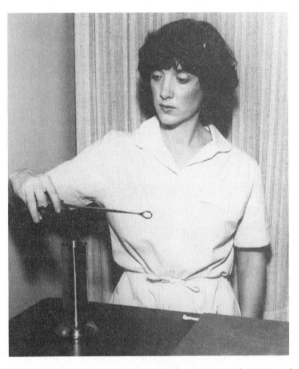

B. When free of the container, hold forceps straight out so that solution will not drip onto forceps handles or back onto the tip of the forceps.

FIGURE 39-3.

Gloving

Gloves are sterilized in double layered packages of cloth or paper. They are arranged so that when opened, the gloves will be on the proper side for gloving. The palms will be up with thumbs pointing to outer edge and the wrist will be cuffed and folded over.

The inside of the glove which comes in contact with the skin, once touched, is considered contaminated. In putting on gloves, the most important principle to remember is that glove surfaces must only touch glove while skin surfaces may only touch skin surfaces.

Procedure

DONNING STERILE GLOVES

Note: Background information is given in Unit 10.

1. Wash hands and dry them thoroughly. Gloves will stick to moist hands making application difficult.
2. Pick up wrapped gloves. Check seal for sterility. Place on clean, flat surface.
3. Open seal and open outer cover touching outside of package only by grasping either side of glove case by pinching outer surface between thumb and forefinger, Figure 39-4A and B.
4. With one hand, remove inner package of gloves and open onto inner surface of outer cover.
5. Lift inner covering—open, exposing gloves and allowing them to remain flat on the inside of inner covering. The gloves will now be flat with palm sides up, Figure 39-4C. The right glove is on the right and left is on the opposite side. If powder packette is included, lift free, without touching gloves. Move away from gloves. Gently sprinkle powder on hands. Rub hands together to spread powder. Drop packette in waste basket.

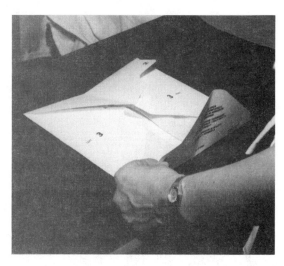

A. Open the outer cover by grasping a corner of the glove case with thumb and forefinger.

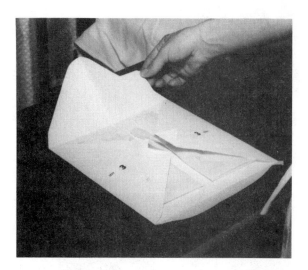

B. Then, grasp the opposite corner with thumb and forefinger.

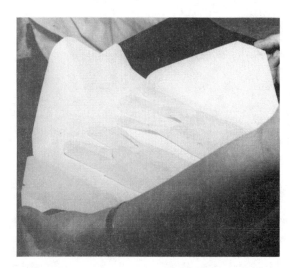

C. Finally, using your thumbs and forefingers again, grasp the sides of the glove case and open them.

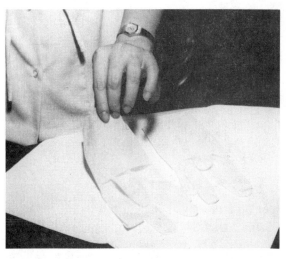

D. Grasp the right glove by the cuff. Do not allow fingers to touch the outside of the glove.

FIGURE 39-4. Procedure for donning sterile gloves

6. With left hand, pick up right glove as shown in Figure 39-4D. Proceed as follows:
   a. Slip thumb of left hand inside edge of right glove at wrist. Grasp glove at edge. Fingers must not extend beyond the cuff or touch outside of glove, Figure 39-4E.
   b. Lift glove free of covering and table and step back. Glove must not touch any unsterile surface.
   c. Curve right hand with thumb toward palm. Insert into glove with a rotating motion. Pull up with left hand.
   d. Once in place, let go with left hand but *do not pull cuff over wrist.*
7. Don left glove as follows:
   a. Holding gloved fingers of right hand together, slide them under cuff of left glove, Figure 39-4F, (your fingers will be pointed toward you). Thumb of right hand may touch only the rim of cuff for control.
   b. Lift glove clear of table and wrapping.
   c. Curve fingers of left hand, bending thumb slightly forward and insert in glove. As hand is inserted, spread fingers to slide into proper areas, Figure 39-4G. Do not let the right gloved thumb touch the left, ungloved hand.
   d. Cuff may be brought slightly down on wrist as long as the gloved hand never touches the inner cuff surface.
8. Adjust cuffs as follows:
   a. Gloved fingers of left hand are slipped into cuff of right glove, adjusting the cuff by pushing downward toward arm, Figure 39-4H.
   b. If gloves only are worn, a small rim of cuff may be left. It is, of course, not to be considered sterile.
9. Adjust fingers with a gentle, rotating motion, working from tips to base of fingers.

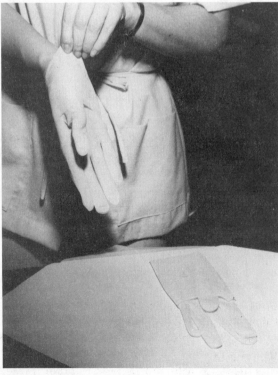

E. Lift the right glove clear of the package. Curve your fingers and insert them into the glove, drawing the glove over your right hand.

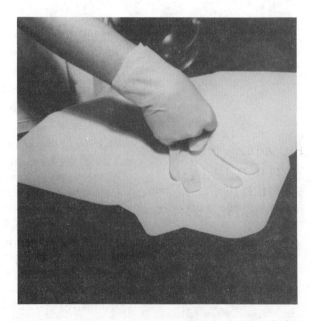

F. Slip gloved fingers under the cuff of the left-hand glove.

FIGURE 39-4. Continued

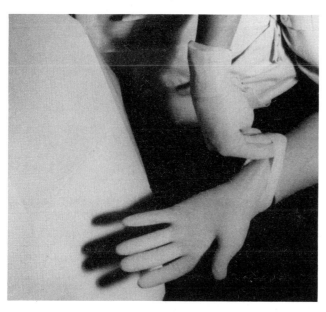

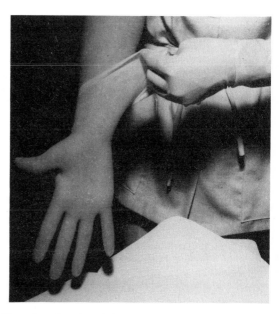

G. Slip your left hand into the glove, being careful not to contaminate it.

H. Note that the gloved fingers touch only the sterile surface of the other glove. Turn the right cuff up with the sterile (left) gloved hand.

FIGURE 39-4. Continued

If gloves are included in a sterile, prepackaged procedure set, proceed as follows:

1. Wash hands.
2. Remove lid, exposing sterile interior.
3. Follow steps 6–9.
4. Sterile supplies within kit may then be handled with sterile, gloved hands.

URINE AND STOOL TESTS

Special tests performed on urine and stool samples that may be part of your responsibility include the following three procedures. Additional information may be found in Unit 24 and Unit 36.

Procedure

TESTING URINE WITH THE HEMACOMBISTIX®

Note: The HemaCombistix® is used to test for the presence of protein, blood, glucose, and for pH (acidity) of urine.
1. Wash hands and assemble the following equipment:
   • Bottle containing HemaCombistix®
   • Fresh sample of urine
2. Take reagent and sample to bathroom.
3. Remove cap and place top side down on table.
4. Shake bottle gently until reagent strips protrude from end.
5. Remove one reagent strip. Do not touch test areas of strip with fingers. Be sure your hands are dry.
6. Dip reagent end of strip in fresh, well-mixed urine—remove immediately or pass through urine stream.
7. Tap edge of strip against container to remove excess urine.
8. Compare reagent side of test areas with corresponding color charts on the bottle at the time intervals specified. See Figure 39-5.

Blood	30 sec.	Lt. blue green	— Deep blue
Glucose	10 sec. qualitative	Lt. blue	— Dark brown
	30 sec. qualitative		
Protein	Immediately	Yellow	— Green
pH	Immediately	Orange	— Blue

FIGURE 39-5. HemaCombistix® results

9. Wash hands.
10. Report and chart:
    • Date and Time
    • Procedure: HemaCombistix® Reactions
    • Findings or reaction: Positive/Negative

Procedure

TESTING FOR OCCULT BLOOD USING HEMOCCULT® AND DEVELOPER

1. Wash hands and assemble the following equipment:
   • Bedpan with fresh specimen
   • Hemoccult® slide packette and
   • Hemoccult® developer
   • Tongue blade
   • Paper towel
2. Place paper towel on flat surface and open flap of Hemoccult® packette, exposing **guairac paper**.
3. Using a tongue blade, take small sample of feces and smear on paper marked A, Figure 39-6.

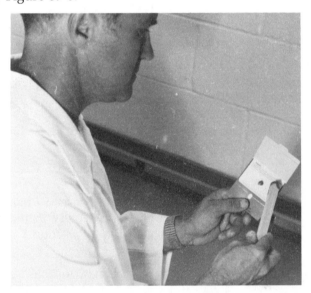

FIGURE 39-6.   A small specimen of stool is placed on a special area of the card for an occult blood test on stool. *(From Simmers,* Diversified Health Occupations, *1983, Delmar Publishers Inc.)*

4. Repeat the procedure, taking fecal sample from a different part of the specimen and making smear in area B.
5. Close tab and turn packette over.
6. Open back tab.
7. Apply two drops of Hemoccult® developer directly over each smear. Time reaction.
8. Read results 30–60 seconds later.
9. Presence of blood is indicated by a blue discoloration around perimeters of smear.

10. Dispose of specimen.
11. Clean bedpan per hospital policy and dispose of paper towel, packette and tongue blade.
12. Wash hands.
13. Report findings to nurse.
14. Chart:
    • Date and Time
    • Procedure: Hemoccult® test
    • Findings: Positive/Negative

Procedure

TESTING FOR OCCULT BLOOD USING HEMATEST® REAGENT TABLETS

1. Place Hematest® filter paper on a glass or porcelain plate. Smear a thin streak of fecal material lightly on the filter paper. Do not use an emulsion or suspension.
2. Place the Hematest® Reagent tablet on smear.
3. Place one drop of distilled water on the Hematest® Reagent tablet and allow 5–10 seconds for the water to penetrate the tablet. Then add a second drop so that the water runs down the side of the tablet onto the specimen and filter paper. Gently tap side of plate once or twice to knock off water droplets from top of tablet. For up to 2 minutes, observe filter paper for color change.
4. Read reaction. A positive reaction is indicated by a blue halo forming on the paper towel around the smear.
5. Dispose of specimen and equipment per hospital policy.
6. Wash hands.
7. Report findings to nurse.
8. Chart:
    • Date and Time
    • Procedure: Hematest®
    • Findings: Positive/Negative

RECTAL SUPPOSITORIES

Suppositories are given to stimulate bowel evacuation or to instill medications. Medicinal suppositories must be inserted by the nurse. You may be asked to insert suppositories that soften the stool and promote elimination.

Procedure

INSERTING A RECTAL SUPPOSITORY

Note: Background information is given in Unit 35.
1. Wash hands and assemble the following equipment:
    • Suppository as ordered
    • Lubricant
    • Toilet tissue
    • Gloves
    • Bedpan and cover if needed
2. Identify patient and explain what you plan to do.
3. Help patient assume the left Sims' position.
4. Expose buttocks only, Figure 39–7.
5. Put on gloves and unwrap suppository.
6. With left hand, separate the buttocks exposing the anus.
7. Apply a small amount of lubricant to anus and insert the suppository. Suppository must be inserted deeply enough to enter the rectum beyond the sphincter (approximately 2 inches).

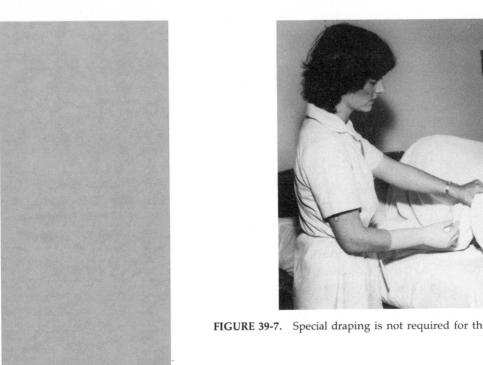

FIGURE 39-7.   Special draping is not required for the insertion of a suppository.

8. Encourage patient to take deep breaths and relax until the need to defecate is experienced, approximately 5–15 minutes.
9. Remove gloves and dispose per hospital policy.
10. Adjust the bedding, helping patient assume a comfortable position.
11. Place call bell near patient's hand but check every 5 minutes.
12. Assist patient to bathroom or position on bedpan.
13. Record time of insertion, type of suppository and results.
14. Wash hands.

CARE OF THE PATIENT WITH A COLOSTOMY

Since the normal sphincter control has been lost because of the surgery, there may be problems of leakage, odor control and irritation of the surrounding area. It is very important to keep the area clean and dry. To collect the drainage, a disposable colostomy bag covers the stoma and is held in place with a belt. Irrigation of the fresh colostomy is done by the nurse. If this procedure is to be permanent, patients are taught to carry out this procedure for themselves. You may be assigned to give routine stoma care. Further detailed information is given in Unit 35.

Procedure

GIVING ROUTINE STOMA CARE (COLOSTOMY)

1. Wash your hands and assemble the following equipment:
   • Wash cloth and towel
   • Basin of warm water
   • Bed protector
   • Bath blanket
   • Disposable colostomy bag and belt
   • Bedpan
   • Disposable gloves
   • Skin lotion as directed
2. Take equipment to bedside.
3. Identify the patient and explain what you plan to do.
4. Replace top bedding with the bath blanket.
5. Place bed protector under the patient's hips.

6. Put on disposable gloves.
7. Remove the soiled disposable stoma bag and place in bedpan—note amount and type of drainage.
8. Remove belt which holds stoma bag and save if clean.
9. Gently clean area around stoma with toilet tissue to remove feces and drainage. Dispose of tissue in bedpan.
10. Wash area around stoma with soap and water. Rinse thoroughly and dry.
11. If ordered, apply skin lotion lightly around the stoma—too much lotion may interfere with proper adhesion of fresh ostomy bag.
12. Position clean belt around patient—inspect area for irritation or breakdown.
13. If necessary, remove and replace adhesive wafer. Place clean ostomy bag over stoma and secure belt.
14. Remove bed protector. Check to be sure bottom bedding is not wet. Change if necessary.
15. Replace bath blanket with top bedding, making patient comfortable.
16. Gather soiled equipment and dispose according to hospital policy.
17. Clean bedpan and basin and return to unit.
18. Wash hands.
19. Chart:
    - Date and time
    - Procedure: ostomy care
    - Lotion, if any, applied
    - Type and amount of drainage
    - Signs of irritation
    - Patient's reaction to the procedure

CARE OF THE PATIENT WITH AN ILEOSTOMY

Care of the patient with a fresh ileostomy is given by the professional nurse. Routine care may be given by health care assistants. It is similar to the routine care that is given to the colostomy patient. Since the ileostomy creates an opening in the ileum, the drainage contains digestive enzymes and is in a liquid form. The drainage is very irritating to the skin so careful care of the skin surrounding the stoma is mandatory. The fit of the ileostomy ring is important so that leakage doesn't occur. This is true for both the disposable and reuseable types of appliances.

Procedure

ROUTINE CARE OF AN ILEOSTOMY (WITH PATIENT IN BED)

1. Wash hands, assemble the following equipment, and take to bedside:
   - Basin of warm water
   - Bed protector
   - Bath blanket
   - Bedpan/cover
   - Disposable gloves
   - Fresh appliance and belt
   - Clamp for appliance
   - Prescribed solvent/dropper
   - Cotton balls
   - Deodorant (if permitted)
   - Soap or cleansing agent
   - Karaya ring
   - 4 × 4 gauze squares
   - Toilet tissue
   - Paper towels
2. Identify patient and explain what you plan to do.
3. Screen unit. Raise opposite siderail for safety. Elevate head of bed and assist patient to turn on side toward you.
4. Replace bedding with bath blanket.
5. Place bed protector under the patient.
6. Put on disposable gloves.
7. Place bedpan on bed protector against patient.

8. Place end of ileostomy bag in bedpan. Open clamp and allow to drain. Note amount and character of drainage.
9. Wipe end of drainage sheath with toilet paper and move out of drainage. Place tissue in bedpan.
10. Disconnect belt from appliance and remove from patient. Place on paper towels.
11. With dropper, apply a small amount of solvent around the ring of the appliance. This will loosen it so it can be removed. Wait a few seconds; do not force the appliance free.
12. Cover stoma with gauze. Carefully inspect skin area around stoma. If the area is irritated or skin broken, cover patient with bath blanket, raise siderail, and lower bed. Wash hands and report to the nurse for instructions.
13. Cleanse the area around the stoma gently with cotton balls. Use soap or other cleansing agent. Pat dry gently.
14. Remove gauze from stoma and place in paper towels.
15. If appliance is used with a Karaya ring, moisten ring and allow it to become sticky and position around stoma (peel paper from stoma opening of bag).
16. Clamp appliance bag, add deodorant, and apply to ring.
17. Adjust a clean belt in position around the patient and connect it to the appliance.
18. Remove covered bedpan and place on chair on paper towels.
19. Remove bed protector and disposable gloves and place on bedpan. Check bottom bedding and make sure it is dry. Change, if necessary.
20. Replace bath blanket with top bedding, making patient comfortable. Leave call bell within easy reach.
21. Lower bed to lowest position. Leave unit tidy.
22. Gather soiled materials and bedpan. Take to utility room. Dispose of according to hospital policy. If belt and bag are reuseable, wash and allow to dry.
23. Empty, wash, and dry bedpan. Return to patient's unit.
24. Wash hands.
25. Record and report:
    - Procedure: Ileostomy care
    - Character and amount of drainage
    - Any observations you have made

Procedure

ROUTINE CARE OF AN ILEOSTOMY (IN BATHROOM)

1. Wash hands, assemble the following equipment and take to the patient's bathroom:
   - Disposable gloves
   - Fresh appliance and belt
   - Bath blanket
   - Clamp for appliance
   - Cotton balls
   - Solvent/dropper
   - Deodorant
   - Soap and cleansing agent
   - Karaya ring
   - 4 × 4 gauze squares
   - Paper towels
2. Identify patient and explain what you plan to do.
3. Screen unit and assist patient into robe and slippers.
4. Assist patient into bathroom. Position on toilet.
5. Place bath blanket over patient's legs. Raise gown and roll at waist exposing appliance. Instruct patient to separate legs.
6. Put on gloves. Open ileostomy appliance, directing drainage into toilet. Note character and amount of drainage.
7. With dropper, apply a small amount of solvent around the Karaya gum ring to loosen from skin. Do not force from skin.

8. Cover stoma with gauze sponge to collect drainage.
9. With cotton balls, cleanse area around stoma with warm water and soap or cleansing agent (if skin area is broken, report to nurse for instructions). Pat area dry.
10. Remove gauze from stoma and place in paper towels.
11. If appliance is used with a Karaya ring, moisten ring, allow to become sticky and apply to stoma (if appliance uses paper-covered adhesive strip around the stoma opening, remove paper and apply around stoma).
12. Clamp appliance bag and apply to ring.
13. Remove gloves, adjust clean belt in position around the patient, and connect it to the appliance.
14. Remove bath blanket, assist patient to wash his hands and return to bed. Make comfortable with signal bell at hand and leave unit tidy.
15. Clean patient's bathroom by handling disposables according to hospital policy. Wash belt and appliance, if reusable, and allow to dry.
16. Wash hands.
17. Record and report:
    • Procedure: Ileostomy care
    • Character and amount of drainage
    • Any observations you have made

Remember, all the procedures presented in this unit require advanced training and close supervision before you attempt to perform them. In addition, you must do so only when properly authorized to do so.

Summary

Material in the unit introduces techniques that may be assigned to the experienced health care assistant who has received advanced training and who has demonstrated skill and proficiency.

These procedures must be carried out under proper supervision and authorization, since any errors might result in a greater likelihood of injury to the patient or inaccuracy of test results.

You should be willing to learn and grow in your chosen field, always bearing in mind your ethical and legal limitations.

SUGGESTED ACTIVITIES

1. Practice carrying out the procedures for occult blood.

2. Practice carrying out sterile procedures such as opening packages, using transfer forceps and donning sterile gloves.

3. Practice inserting a rectal suppository.

4. Practice giving routine stoma care.

5. Practice giving routine ileostomy care.

Note: Practices should be carried out on a mannequin until you become skillful and only with the closest supervision on patients.

VOCABULARY

Learn the meaning and correct spelling of the following words.

colostomy	ostomy	stoma
contamination	sterile field	suppository
ileostomy	sterilization	tongue blade
occult		

UNIT REVIEW **A. Clinical Situations.** Briefly describe how a health care assistant should react to the following situations.

1. You touched the side of the container while removing transfer forceps.

2. You were helping with a dressing and you touched the sterile field.

3. You are setting up a sterile field and touch it as you add sterile equipment.

4. You are giving stoma care to a patient with an ileostomy. What are your primary responsibilities?

B. Completion. Complete the following sentences.

1. The rectal suppository is inserted _____ inches.
2. To make insertion of the rectal suppository easier, the patient should be instructed to _____.
3. A colostomy is an artificial opening in the _____.
4. Transfer forceps are used to _____ sterile equipment.
5. Sterile articles should not be opened until _____.
6. When opening a sterile package, the final flap to be opened is _____ to you.
7. Articles to be sterilized are wrapped in _____ layers of packaging.
8. The HemaCombistix® is a test to detect the presence of protein, blood, and glucose and to check the _____.
9. Drainage of an ileostomy is particularly irritating because it _____ and is in a liquid form.

Unit 40 Response to Basic Emergencies

OBJECTIVES

As a result of this unit, you will be able to:

- Recognize emergency situations.
- Be able to assess the situation and determine the sequence of appropriate action needed.
- Give immediate care to prevent death or additional injury.

INTRODUCTION

Emergency situations can occur at any time to anyone: an automobile accident, a stroke, a patient suddenly feeling weak, then fainting and falling are just a few examples. All are emergency situations that develop rapidly and unpredictably.

If you are the first person to witness an accident or arrive on the scene, your action could save a life or prevent serious additional injury, so be prepared to offer assistance in any emergency situation but always defer to someone who has the greater training and experience.

First aid techniques are taught by the American Red Cross as a specific course. You should avail yourself of the opportunity to be thoroughly and properly trained in these skills. In addition, the American Heart Association provides instruction and certification in Cardio Pulmonary Resuscitation (CPR); you are encouraged to sign up to learn this life saving technique.

If you are able to react in an emergency situation remember: (1) always keep calm so that your actions reflect clear thinking; (2) use a calm voice to talk to the victim and to instruct others in the area; and (3) keep onlookers away and proceed in a methodic, quiet way.

Working in the hospital or long-term care facility, you are always close to professional medical help but when you witness an accident away from the medical facility, that help is not always readily available. Whatever course of action you choose, the victim should not be placed in additional jeopardy.

In certain areas of the country an emergency number which can be contacted for help in case of an accident is 911. In other areas the closest sources of help are the police, local rescue squads, or the telephone operator who can complete the call for you. When calling the number, give your name, location, and a brief description of the scene. Be sure to include information about the type of injury and possible help you may need.

FIRST AID

First aid is immediate care for victims of injuries or sudden illness. These conditions can range from the minor to the very severe. When you give first aid, you deal with the victim's emotional state, physical injuries, and the whole accident situation. First aid also includes care needed later if medical help is delayed or is not available. There are actions which you may take which can effectively help each of these victims but be sure to take care of life-threatening situations first.

The first step is to determine if life is in danger. A person who has stopped breathing, who has had a heart attack, or who is bleeding heavily is in danger of imminent death. Shock, poisoning, and choking are also life-threatening situations. *Persons in life-threatening situations must be given immediate attention.*

Assessing the Situation

Your first task, as just mentioned, is to assess the situation and determine the extent of injuries. Quickly take into account the number of victims, their potential injuries, and any dangerous factors at the scene.

For example, at the scene of an auto accident there may be several victims. Some may be trapped in their vehicles, others may be strewn on the highway. There may be cars burning and the danger of explosion. In this situation, it becomes imperative to get yourself and the victims away from further danger first.

In the medical facility, unless there is a fire, usually you will be dealing with a single victim and you will be able to focus on the needs of that individual person.

If you are close to the call bell, summon help or ask someone close by (such as another patient) to signal. Give your name, location, and name of the patient to the person on the other end of the line. Clearly, but briefly, state what you believe to be the situation or extent of injury.

For example, you might enter a patient's room and, despite the fact that siderails are up at the bed, a patient is lying on the floor. Make a quick assessment as you signal for help, giving your name, the patient's name and location, and describing the scene.

Do not move the victim if professional help is available. Keep the person quiet and calm until help arrives. Try to maintain an even body temperature and provide urgent care if it is needed.

URGENT CARE

Urgent care is care that must be given right away to prevent loss of life. If you are out in the community ask someone nearby to summon help. Do not leave people who need urgent care to get help yourself.

As help is on the way, make your assessment of the patient. Check for degree of consciousness, Figure 40-1, breathing capability, rate of heart beat, and signs of bleeding—in that order. Do not move the person if you do not have to and do not allow the conscious person to get up and walk around. The conscious person will also be able to communicate a response to your questions. You should now check for other injuries.

In the health facility or out in the community the same rule applies; your basic role is to reassure the victim and keep the person warm.

THE UNCONSCIOUS PATIENT

If the patient is unconscious and breathing laboriously, or if breathing has ceased, immediate appropriate action must be taken.

Breathing brings vital oxygen into the body. All organs require it to maintain life. Of all the organs in the body, the brain is the most sensitive to oxygen deprivation. Permanent damage to the brain and other vital organs occurs when oxygen is denied. Therefore, breathing must be rapidly restored.

To check for breathing, *look* at the chest for movement. *Listen* and *feel*

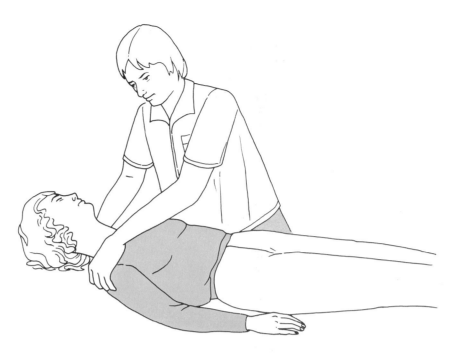

FIGURE 40-1. Determine if the patient is conscious and check for breathing.

for breathing by putting your ear near the mouth and nose. Check for about 5 seconds.

If the person is lying on the stomach, and there may be back injuries or other injuries that could be made worse by moving the person, check by looking at the back for movement. Hold your hand near the mouth and nose to feel for breathing.

Opening An Airway

The airway must be open for air to enter and leave the lungs. Sometimes just opening the airway allows respirations to resume. One way to do this is as follows:

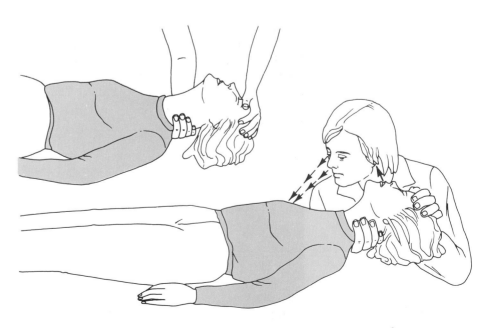

FIGURE 40-2.

1. Place one hand under the neck and lift gently.
2. Push down on the forehead with the other hand, Figure 40-2A.
3. Tip the head back as far as you can. *Look* at the chest to see if it is moving.
4. Place your ear and cheek near the mouth and *listen* and *feel* for air going in and out, Figure 40-2B.

ALTERNATE METHOD. Another way to open the airway is to tip the head and lift the chin without pressure on the neck. To follow this method:

1. Place one hand on the forehead and apply backward pressure with your palm.
2. To help tip the head way back, gently lift the chin with your other hand by placing your fingertips under the bony part of the jaw near the chin.
3. Support and lift the jaw with your fingertips. Be careful not to close the mouth, Figure 40-3.
4. Pull upward so as not to put pressure on the soft tissues of the throat.

Steps to Follow

If the person is not breathing, give four quick, full breaths, Figure 40-4. Keep the head tipped. Pinch the nose so air will not escape and blow into mouth. Make sure your mouth covers victim's mouth so there is a good seal. Watch to see the victim's chest rise as you blow into the mouth. Be-

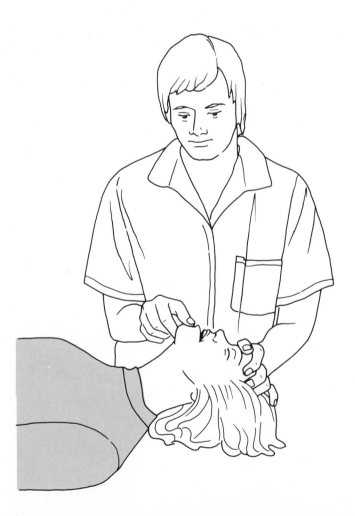

FIGURE 40-3.   Press down on forehead while lifting chin up with fingertips of other hand.

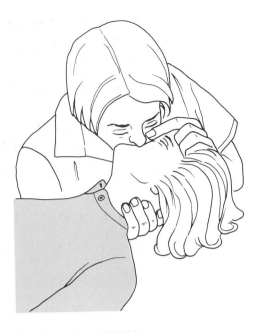

FIGURE 40-4.

tween each breath, remove your mouth, then inhale deeply and quickly. Check for air exchange, Figure 40-5. If breathing has not been restored, continue the technique but do so at a rate of one breath every five seconds.

Infants who have stopped breathing need emergency assistance also. You must be very gentle with them. Do not tilt the head back as far as with an adult, Figure 40-6, and cover both the nose and mouth of the infant. Use small puffs instead of deep breaths. If breathing is not resumed after the initial puffs, continue the technique at a rate of one gentle puff every 3 seconds.

After the initial four quick inflations, check for a pulse. The easiest place to check is the carotid artery found on either side of the trachea in the neck. If there is no pulse, then cardiopulmonary resuscitation is needed.

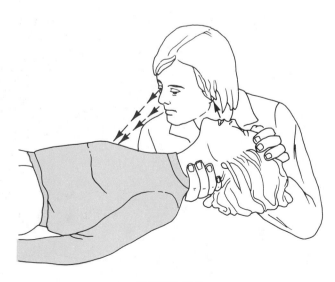

FIGURE 40-5.

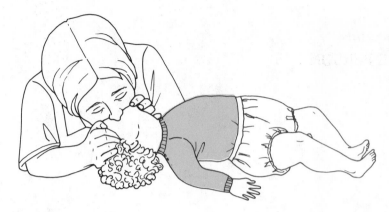

FIGURE 40-6.   Note that head is not as extended as in an adult. Mouth covers both nose and mouth of infant.

CARDIOPULMONARY RESUSCITATION (CPR)

Cardiopulmonary resuscitation combines the techniques of artificial respiration and cardiac stimulation to restore circulation.

CPR is needed when the heart and circulation fails. This is seen following heart attacks, severe injury, drug overdoses, electrocution, drowning, inhalation of toxic gases, and strangulation.

You must recognize the need for cardiopulmonary resuscitation quickly and take action promptly. The patient willl be unconscious, with no respiratory movements or pulse. The skin is pale to cyanotic and cool to touch. Patients who are in shock, or those who have fainted or suffered a stroke will also be unconscious but may not need CPR.

If you have been properly trained and certified, you can perform this life-saving technique. Your instructor or supervisor, who is certified, can teach you this technique and supervise your practice until you become proficient.

The term *cardio* refers to the heart and *pulmonary* refers to the lungs, so in *cardiopulmonary resuscitation* the heart and lungs are revised or restored to action. CPR is the combination of mouth-to-mouth breathing, which supplies oxygen to the lungs, and chest compressions, which circulate the blood. By giving CPR, you breathe and circulate blood for a person whose heart and lungs have stopped working (cardiac and respiratory arrest).

When you give CPR, the victim's head should be at the level of the heart or slightly lower than the heart. If the head is higher than the heart, blood will not flow up to the brain.

The person must be on a firm surface because on a soft one, chest compressions will not press the heart between the backbone and the sternum. Either get the person onto a firm surface such as the ground or floor or, if the person is in a bed and difficult to move put something firm, such as a board, under the back below the heart area. In the health care facility, the chest board will be on the emergency cart or attached to the bed.

As soon as possible, elevate (raise) the feet and legs of a person being given CPR. This helps blood return to the heart. Do not stop giving CPR to elevate the legs—have another person do it.

Remember, you must be trained to give CPR before attempting this technique. CPR may be administered by one person or two persons and may be done with adults and children. A slightly different technique is used in each of these situations.

Procedure

ONE PERSON CPR

1. Check for consciousness.
2. Signal for assistance.
3. Position person on back. Lift neck and tilt head.
4. Check for breathing by placing your ear close to the person's mouth and watch chest for 5 seconds, Figure 40-7.

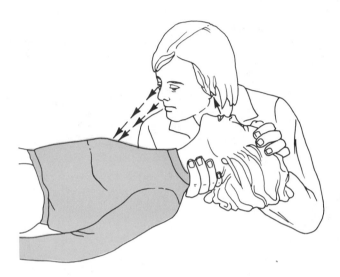

FIGURE 40-7.   Check for breathing. Listen, feel, look.

5. Give 4 quick, full breaths while pinching the nose closed and blowing into the person's mouth, Figure 40-8.

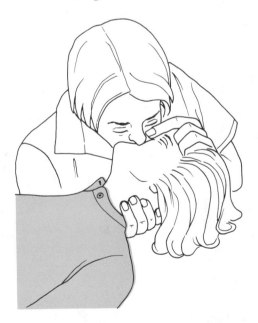

FIGURE 40-8.   Seal mouth and give 4 quick breaths.

6. Check the pulse and check for breathing again. Use the carotid pulse located on the side of the windpipe, Figure 40-9. Check for no less than 5 seconds and no more than 10 seconds. If there is no pulse or breathing, continue on with the CPR.

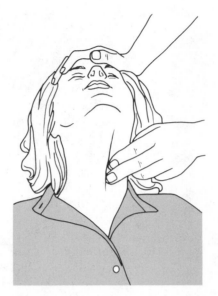

FIGURE 40-9.   Locate the carotid pulse.

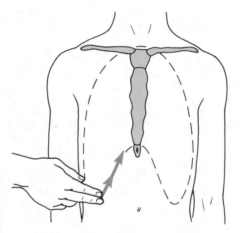

A. Trace along rib cage to notch.

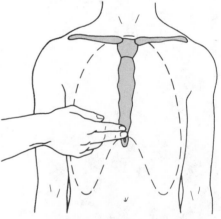

B. Place middle finger on notch with index finger beside it.

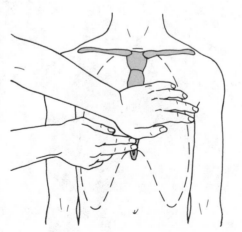

C. Measure by placing one hand beside the index finger of the other hand.

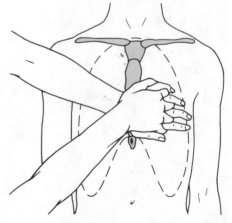

D. Lace fingers and keep them up off the chest.

FIGURE 40-10.

7. Give breaths at rate of one every 5 seconds as follows:
   a. Be sure the head is still tipped.
   b. Pinch the nose closed again.
   c. Take a deep breath, open your mouth wide and make a tight seal over the person's mouth. Say to yourself between breaths, "one thousand and one; one thousand and two; one thousand and three; one thousand and four." This will help you gauge the proper amount of time between breaths.
   d. Turn your head to look at the person's chest while you take another breath. If it fails to rise check for obstruction. If necessary, clear the obstruction and go back to the CPR.
8. Check for pulse. If absent, start external chest compressions.
9. Locate proper position for placement of heels of hands on sternum. (See Figure 40-10.)
10. Administer 15 chest compressions as follows:
    a. Get on your knees—don't rest on heels.
    b. Place knees about a shoulder width apart.
    c. Keep arms straight.
    d. Bending forward, use heels of hands to push straight down about 1 1/2 inches. Keep fingers clear of the chest, Figure 40-11.

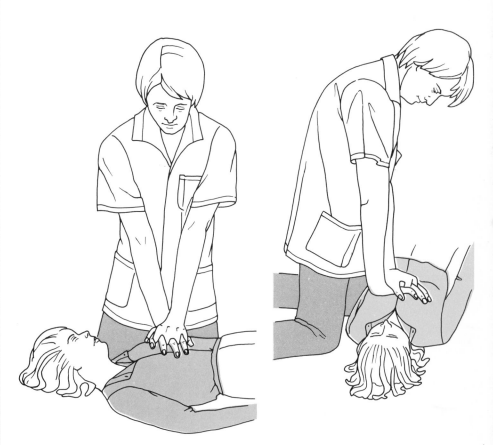

FIGURE 40-11. Get on your knees while compressing.

   e. Compress the adult chest at the rate of 80 compressions per minute. Count in your mind, "one and two and," with each compression to help you keep count. Note: four cycles of 15 compressions and two ventilations are given per minute.

11. Open airway and give two quick breaths.
12. Repeat steps 10 and 11 for four cycles.
13. Check for pulse and breathing.
14. If pulseless and breathless repeat steps 10 and 11.
15. Once you have started CPR, check the pulse and breathing after the first minute and every few minutes after that. Check right after you give breaths. Do not stop CPR for more than 5 seconds to check the pulse and breathing. Also check the pulse if you see signs of recovery, such as small movements, return of reflexes such as swallowing, and improved skin color in persons who have light skin.
    • If you find no pulse, continue CPR. When you start one-rescuer CPR again after checking the pulse, give two breaths first, then compressions.
    • If you find a pulse but no breathing, give mouth-to-mouth breathing. Check the pulse and breathing frequently.
    • If you find a pulse and breathing, keep checking the pulse and breathing. Get the person to a hospital or life-support unit quickly.

Procedure
TWO PERSON CPR

1. Give CPR according to one man procedure until qualified assistant arrives.
2. Person to assist will check for pulse and will take over mouth-to-mouth resuscitation.
3. At signal from assistant, stop compressions briefly while he checks for pulse and breath.
4. If CPR needs to be continued, the assistant will give one breath.
5. You give chest compressions at the rate of 60 per minute, counting out loud as you previously did mentally.
6. At the fifth compression assistant gives one breath.
7. Continue compressions and repeat counting out loud.
8. Change position with assistant about every two minutes to prevent fatigue as follows:
    a. Count "change one-thousand," as you compress, to alert assistant that position is to be changed.
    b. Continue compressing and counting as before until you say five-one thousand.
    c. Assistant gives one breath and moves to assume chest compression position.
    d. You assume assistant's position; check for pulse. Signal need for continued CPR.
    e. Give one mouth-to-mouth breath.
9. Assistant begins compression and counting.
10. Continue two person CPR until help arrives.

Procedure
CPR ON AN INFANT

Note: remember the following special points.
1. Do not hyperextend the infant's neck.
2. Cover both nose and mouth when giving breaths.
3. Breaths should be "puffs" rather than full blows.
4. Use fingertips to compress sternum.
5. Compress sternum only one-half to one inch.
6. Give compression at a rate of 100 per minute with ventilations after each 5 compressions. (This is a rate of 20 ventilations per minute.)
7. Count with no pause between numbers: eg. one, two, three, four, five, etc.
8. Follow basic procedure for CPR.

Procedure **CPR ON A CHILD**	Note: remember the following points. 1. Compress the sternum one-half to one inch. 2. Give 80 compressions per minute. 3. Count "one and two and." 4. Give 15 ventilations per minute. (This is one after each 5 compressions.) 5. Follow basic procedure for CPR.

CHOKING

A person chokes when the throat is occluded and air cannot get into the airway. Food, vomitus, or blood can accumulate in the back of the throat, blocking the airway, especially in an unconscious person. Tilting the head can sometimes clear the airway since positioning in this way pulls the tongue forward.

If the person can speak and is coughing vigorously, do not intervene. Coughing is the most effective way to dislodge materials from the airway. Stay close by and encourage coughing.

A complete blockage is signalled by the person being unable to speak, high-pitched sounds on inhalation, and grasping the throat, Figure 40-12. In this situation, you must take quick, decisive action.

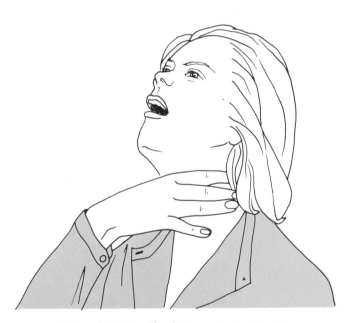

FIGURE 40-12. The distress signal of choking.

Procedure **ASSISTING THE CONSCIOUS CHOKING PERSON**	1. Stand behind and to one side of the victim. 2. Place one hand on the victim's chest for support. 3. Tilt person forward so that head is below chest if possible. 4. Give 4 sharp blows over the spine between the shoulder blades, Figure 40-13. Use the heel of your open hand. Strike hard enough to knock the object loose. 5. If the patient starts to cough, wait. 6. If blows do not discharge object, give 4 thrusts to the abdomen as follows:

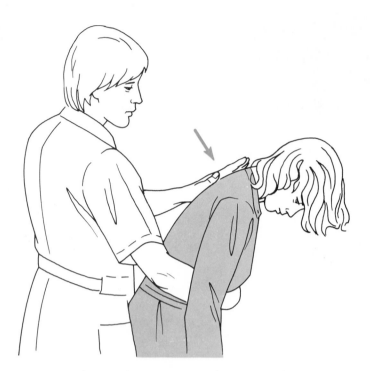

FIGURE 40-13.   Sharp blows may dislodge object.

a. Clench fist, keeping thumb straight, Figure 40-14A.
b. Place fist, thumb side in, against abdomen.
c. Grasp clenched fist with opposite hand, Figure 40-14B.
d. Push forcefully with thumbside of fist against midline of abdomen, between ribcage and the waist, inward and upward, Figure 40-14C. Be sure you are below the tip of the sternum (xiphoid process).

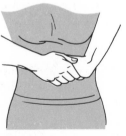

A

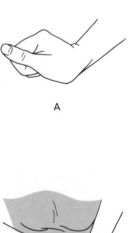

B

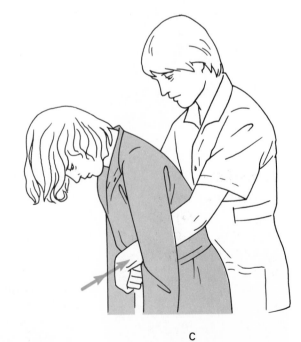

C

FIGURE 40-14.

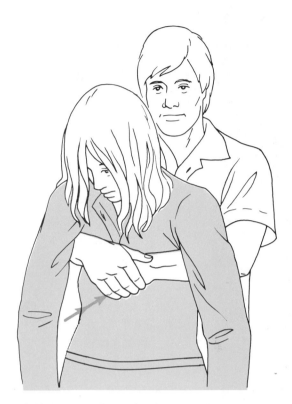

FIGURE 40-15.   Grasp the person under the armpits.

7. Repeat steps four and five if object has not been dislodged, but if the person begins to cough forcefully, wait.

Note: chest thrusts are used when pressure to the abdomen would be harmful. This would be if the choking person is pregnant or if the victim is so large you are unable to get your arms around them. Follow steps one through four, then:

5. Stand behind victim.
6. Place arms around victim directly under the victim's armpits.
7. Form fist as previously described and place thumbside of fist against breastbone (sternum), level with the armpits.
8. Grasp fist in opposite hand and administer thrusts, pulling straight back toward you, Figure 40-15.

Procedure

ASSISTING THE UNCONSCIOUS PERSON WHO HAS AN OBSTRUCTED AIRWAY

1. Tip the head and check for signs of breathing.
2. Try to give breaths by inhaling and then placing your mouth over the mouth of the victim and blowing into the victim's mouth.
3. If air will go into the lungs, give 4 quick breaths.
4. Check for pulse and breathing.
5. If air will not go in and lungs do not inflate, retip head and try again. If second attempt fails, proceed as follows.
   a. Kneel down beside the victim.
   b. Place one hand on the victim's hip and one on his shoulder. Roll the victim on their side toward you.
   c. Strike the victim with the heel of your open hand 4 times rapidly and hard, over the spine between the shoulder blades, Figure 40-16.

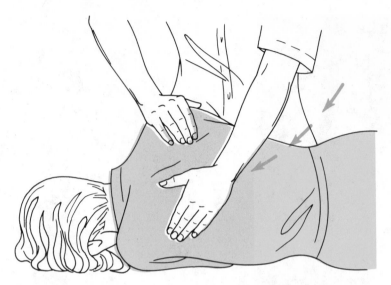

FIGURE 40-16.   Roll person toward you and strike the victim's back.

Note: The next two steps cover abdominal and chest thrusts. Chest thrusts may be substituted for abdominal thrusts when the person is unconscious. Either can be given without being astride the person's body.

6. Immediately roll the person onto his back, straddle his body with your legs and administer 4 abdominal thrusts as follows.
   a. Place the heel of one hand on the victim's abdomen between ribcage and waist. Hand should be flat with fingers pointing toward victim's head.
   b. Place your other hand in a similar position over the first.
   c. Keep your elbows straight with your shoulders directly over the victim's abdomen. Press inward and upward with 4 quick thrusts, Figure 40-17. Keep hands centered on person's abdomen.
7. To give chest thrusts, proceed as follows. (See page 462.)
   a. Locate the lower edge of the victim's rib cage on the side near you. Use the hand that is nearest the victim's feet.
   b. Using the middle and index finger, trace the ribs up to the notch where the sternum and ribs meet. Keep your finger on the notch and place your finger next to it on the lower end of the sternum.
   c. Place the heel of your other hand on the sternum next to the index finger. Keep fingers separated and off the chest.
   d. Put the hand you measured with on the hand which is on the breast bone.
   e. Interlace fingers—keep off chest.
   f. Keep elbows straight and push straight down with heels of hands.
8. Grasp the tongue and lower jaw between thumb and fingers. Pull upward. With the index finger of your other hand, follow down along the inside of one cheek, deep into the throat to the base of the tongue. Sweep in from the side. Do not poke straight in because that may push the object down. Use a hooking action, across toward the other cheek, to loosen and remove the object.

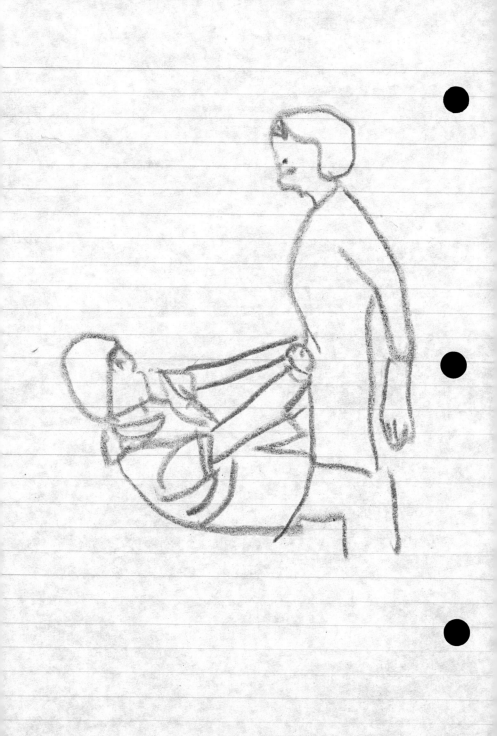

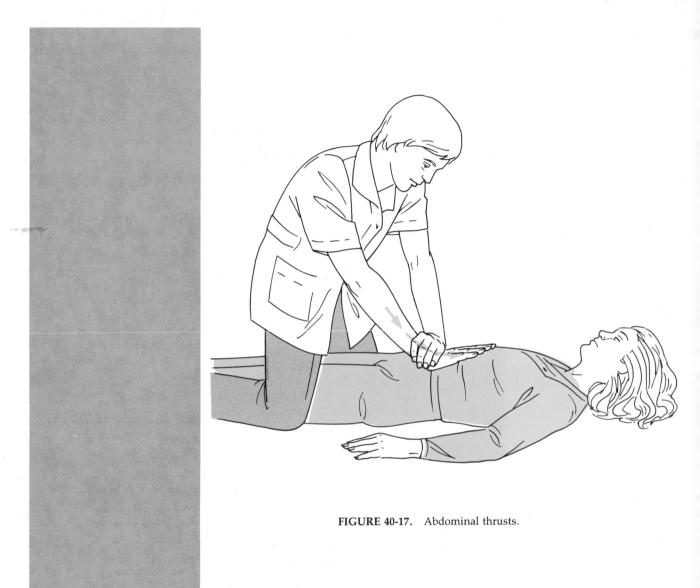

FIGURE 40-17.   Abdominal thrusts.

9. After sweeping in the mouth, whether or not you remove the object, tip the head and try to give breaths. If air will not go into the lungs, repeat 4 back blows, 4 thrusts and sweeping. Then try again to give breaths.

Note: A victim who is given mouth-to-mouth breathing, back blows, or thrusts may vomit. Roll a victim who vomits toward you on one side and clean out the mouth with your fingers. Then roll the victim back and continue repeating the sequence of breaths, blows, thrusts, and sweep.

BLEEDING

Remember that if the person is conscious the extent of injuries is likely to be far less severe. With the unconscious person, however, the next imminent threat to life is the loss of blood. Bleeding is usually easy to see but sometimes the bleeding is internal and will only be evidenced by the

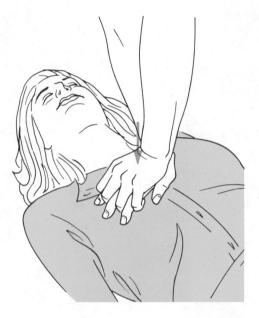

FIGURE 40-18.   Chest thrusts.

signs of shock as they are described in the next section. Examine the person for evidence of bleeding and take the following steps to prevent additional loss:

1. Identify the location of bleeding area.
2. Apply continuous, direct pressure over bleeding area with a pad or even your hand, if necessary.
3. If seepage occurs, increase the padding and pressure.
4. If there are no broken bones and no pain, raise the wounded area above the level of the heart. This will help to reduce bleeding but do not release pressure.
5. Support the elevated area.
6. Use binding of some kind to hold the padded pressure if there is bleeding from more than one area.
7. If you have learned the location of the major blood vessels which control blood flow to an area and direct pressure seems ineffective, apply pressure over the appropriate vessel to stem hemorrhage.
8. Keep the person comfortably warm and quiet until help arrives.

Note: People who are bleeding are often very frightened and the anxiety contributes to the development of shock. Continuous reassurance is essential.

SHOCK

Shock is defined as a disturbance of the oxygen supply to the tissues and return of blood to the heart. It can follow any severe injury: cardiac standstill, hemorrhage, severe pain, or excessive loss of body fluids as seen in severe burns. Anxiety contributes to the situation, but shock can be prevented if steps are taken early. Prevention of shock includes situations that could trigger it. These include: keeping the person lying down and quiet and maintaining the normal body temperature. If burn areas are involved, however, the area should be elevated unless it causes the person pain.

Unless contraindicated by specific injury, position the person with the feet and legs slightly higher than the body and head. This assures improved circulation to the vital organs. If fractures are involved, make sure they are splinted (braced) before positioning the person to prevent shock.

In the health care facility, fluids to improve circulatory volume will be started and low volumes of oxygen will be given; this equipment is readily at hand. In the community, the emergency personnel answering the call will bring with them the supplies necessary to manage fluid and oxygenation.

If help is delayed over an hour and the person's condition seems to be deteriorating, small amounts of fluids may be given by mouth. Fluids should not be given if surgery is possible, if there is abdominal injury, if the person is likely to vomit, convulse, or is unconscious. A solution of tepid water, salt and baking soda can be given.

Signs and Symptoms

The early signs and symptoms of shock include skin that is pale, cold, and moist to the touch. The person probably complains of feeling weak and, when checked, the pulse is weak and rapid. Breathing is increased and irregular. Usually the person is restless and anxious. Later signs include mottled skin, apathy, and lack of response. The eyes become sunken, pupils are dilated with a vacant expression. Loss of consciousness follows, body temperature falls, and death can occur. Until help arrives, your care can often make the difference between life and death.

FAINTING

When the blood supply to the brain is reduced for a short time, the person loses consciousness: called fainting. Fainting is usually a temporary condition which is corrected as soon as blood flow to the brain is restored.

Unfortunately, when consciousness is lost, the person is likely to fall and injuries can occur. Patients who are ambulating for the first time should be assisted, but if fainting occurs, assist the patient to the floor so they won't be injured in a fall. Assist patients who are *feeling* faint to a safe position.

The patient who is sitting and feels faint, light-headed, dizzy, and nauseated should be encouraged to lower his or her head between their knees. Pallor, cold skin, perspiration, or visual changes also signal fainting. Your assistance means that you should:

1. Help the patient to assume a protected position sitting or lying down.
2. Loosen tight clothing.
3. Position head lower than heart to encourage cerebral blood flow.
4. Allow person to rest for at least 10 minutes.
5. Maintain normal body temperature.

HEART ATTACK

Heart attacks can occur in any age group but the high risk group includes those who are overweight and those persons who smoke. Even persons already hospitalized can have them. Heart attacks can fall at either end of the symptom spectrum. They may be a dramatic event with the person grasping the chest, complaining of a crushing pain that can radiate up the jaw and down the arm. The face may be pale to greyish and perspiring. The attack may be so severe that the victim stops breathing, loses consciousness and his heart function ceases. The loss of heart function is called cardiac arrest.

At other times, the pain of the attack may resemble indigestion and the person remains conscious. Do not be fooled into thinking that the degree of pain indicates the severity of the attack. Both victims need immediate attention.

In the health care facility, immediately signal for help. If the patient is conscious, stay with him and help keep him calm. Elevate the head of the bed to assist breathing and provide O_2 if available.

If the patient is unconscious, check for breathing and heart beat. If necessary, institute CPR, if you have been trained, until a professional takes charge.

In the community and if the person is conscious proceed as follows.

1. Assess the situation.
2. If possible, send someone to call for an ambulance equipped with oxygen and emergency care heart equipment.
3. Allow the person to sit up or raise the head and shoulders—loosen clothing about neck.
4. Keep onlookers away.
5. Provide fresh air but keep the person comfortably warm.

In the community, if the person is unconscious follow steps 1 and 2. Then:

3. Check for breathing and heart beat.
4. If heart beat is present but breathing has ceased, institute mouth-to-mouth resuscitation.
5. If breathing and heart beat have ceased (cardiac arrest) institute CPR until a professional takes charge.

STROKE

A stroke (cerebral vascular accident or CVA) occurs when there is an interference to the normal blood circulation to the brain. It usually is caused by a clot that has lodged in a cerebral vessel or by a blood vessel that has ruptured.

The severe stroke victim usually loses consciousness, experiences difficulty breathing, and develops paralysis on one side of the body and of the muscles of either side of the face. The pulse of the eyes becomes unequal. If consciousness is not lost in a minor stroke, speech may become slurred and confusion, dizziness, and headache are commonly experienced.

Later memory, speech, and personality may be altered, as well as the development of weakness in the affected limbs. First aid includes maintaining an airway, providing mouth-to-mouth breathing, and CPR as needed. Position the person on one side so fluids will drain from the mouth. Maintain normal body temperature and keep the person quiet until help arrives or transportation to a medical facility can be arranged.

SEIZURES (CONVULSIONS)

Seizures or convulsions are sometimes seen when there is head injury, stroke, poisoning, infectious disease, and in neurologic conditions such as seizure syndrome (epilepsy).

Seizure syndrome is largely controlled today with medication but unusual stress, medication omission, and other factors can precipitate a convulsion. Seizures do not always follow the same pattern. They range from a momentary loss of contact (petite mal), in which there are no random or uncontrolled movements, to the more dramatic form (grand mal), in which consciousness is lost, the person falls, becomes rigid, and then uncontrolled voluntary movements and frothing at the mouth occurs and the person becomes cyanotic.

Gradually the seizure lessens and the person recovers. The person is usually confused, may be disoriented for a period of time, and feels very tired. If you witness a seizure, take the following steps:

1. Do not restrain the movements.
2. Move any objects that might cause injury out of the way.
3. Loosen clothing around the neck.
4. Maintain an airway.
5. Turn person to the side so fluid or vomitus can drain freely after the movements subside.
6. Give mouth-to-mouth resuscitation if breathing is not resumed following the seizure.
7. Allow the person to rest undisturbed.
8. Summon medical assistance.

ELECTRIC SHOCK

Electric shock can occur in the community when high-tension wires are knocked down in accidents or storms. In the health facility, frayed wires, and faulty outlets or fixtures can cause electrical shock. Severe burns and cardiac and respiratory arrest can result from electric shock. You must protect yourself as you try to rescue the victim.

1. Turn off the source of electricity from the terminal source, such as at a fuse box before touching the person.
2. If the source of electricity cannot be controlled, try to move the victim away with some non-conductive material. Dry wood is a good non-conductor.
3. Once free of electrical source, check victim for breathing and pulse.
4. Administer CPR if necessary.
5. Once breathing and heart function is restored, check for burns and other injury. Keep person lying down and comfortable.
6. Give first aid for burns or other injuries.
7. Try to get medical help.

Summary

Emergency situations can occur without warning at any time. A person who has been specially trained in the techniques of first aid can be in a position to be of great service. Never overestimate your abilities but use the special skills you have been taught wisely.

Special training will enable you to assess injuries, know the proper steps to follow in summoning help, and to carry out life-saving skills such as mouth-to-mouth resuscitation, bleeding control and CPR.

VOCABULARY

Learn the meaning and correct spelling of the following words.

arrest	first aid	stroke
CPR	hemorrhage	urgent care
chest thrust	seizure syndrome	victim
compression	shock	
contraindicated	splintered	

UNIT REVIEW

A. Completion. Complete the following sentences.

1. An organization which teaches specific first aid courses is the _____ _____.

2. The American Heart Association teaches a course to certify people in the life-saving technique called _____.

3. First aid provides _____ care for the sick and injured.
4. The special emergency number to call to contact emergency help is _____ .
5. Your first step in accessing an emergency situation is to determine if _____ .
6. Urgent care is given to prevent loss of _____ .
7. To check for breathing, look at _____ .
8. When giving mouth-to-mouth breathing, inhale and give an initial _____ quick full breaths.
9. In mouth-to-mouth breathing, after the initial breaths, check for _____ .
10. To insure adequate chest compression in CPR, always place the person on a _____ surface.

B. **Clinical Situations.** Briefly describe how a health care assistant should react to the following situations.
   1. You are the first person on the scene of an auto accident. One person has been thrown out of the car and is lying beside the car, which is on fire. Describe your first action.

   2. You have been trained in mouth-to-mouth resuscitation. The person you found is unconscious. What do you check first?

   3. You are in a dining area and an ambulatory patient grasps his throat, high pitched sounds are heard, and the person is unable to speak. Describe your actions.

Section Twelve
Self-evaluation

A. Match the term in Column I with the statement in Column II.

Column I

1. Occult
2. Leboyer method
3. Ostomy
4. Episiotomy
5. Lochia
6. Excessive blood loss
7. Colostrum
8. Suppository
9. Postpartum
10. Stoppage

Column II

a. arrest
b. hemorrhage
c. incision in perineum
d. first breast milk
e. birth without violence
f. vaginal discharge
g. hidden
h. a cone-shaped solid mass inserted into the rectum for lubrication
i. after birth
j. artificial opening

B. Choose the answer that best completes each statement by circling the letter.

11. You observe someone having a convulsion. You should
    a. restrain the movements.
    b. force something between the teeth to prevent injury to the tongue.
    c. move articles away that the patient might strike.
    d. encourage the patient to be active following the attack.
    e. keep the person flat on his back following the attack.

12. Your patient has just returned from delivery, looks pale, complains of feeling cold and begins to shiver. You suspect
    a. she is excited about the delivery.
    b. she is just tired.
    c. she needs something to eat.
    d. she is in danger of shock.
    e. she is really all right and can safely be left alone.

13. The newborn has just been admitted to the nursery. You will
    a. leave him undressed so he can be examined.
    b. tilt the crib with head down.
    c. tilt the crib with head up.
    d. start feeding with milk substitute.
    e. detach the name band and affix to the crib.

14. When administering CPR, the patient should be
    a. on his stomach.
    b. on a soft bed.
    c. with his head raised.
    d. on a flat, firm surface.
    e. Any position is correct.

15. When giving routine ileostomy care you should
    a. not wear gloves.
    b. leave unit unscreened.
    c. dry area around stoma briskly.
    d. not examine drainage.
    e. No answer applies.

16. You are assigned to insert a suppository as a stool softener. You will insert it
    a. 1 inch.
    b. 2 inches.
    c. 3 inches.
    d. 4 inches.
    e. 5 inches.

17. When doing a Hematest® Reagent tablet to check feces for occult blood, add to the tablet and fecal smear
    a. 1 drop of water
    b. 2 drops of water.
    c. 3 drops of water.
    d. 4 drops of water.
    e. 5 drops of water.
18. When putting on sterile gloves,
    a. leave hands a little moist.
    b. set up a sterile field to open the gloves.
    c. pick both gloves up at the same time.
    d. touch only the inside cuff of the glove with your bare hands.
    e. spread fingers and slip into first glove.
19. A sterile field has been set up and you are to add some 4 × 4 sponges. You
    a. may reach over the sterile field as long as you don't touch it.
    b. place sponges at least 1/2 inch from the edge.
    c. may place the unopened package on the field.
    d. place sponges at least 2 inches away from the edge of the field.
    e. No answer applies.
20. Shock is a life-threatening situation. You would do which of the following?
    a. Elevate the head.
    b. Apply external heat in the form of hot water bags.
    c. Raise the feet and legs.
    d. Restrict all fluids.
    e. Give ice water.
21. Your first task in an emergency is to
    a. move the victims.
    b. assess the situation.
    c. call for help.
    d. ask the victim what happened.
    e. No answer applies.
22. To provide an open airway,
    a. place one hand on the throat and one on the forehead.
    b. lift the neck gently and push down on the chin.
    c. lift the neck gently and push down on the forehead.
    d. put both hands under the shoulders.
    e. raise the arms over the head.
23. When performing CPR on an adult, perform 4 cycles of 15 compressions and how many ventilations per minute?
    a. 1
    b. 2
    c. 3
    d. 4
    e. 5
24. Once you have started CPR and stop to check pulse and breathing, do not stop longer than
    a. 1 second.
    b. 5 seconds.
    c. 10 seconds.
    d. 15 seconds.
    e. 1 minute.
25. A patient who is choking begins to cough. You had best
    a. administer chest thrusts.
    b. sweep his mouth.
    c. strike him sharply on the back between the shoulder blades.
    d. encourage him to continue coughing.
    e. encourage him to drink water.

Comprehensive Final Evaluation

A. In each question, select the best answer.

1. Special health services offered in the community include
   - a. safe drinking water.
   - b. statistical services.
   - c. immunization procedures.
   - d. X-rays.
   - e. All of the above.

2. The national health agency is called
   - a. WHO.
   - b. The Federal Bureau of Health.
   - c. The U.S. Statistical Bureau.
   - d. The U.S. Public Health Service.
   - e. The National Public Health Agency.

3. Health care assistants are most often employed in
   - a. homes for the aged.
   - b. local health departments.
   - c. The World Health Organization.
   - d. state sanitation departments.
   - e. statistical gathering agencies.

4. The *immediate supervisor* of the health care assistant is
   - a. another health care assistant.
   - b. an RN.
   - c. an orderly.
   - d. an M.D.
   - e. None of the above.

5. A health care assistant failed to check the temperature of an enema solution and the patient was burned. This is a case of
   - a. malpractice.
   - b. negligence.
   - c. carelessness.
   - d. aiding and abetting.
   - e. dishonesty.

6. The health care assistant starts an intravenous infusion and the patient develops an infection. This is a case of
   - a. malpractice.
   - b. negligence.
   - c. carelessness.
   - d. aiding and abetting.
   - e. dishonesty.

7. The health care assistant feels unsure of how to manipulate the circle bed. She should
   - a. ask another assistant for instruction.
   - b. try anyway.
   - c. omit turning the patient.
   - d. ask help of the team leader.
   - e. tell the patient she doesn't know how.

8. The patient offers the health care assistant a little extra money for the care received. The health care assistant should
   - a. accept and say nothing.
   - b. accept and share with the other team members.
   - c. refuse courteously.
   - d. refuse and abruptly walk out of the room.
   - e. pretend that the offer wasn't heard.

9. The health care assistant learns that the patient has several bank accounts. The assistant should
   - a. inform the charge nurse.
   - b. share the information with co-workers.
   - c. tell the family this information.
   - d. keep this information secret.
   - e. let only her family know this information.

10. The health care assistant learns that the patient is concerned about the cost of hospitalization. The assistant should
    - a. inform the charge nurse.

    b. share the information with co-workers.

    c. tell the family this information.

    d. keep this information secret.

    e. let only her family know this information.

11. The patient is terminal and begs the health assistant to pull the plug. The assistant should

    a. do as asked so the patient will not suffer longer.

    b. explain God makes those decisions and tell the patient to pray.

    c. report incident to team leader.

    d. tell the family.

    e. call a clergy of the health care assistant's faith to talk to the patient.

12. Good grooming is seen when the health care assistant has

    a. long, flowing hair.

    b. short, well-kept, clean nails.

    c. bright red nail polish.

    d. dirty shoes and laces.

    e. failed to use a deodorant.

13. Another health care assistant asks you to help move a patient up in bed. You should

    a. refuse. It's not your assignment.

    b. agree to help but be annoyed.

    c. say you are doing more than your share already.

    d. agree in a courteous manner.

    e. say you can only help if the other health care assistant will do part of your assignment.

14. Your team leader needs a specimen taken to the laboratory "stat" and asks you to do so.

    a. You tell her you can't; you are too busy.

    b. You ask another health care assistant to take the specimen.

    c. You follow directions but give a patient status report to your team leader before leaving.

    d. You take the specimen and deliver it upon completion of your assignment.

    e. You take the specimen and leave the floor immediately without reporting.

15. Your patient is very irritable this morning and complains about how slow you are. You know that

    a. illness brings out the best in people.

    b. people sometimes direct their frustrations about their illness toward other people.

    c. you had better rush the care.

    d. you had better get help to finish the care.

    e. that the patient is being unfair and you tell him so.

16. Which of the following could act as a fomite?

    a. Drinking cup

    b. Bedpan

    c. Instruments

    d. Dressings

    e. All of the above.

17. In carrying out the hand washing procedure,

    a. it is all right to leave suds on the soap.

    b. rinse hands with fingertips down.

    c. rinse hands with fingertips straight up.

    d. use very hot water.

    e. turn faucets on and off with your bare hands.

18. The best temperature for the patient's room is about

    a. 65°.

    b. 68°.

    c. 70°.

    d. 75°.

    e. 80°.

19. A patient is being visited by his clergy. You should provide privacy by

    a. drawing the curtains.

    b. asking the other patients to leave.

    c. asking the other patients not to listen.

    d. tell the cleric to speak softly.

    e. doing nothing.

20. You are assigned to do terminal cleaning after patient discharge. Which of the following factors would *not* be part of that procedure?

    a. Remove all special equipment and clean.
    b. Wrap all disposable materials to be burned.
    c. Clean all bedside equipment and sterilize.
    d. Strip bed and dispose of linen per hospital policy.
    e. Remake the bed as an open bed.

21. The health care assistants communicate their feelings by
    a. facial expression.   d. body language.
    b. choice of words.   e. All of the above.
    c. touch.

22. Your patient has difficulty sleeping. You should consider
    a. noise in the unit.   d. All of the above.
    b. pain.   e. None of the above.
    c. worry and anxiety.

23. The health care assistant can increase the patient's sense of security by
    a. hanging his clothes away in the closet.
    b. responding angrily to a refusal to cooperate.
    c. providing opportunities for the patient to talk.
    d. taking every remark by the patient personally.
    e. doing every aspect of care that the patient could do.

24. The health care assistant demonstrates proper body mechanics by
    a. having sloping shoulders.
    b. using the right muscles to do the job.
    c. using the smaller back muscles to lift heavy objects.
    d. bending from the waist when picking up objects.
    e. keeping feet close together when picking up an object.

25. The health care assistant will turn patients frequently when they are unable to change their own position
    a. to prevent contractures.   d. All of the above.
    b. to improve circulation.   e. None of the above.
    c. to prevent decubitus ulcers.

26. The patient is severely burned and unable to turn himself. Which type of bed would most likely be used for such a patient?
    a. Closed bed   d. Open bed
    b. Circo-electric bed   e. Gatch bed
    c. Orthopedic bed

27. Toepleats are put in the occupied bed to prevent
    a. decubitus.   d. pressure on the chest.
    b. footdrop.   e. None of the above.
    c. wristdrop.

28. The proper temperature for bath water is
    a. 85°F.   d. 115°F.
    b. 95°F.   e. 125°F.
    c. 105°F.

29. During the bath procedure, other care is given which includes
    a. care of teeth.   d. range of motion exercises.
    b. care of nails.   e. All of the above.
    c. care of hair.

30. Your patient will be most apt to require special mouth care if
    a. he is unconscious.   d. he can't get out of bed.
    b. he drinks lots of fluids.   e. None of the above.
    c. he is receiving an IV.

31. To protect the patient's dentures,
    a. leave uncovered in the bedside table.
    b. use hot water to cleanse dentures.
    c. use a heavy stream of water and toothpaste.
    d. store in a denture cup.
    e. wash only the front surfaces.

32. Your adult patient on a house select diet should have included in the diet
    a. five or more servings of vegetables and fruits.
    b. two or more servings of milk or milk substitutes.
    c. four or more servings of meat.
    d. two or more servings of breads and cereals.
    e. None of the above are correct.

33. The patient orders read NPO after 4 PM. This means that the health care assistant will
    a. withhold dinner.
    b. force fluids.
    c. encourage the patient to ambulate.
    d. do range of motion exercises.
    e. change the patient's diet.

34. The patient has an order for a clear liquid diet. Which of the following would you omit from the tray?
    a. Coffee with cream
    b. Gingerale
    c. Strained carrot juice
    d. Tea with sugar
    e. None of these.

35. The patient has dentures and a soft diet has been ordered. What should be omitted from the tray?
    a. Coffee with cream and sugar
    b. Cooked, sieved peaches
    c. Fried eggs
    d. Toast
    e. Cream of wheat.

36. You are assigned to give postmortem care. You assemble equipment to
    a. give a bed bath.
    b. give afternoon (PM) care.
    c. determine vital signs.
    d. care for the body after death.
    e. None of the above.

37. The most accurate temperature reading is taken
    a. orally.
    b. rectally.
    c. vaginally.
    d. axillary.
    e. under the breast.

38. A temperature of 98.6°F is equal to
    a. 32°C.
    b. 35°C.
    c. 37°C.
    d. 39°C.
    e. 41°C.

39. An oral thermometer should be left in place before reading for
    a. 1 minute.
    b. 2 minutes.
    c. 3 minutes.
    d. 4 minutes.
    e. 5 minutes.

40. When inflating a blood pressure cuff, close the valve and
    a. pump up to 200 mm rapidly.
    b. pump 20 mm above last pulse sound heard.
    c. pump up slowly to 200 mm.
    d. pump 40 mm above last pulse sound heard.
    e. pump up up to 150 mm.

41. A blood pressure of 80/30 should be reported since the patient is probably suffering from
    a. bradycardia.
    b. tachycardia.
    c. hypertension.
    d. hypotension.
    e. None of the above.

42. The health care assistant would record vital signs on the
    a. doctor's progress report.
    b. graphic chart.
    c. physical and history.
    d. operative record.
    e. X-ray record.

43. Your patient is to be transferred to ICU. You would assist in transporting him to
    a. isolation care unit.
    b. intermediate care unit.
    c. intensive care unit.
    d. isotope unit.
    e. None of the above.

44. Your patient is to have f.f. and receive solids ad.lib. You will
    a. encourage the patient to eat but withhold liquids.

    b. place an NPO sign on the bed.

    c. caution the patient to limit his drinking to two glasses of water every 8 hours.

    d. encourage fluids and let the patient eat what he wished.

    e. let the patient drink anything he wants but restrict solid food.

45. When giving an oral report include the patient's
    a. name, age, weight.
    b. name, marital status, diagnosis.
    c. name, location, dependents.
    d. location, diagnosis, age.
    e. name, location, diagnosis.

46. SOAPE charting is
    a. procedurally oriented.
    b. problem oriented.
    c. order oriented.
    d. using only the graphic chart.
    e. only valid if block printed.

47. Important rules to remember about charting include
    a. erasures are permitted.
    b. each entry must be signed.
    c. spaces may be safely left.
    d. entries need not be dated or timed.
    e. All are correct.

48. The time 1 PM is expressed in international time as
    a. 0100.
    b. 0101.
    c. 1000.
    d. 1100.
    e. 1300.

49. Locate the appendix in its proper quadrant.
    a. Upper right.
    b. Upper left.
    c. Lower right.
    d. Lower left.
    e. Retroperitoneal space

50. Which of the following represents normal body defenses?
    a. Unbroken skin
    b. Gastric juice
    c. Saliva
    d. White blood cells
    e. All of the above.

51. The patient is on her abdomen with arms flexed and hands under her face which is turned to one side. This position is
    a. semi-Fowlers.
    b. Sims'.
    c. prone.
    d. trendelenburg.
    e. dorsal lithotomy.

52. The patient is going to surgery. Which of the following would you check?
    a. The chart for proper records
    b. Presence of prosthesis
    c. Removal of makeup including nail polish
    d. Bed rails up and in high position
    e. All of the above.

53. TED hose or elastic bandages are used postoperatively to
    a. support the neck.
    b. support the leg veins.
    c. reduce the flow of blood to the legs.
    d. reduce the flow of blood to the arms.
    e. support the joints during initial ambulation.

54. The patient has small solid raised red spots all over the chest. These are best described as
    a. decubiti.
    b. pustules.
    c. papules.
    d. macules.
    e. vessicles.

55. The patient with emphysema is receiving oxygen by nasal cannula. Which of the following precautions should be followed?
    a. No smoking allowed.
    b. Use only woolen blankets.
    c. Keep O_2 running while operating electric equipment.
    d. All of the above apply.
    e. None of the above apply.

56. The patient is recovering from an attack of congestive heart failure. Which of the following applies?
    a. Weigh the patient at the same time daily.
    b. Careful I & O
    c. Low salt diet
    d. Assist patient by oxygen and positioning.
    e. All of the above.
57. Your patient has a fractured femur and is currently in traction. Which of the following applies?
    a. Check for areas of pressure or irritation.
    b. Allow feet to press gently against end of bed.
    c. Keep weights balanced on the floor.
    d. Periodically remove traction to relieve pressure.
    e. All of the above apply.
58. Your patient has diabetes mellitus. Which of the following nursing care will you give?
    a. Strain all urine.
    b. Test urine for sugar and acetone.
    c. Serve a high carbohydrate diet.
    d. Restrict fluids.
    e. All of the above.
59. Your patient has had surgery to remove a cataract. You remember the following.
    a. Avoid abrupt movements.
    b. Encourage coughing.
    c. Glasses will no longer be needed.
    d. Hearing will be improved.
    e. Paralysis is a frequent complication.
60. Your patient has an order for a Harris flush. You know the following.
    a. The temperature of solution should be 115°.
    b. Approximately 1500 ml will be needed.
    c. The tube should be inserted 4 inches.
    d. The container should be raised 5 inches above the hips and then lowered the same distance.
    e. No answer applies.
61. Your patient has a douch ordered. You know the following.
    a. The temperature of the solution is 105°.
    b. The procedure is simple and will not require draping.
    c. The perineum should be cleansed.
    d. This is a sterile procedure.
    e. The patient should assume the prone position.

B. I. Match the following.
    62. Solid wastes
    63. Abnormal shortening of muscle fibers
    64. Intravenous infusions
    65. Armpit area
    66. External reproductive organs
    67. Intake & Output
    68. Area around nail beds
    69. An item that can be thrown away
    70. Artificial teeth
    71. Nutrient which provides energy

    a. expendable
    b. genitalia
    c. carbohydrates
    d. contracture
    e. dentures
    f. minerals
    g. feces
    h. I & O
    i. IV
    j. axilla
    k. cuticle

    II. Match the following sets.
    72. Poisons produced by microbes
    73. Bacteria that grow in clusters
    74. Procedures used to prevent germs from spreading
    75. One-celled microbes that cause malaria and diarrhea
    76. Disease-producing microbes
    77. Contaminated articles

    a. anaerobe
    b. fomites
    c. spores
    d. autoclave
    e. aerobes
    f. staphylococci
    g. medical asepsis

78. Machine used to sterilize equipment
79. Organisms that grow best in absence of oxygen
80. Rod-shaped microbe
81. Resistent forms of bacteria

h. pathogens
i. bacteria
j. toxins
k. protozoa

III. Match the following values.
82. 1 minum
83. 16 minums
84. 1 ounce
85. 1 pint
86. 1 quart
87. 2.2 pounds
88. 1 inch
89. 1 foot
90. 3 feet
91. 3 kilograms

a. 500 ml
b. 2.5 centimeters
c. 90 centimeters
d. 1 ml
e. 30 centimeters
f. 6.6 pounds
g. 0.0616 milliliters
h. 1000 milliliters
i. 2 quarts
j. 1 kilogram
k. 30 ml

IV. Match the following.
92. Given to provide moist heat to perineal area
93. Used to listen to body sounds
94. Used to provide continuous, constant temperature
95. A cooling bath
96. Used to determine blood pressure

a. sitz bath
b. sphygmomanometer
c. alcohol sponge
d. stethoscope
e. aqua K-pad

C. You have been asked to prepare an isolation unit. The following statements apply to this assignment.
97. T F   Place the proper color barrier sign on door.
98. T F   Stock a table or cart just inside the door with isolation gowns.
99. T F   Line wastepaper basket inside room with plastic bag.
100. T F   Prepare a basin of disinfectant and leave near sink in room.

Procedure Evaluation

Student _____

PROCEDURE	Satisfactory	Marginal	Unsatisfactory
Admitting a Newborn Infant			
Admitting the Patient			
Applying a Disposable Cold Pack			
Applying a Heat Lamp			
Applying a Hot Water Bag			
Applying a Moist Dressing			
Applying an Ice Bag			
Applying Elasticized Stockings			
Applying the Aquamatic K-pad			
Assisting the Conscious Choking Person			
Assisting the Patient in Initial Ambulation			
Assisting the Patient into a Chair or Wheelchair			
Assisting the Patient into Bed from a Chair or Wheelchair			
Assisting the Patient to Brush His Teeth			
Assisting the Patient to Dangle			
Assisting the Patient to Move to the Head of the Bed			
Assisting the Patient to Sit up in Bed			
Assisting the Patient Who Ambulates with a Cane or Walker			
Assisting the Patient Who Can Feed Himself			
Assisting the Unconscious Choking Person Who Has an Obstructed Airway			
Assisting with Routine Oral Hygiene			
Assisting with Special Oral Hygiene			
Assisting with the Cooling Bath (Alcohol Sponge Bath)			
Assisting With the Hot Arm Soak			
Assisting with the Hot Foot Soak			

476

PROCEDURE	Satisfactory	Marginal	Unsatisfactory
Assisting with the Sitz Bath			
Assisting with the Tub Bath or Shower			
Assisting with the Use of the Bedside Commode			
Care of Eyeglasses			
Care of Laundry in the Isolation Unit			
Care of Patient with an Artificial Eye			
Caring for Dentures			
Collecting a Clean-catch Urine Specimen			
Collecting a Fresh Fractional Urine Specimen			
Collecting a Routine Urine Specimen			
Collecting a Routine Urine Specimen from an Infant			
Collecting a Specimen in the Isolation Unit			
Collecting a Sputum Specimen			
Collecting a Stool Specimen			
Collecting a 24-hour Urine Specimen			
Counting Respirations			
CPR on a Child			
CPR on an Infant			
Disconnecting a Catheter			
Discharging the Patient			
Donning Clean Mask, Gown, and Gloves			
Donning Sterile Gloves			
Emptying a Urinary Drainage Unit			
Feeding the Helpless Patient			
Feeding the Infant in the Nursery			
Footprinting the Infant			
Giving a Back Rub			
Giving a Bed Bath			
Giving a Bed Shampoo			
Giving a Harris Flush (Return-flow Enema)			
Giving a Nonsterile Vaginal Douche			
Giving a Partial Bath			
Giving a Rotating Enema			

PROCEDURE	Satisfactory	Marginal	Unsatisfactory
Giving a Soapsuds Enema			
Giving an Emollient Bath			
Giving an Oil-retention Enema			
Giving and Receiving the Bedpan			
Giving and Receiving the Urinal			
Giving Daily Care of the Hair			
Giving Daily Indwelling Catheter Care			
Giving Eye Care to the Newborn Infant			
Giving Female Perineal Care			
Giving Foot and Nail Care			
Giving Hand and Fingernail Care			
Giving Postmortem Care			
Giving Routine Perineal Care			
Giving Routine Stoma Care			
Handwashing			
Inserting a Rectal Suppository			
Inserting a Rectal Tube and Flatus Bag			
Lifting a Patient Using a Mechanical Lift			
Log Rolling a Patient			
Making a Closed Bed			
Making an Occupied Bed			
Making the Surgical Bed			
Measuring and Recording Fluid Intake			
Measuring and Recording Fluid Output			
Moving a Helpless Patient to the Head of the Bed			
One Person CPR			
Opening a Sterile Package			
Opening the Closed Bed			
Performing Range of Motion Exercises (Following Bath Procedures)			
Preparing the Isolation Unit			
Providing AM Care			
Providing PM Care			

PROCEDURE	Satisfactory	Marginal	Unsatisfactory
Removing Contaminated Gown, Gloves, and Mask			
Removing Gown with IV in Place			
Replacing the Urinary Condom			
Routine Care of an Ileostomy (with Patient in Bed)			
Routine Care of an Ileostomy (in Bathroom)			
Shaving a Patient			
Shaving the Operative Area			
Taking a Radial Pulse			
Taking a Rectal Temperature (Electronic Thermometer)			
Taking a Rectal Temperature (Glass Thermometer)			
Taking an Apical Pulse			
Taking an Axillary or Groin Temperature (Electronic Thermometer)			
Taking an Axillary or Groin Temperature (Glass Thermometer)			
Taking an Oral Temperature (Electronic Thermometer)			
Taking an Oral Temperature (Glass Thermometer)			
Taking an Oral Temperature (Plastic Thermometer)			
Taking Blood Pressure			
Taking the Infant for Feeding			
Terminal Cleaning of Patient Unit			
Testing for Occult Blood Using Hematest® Reagent Tablets			
Testing for Occult Blood Using Hemoccult® and Developer			
Testing Urine for Sugar: Clinitest			
Testing Urine for Sugar: Tes-tape			
Testing Urine for Acetone: Acetetest			
Testing Urine for Acetone: Ketostix Strip Test			
Testing Urine with the Hemacombistix®			
Transferring a Conscious Patient from Bed to Stretcher			
Transferring a Conscious Patient from Stretcher to Bed			
Transferring an Unconscious Patient From Bed to Stretcher			
Transferring an Unconscious Patient From Stretcher to Bed			

PROCEDURE	Satisfactory	Marginal	Unsatisfactory
Transferring Food and Disposable Equipment Outside the Isolation Unit			
Transferring Forceps in Solution			
Transferring Nondisposable Equipment Outside the Isolation Unit			
Transferring the Patient			
Transporting a Patient by Stretcher			
Transporting a Patient by Wheelchair			
Transporting the Patient in Isolation			
Turning the Patient Away from You			
Turning the Patient Toward You			
Two Rescuer CPR			
Using a Peri Light			
Weighing and Measuring the Patient			

Evaluations of Clinical Performance

Student _____   Area/Agency _____

AREAS OF EVALUATION

PERSONAL CHARACTERISTICS	Satisfactory	Marginal	Unsatisfactory
Attendance			
Flexibility			
Grooming			
Interpersonal relationships			
Promptness			
Response to criticism			
EXECUTION OF NURSING CARE			
Acceptance of responsibility			
Accuracy; safety			
Energy level; productivity			
Knows limitations; seeks appropriate guidance			
Observational skills			
Organization; use of time			
Theoretical knowledge			
COMMUNICATION			
Oral			
Written			

COMMENTS: (Strengths and Weaknesses)

Teacher's Signature _____

Student's Signature _____

Clinical Rating:
Satisfactory _____
Marginal _____
Unsatisfactory _____
Date _____

Teacher will initial and date observations of clinical performance. Summary and comments can then be made and the performance record signed by both teacher and student.

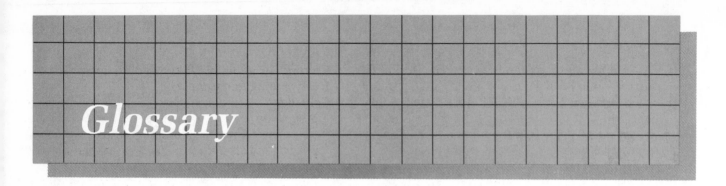

Glossary

Abduction—movement away from midline center.

Accelerated—increased motion as in pulse or respiration.

Accuracy—completing assignments carefully without mistakes.

Adduction—movement toward midline center.

Adenoma—an epithelial tumor composed of glandular tissue.

Adrenalin—proprietary name for epinephrine.

Aerobic—microorganisms that live best where plenty of oxygen is available.

Aiding and Abetting—not reporting dishonest acts that are observed.

Alignment—keeping a patient in proper position.

Allergen—the material that causes sensitivity.

Allergic reaction—presence of an organism which causes the body to react violently.

Allergies—sensitivity reactions.

Alveoli—the tiny air sacs which make up the bulk of the lungs.

Ambulation—the ability to walk.

Amenorrhea—without menstruation.

Amniotic sac—the bag or sac formed by the amnion.

Anaerobic—organisms that grow best where there is little oxygen.

Anaphylactic shock—a severe, sometimes fatal, sensitivity reaction.

Anatomy—the study of the structure of the human body.

Anemia—a deficiency of red blood cells in the blood.

Anesthesia—loss of feeling or sensation.

Angina pectoris—acute pain in the chest caused by interference with the supply of oxygen to the heart.

Annointing of the Sick—a Sacrament given to Catholic patients who are in danger of dying (they are given time for confession and the receiving of the Eucharist).

Anterior—body parts in front of the line (ventral).

Antitoxin—a particular kind of antibody produced in the body in response to the presence of a toxin.

Anus—the outlet of the rectum lying in the fold between the nates.

Aorta—the great artery arising from the left ventricle.

Apical—pertaining to the apex.

Apnea—period of no respirations.

Arachnoid mater—the middle layer of the brain and spinal cord.

Arrested—a patient's illness can no longer spread the germs.

Arteriole—a minute arterial branch.

Arteriosclerosis—thickening and loss of elasticity of the coats of the arteries, with inflammatory changes.

Artery—a vessel through which the blood, carrying oxygen, passes away from the heart to various parts of the body.

Arthritis—an inflammatory condition which affects the joints.

Aspiration—to draw in or out as by suction.

Asthma—paroxysmal dyspnea accompanied by the adventitious sounds caused by a spasm of the bronchial tubes or due to swelling of their mucous membrane.

Atria—plural of atrium.

Auditory—hearing.

Autoclave—a machine that steam sterilizes articles.

Axilla—the armpit.

Axillary—pertaining to the axilla.

BMR—abbreviation for basal metabolism rate.

Bacilli—rod-shaped bacteria.

Bacteria—a form of simple microbes.

Benign—a non-malignant tumor.

Bile—a secretion of the liver.

Body mechanics—using the right muscles to move or lift heavy objects properly.

Box (square) corner—one type of corner used in the making of a hospital bed.

Brachial artery—the main artery of the arm.

Bradycardia—an unusually slow heartbeat.

Bronchi—the primary divisions of the trachea.

Bronchioles—the tiny branches of the bronchi.

Bursae—small sacs of fluid found around joints.

Bursitis—a condition in which the bursae become inflamed and the joint becomes very painful.

482

CVA—abbreviation for cerebral vascular accident.

Capillary—one of the minute blood vessels interposed between arterioles and venules conveying lymph.

Carbohydrates—energy foods; the body uses them to produce heat.

Carbon dioxide—a colorless, pungent, and acid-tasting gas (CO_2) that is heavier than air.

Cardiac—pertaining to the heart.

Cardiac decompensation—another name for congestive heart failure.

Cardiocele—hernial protrusion of the heart through the diaphragm.

Cardiopneumatic—pertaining to the heart and the lungs.

Caries—tooth decay or cavities.

Cartilage—small discs (pads) found between bones (as in the back).

Cataract—opacity of lens of eye or its capsule or both.

Catheter (foley, French)—a tube for evacuating or injecting fluids.

Cellulose—carbohydrate foods which supply the body with roughage.

Celsius—the other name for the centigrade scale.

Cerebellum—the portion of the brain lying beneath the occipital lobe. It coordinates muscular activities and balance.

Cerebrospinal fluid—a water cushion protecting the brain and spinal cord from shock.

Cerebrum—the largest part of the brain consisting of two hemispheres separated by a deep longitudinal fissure. It controls all mental activities.

Cervical—pertaining to the neck.

Cervix—the neck of the uterus.

Character—the rhythm and volume of the pulse.

Cheyne-Stokes respirations—these are periods of labored respirations followed by apnea.

Cholecystectomy—the surgical removal of a diseased gallbladder and stones.

Cholelithiasis—the formation of stones in the gallbladder.

Choleystitis—inflammation of the gallbladder.

Choroid—vascular layer beneath the sclera of the eye.

Chyme—the semi-liquid form of food as it leaves the stomach.

Circle® electric bed—a special kind of bed which is used when a patient can't be turned within the bed.

Circumcision—removal of the end of the prepuce by a circular incision.

Cocci—round bacteria.

Cochlea—a winding cone-shaped tube forming a portion of the inner ear.

Colloidal—pertaining to a colloid (gelatinous).

Colon—another name for the large intestine.

Colony—organisms that tend to group themselves into communities.

Colostomy—incision of the colon for the purpose of making a more or less permanent fistula in treatment of carcinomatous stenosis of lower portion of colon and in cases of inoperable carcinoma of rectum.

Colostrum—secretion from the lactiferous glands before the onset of true lactation 2 or 3 days after delivery.

Comminuted fracture—splintered fractures.

Commode—a movable toilet.

Communicable—a disease which may be transferred from one person to another directly or indirectly.

Complete fracture—the separation of the ends of bone at the fracture site.

Compound fracture—the breaking of a bone that protrudes the skin.

Concurrent cleaning—daily cleaning of equipment.

Congestive heart failure—a condition resulting from cardiac output inadequate for physiologic needs, with shortness of breath, edema and abnormal retention of sodium and water in body tissues.

Conjunctiva—a mucous membrane that lines the eyelids and covers the eye.

Connective tissue—tissue that holds other tissues together.

Constrict—to bind or restrict a part.

Contaminate—to make impure, unclean, or corrupt by contact: to transfer germs.

Contamination—contaminating or being contaminated.

Contractures—permanent contraction of a muscle due to spasm or paralysis.

Convulsion—paroxysms of involuntary muscular contractions and relaxations seen in epilepsy and some diseases or cases of poisoning.

Cornea—transparent portion of the eye through which we see.

Coronary occlusion—the closing off of a coronary artery.

Coronary thrombosis—a blood clot within the vessel.

Cortex—the outer portion of the kidney.

Cortisone—a hormone from the cortex of the adrenal gland.

Cranial—pertaining to the cranium.

Creatinine—one of the nonprotein constituents of blood. Increased quantities of it are found in advanced stages of renal disease.

Critical list—a list that patients are placed on when they are dangerously or terminally ill.

Culture—sample taken from the affected area to discover the cause of infection.

Cuticle—the base of fingernails.
Cyanosis—slightly bluish, grayish, slate-like, or dark purple discoloration of the skin. It is due to abnormally low levels of hemoglobin in the blood.
Cyanotic—bluish appearance of the skin.
Cystitis—inflammation of the urinary bladder.
Cystocele—a bladder hernia.
Cystoscopy—a test performed during surgery which enables the doctor to look inside the bladder.
Cytoplasm—protoplasm of a cell outside the nucleus.

D & C—means dilation and curettage where the opening of the cervix is made larger and the uterus is scraped with a surgical instrument called a curette.
Decubitus ulcers—another term for bedsores.
Defecate—to expel feces from the bowel.
Defecation—bowel movement which expels feces.
Dehydration—excessive fluid loss.
Dentures—artificial teeth.
Dependability—reporting to duty on time.
Depressants—drugs which slow down body functions.
Dermis—the true skin.
Diabetes mellitus—a disease of metabolism involving inadequate production or utilization of insulin.
Diaphragm—a musculomembraneous wall separating the abdomen from the thoracic cavity with its convexity upward.
Diastolic—pertaining to the diastole. The point of least pressure in the arterial vascular system.
Dilate—to get bigger as in capillaries.
Disinfect—to destroy pathogens. Usually done with chemicals.
Distal—a term used to show the relationship of the part to first point of attachment to the body.
Diuresis—increase of output of fluids by the kidneys.
Dorsal—pertaining to the back.
Dorsi flexion—toes pointed up.
Drawsheet—one folded under patient so it may be withdrawn without lifting the patient.
Duodenal ulcers—ulcers on the mucosa of the duodenum due to the action of gastric juice.
Dura mater—the outer layer of the brain and spinal cord.
Dysmenorrhea—painful menstruation.
Dyspnea—periods of labored respirations.
Dysuria—painful voiding.

Edema—retention of fluid in the tissues.
Efface—the thinning out of the cervix during labor.

Elasticity—the ability to stretch.
Embolic—pertaining to embolism or embolus.
Embolus—a mass of undissolved material carried in the bloodstream and frequently causing obstruction of a vessel.
Emollient—an agent that will soften and soothe the part when applied locally.
Emphysema—distension of tissues by gas or air in the interstices.
Endocrine gland—a ductless gland which produces an internal secretion discharged into the blood and lymph and circulated to all parts of the body.
Endometrium—the mucous membrane lining the inner surface of the uterus.
Enema—The injection of water into the rectum and colon used to help the bowels eliminate feces.
Environment—all the conditions, circumstances, and influences surrounding and affecting the development of an organism or group of organisms.
Enzymes—organic catalysts produced by living cells but capable of acting independently of the cells producing them.
Epidermis—the top layer of skin.
Epilepsy—an episodic disturbance of brain function or consciousness during which generalized convulsions may occur.
Episiotomy—incision of perineum at end of second stage of labor to avoid laceration of perineum.
Epithelial tissue—covers the body as skin and lines the body cavities as membranes.
Erythema—congestive redness of the skin caused by engorgement of the capillaries in the lower layers of the skin, e.g., sunburn.
Erythrocyte—red blood cell.
Estrogen—the hormone produced by the ovarian follicle and other structures.
Ethics—a system of moral principles or standards governing conduct.
Etiology—the cause of a disease.
Eustachian tube—the auditory tube. Leads from the middle ear to the pharynx.
Expectorate—to spit (to bring up sputum).
Expendable—equipment that is not reuseable: (throw-away items).
Expiration—the forcing of air out of the lungs.
Extension—straightening the angle of a joint.
External urinary meatus—the opening to the outside of the urethra.
Extremities—the terminal part of anything such as arms and legs.

Fahrenheit—the scale used in the United States and England to determine temperature.
Fanfold—procedure for folding a sheet.

Fasting—the act of not eating.

Fats—the body uses them to produce heat; energy foods.

Feces—stool eliminated from the bowel.

Fetus—the child in utero from the third month to birth.

Flexible—the ability to bend in different directions.

Flexion—decreasing the angle between two bones.

Fomites—objects with germs on them.

Forced fluids—the patient must be encouraged to take as much fluid as possible.

Fundus—the body of the uterus from the internal os of the cervix upward above the fallopian tubes.

Gallbladder—a small, saclike organ found on the underside of the liver.

Gastrectomy—surgical removal of a part or the whole of the stomach.

Gastric—pertaining to the stomach.

Gastric ulcers—ulcers of the stomach.

Gavage—feeding through a tube.

General anesthetic—a gas which induces a state of unconsciousness and insusceptibility to pain.

Genitalia—reproductive organs. Usually used to refer to the external portions.

Glomeruli—blood vessels that branch to form balls of capillaries in the cortex.

Gonorrhea—a specific, contagious, catarrhal inflammation of the genital mucous membrane of either sex.

Gossip—temptation to discuss patients' conditions during lunch breaks.

Greenstick fracture—the breaking of a bone on one side only. More likely to be seen in children.

Groin—the depression between the thigh and trunk.

Gurney—equipment used to transport a patient; a stretcher.

Halitosis—bad breath.

Hematuria—blood in the urine.

Hemiparalysis—paralysis of one side of the body.

Hemiplegia—paralysis of one side of the body.

Hemoptysis—the spitting of blood. Blood comes from larynx, trachea, bronchi, or lungs.

Hemorrhage—another name for bleeding. Usually used to denote an abnormal amount.

Hernia—the protrusion or projection of an organ or a part of an organ through the wall of the cavity which normally contains it.

Herniorrhaphy—surgical operation for hernia.

Hormone—a chemical substance originating in an organ, gland, or part which stimulates body parts to increased functional activity.

Hydrochloric acid (HCl)—an aqueous solution of hydrogen chloride containing 35 to 38% (HCl).

Produced by the parietal cells of the gastric glands.

Hydronephrosis—the increasing pressure of urine causing pressure on the kidney cells which results in their destruction.

Hyperadenosis—enlargement of glands.

Hypertension—high blood pressure.

Hyperthyroidism—a condition caused by excessive secretion of the thyroid glands which overstimulates the basal metabolism, causing an increased demand for food to prevent oxidization of body tissues.

Hypertrophy—increase in size of an organ or structure which does not involve tumor formation.

Hypofunction—diminished functioning of a part or organ.

Hypotension—low blood pressure.

Hypothyroidism—a condition due to deficiency of the thyroid secretion, resulting in a lowered basal metabolism.

Hysteralgia—pain in the uterus.

Hysterectomy—surgical removal of the uterus.

Immobilization—the making of a part or limb immovable, usually in a cast.

Impaction—condition of being tightly wedged into a part (as the feces in a bowel).

Inflammation—tissue reaction to injury either direct or referred.

Infrared—invisible heat rays beyond the red end of the spectrum: heat lamps.

Inspiration—the drawing of air into the lungs.

Insulin—a hormone secreted by the beta cells of the islets of Langerhans of the pancreas.

Intake & Output—the recording of the amount of fluid ingested and the amount of fluid expelled by a patient.

Interpersonal relationships—method in which people interact with each other.

Intracranial—within the cranium or skull.

Intravenous infusion (IV)—nourishment given through a sterile tube into the veins. Also the injection of a solution—such as medicine—to secure an immediate result.

Involuntary muscle—these operate without our conscious control.

Involution—the reduction in the size of the uterus following delivery.

Iodine—a nonmetallic element belonging to the halogen group. Needed for proper function of the thyroid gland.

Iris—the colored portion of the eye.

Isolation technique—the name given to the method of caring for patients with easily transmitted diseases.

IV standard—poles usually made of stainless steel which can be attached to the bed or stand on the floor.

Jaundice—the yellowing of the skin due to the obstruction of the flow of bile.

Kidneys—two glandular, bean-shaped bodies, purplish-brown in color, situated in back of the abdominal cavity, one on each side of the spinal column, which excrete waste matter in the form of urine.

Labia majora—the two folds of cellular adipose tissue lying on either side of the vaginal opening and forming the lateral borders of the vulva.

Labia minora—two thin folds of integument which lie within the labia majora and enclose the vestibule.

Labor—the physiological process by which the fetus is expelled from the uterus at term.

Lacrimal gland—manufactures tears.

Lactation—the function of secreting milk.

Larynx—the organ of voice.

Lateral—body parts away from the midline.

Lavage—washing out of the stomach.

Lens—the portion of the eye behind the iris.

Lesions—morbid changes in tissue formation locally.

Leukemia—malignant disease of the tissues in the bone marrow, spleen, and lymph nodes.

Leukocyte—white blood cell.

Ligament—bands of fibrous tissue that holds joints together.

Litter—equipment used to transport a patient. Also called a gurney or stretcher.

Living Will—request by a person in the event of a terminal illness who wishes that no extraordinary means be employed to prolong life.

Lobe—a globular part of an organ separated by boundaries.

Local anesthetic—a type of anesthetic usually injected, that is confined to a limited area. The patient remains awake.

Lochia—the discharge from the uterus of blood, mucus, and tissue during the puerperal period.

Lubricant—agent which makes smooth. A cream.

Lymph—colorless, odorless fluid slightly alkaline and with a salty taste circulating within the lymphatic system.

Lymphatic vessels—vessels which collect lymph from the tissues and carry it to the blood.

Malignant—another term for a cancerous growth.

Malnutrition—the lack of necessary food substances in the body or improper absorption and distribution of them.

Malpractice—occurs when an assistant improperly gives care or gives care in which he/she has not been instructed.

Mastectomy—surgical removal of the breast.

Masticate—the act of chewing food with the teeth in preparation for swallowing.

Meconium—first feces of the newborn infant made up of salts, liquor amnii, mucus, bile and epithalial cells. The color is greenish black to light brown.

Medical asepsis—procedures followed to keep germs from being spread from one person to another.

Medulla—forms the brain stem.

Medulla (of kidney)—renal pyramids.

Membranes—tissue sheets that line the cavities.

Meninges—the three membranes investing the spinal cord and brain.

Meningitis—inflammation of the membranes of spinal cord or brain.

Menorrhagia—excessive bleeding during menstruation.

Menstruation—the loss of an unneeded part of the endometrium.

Metastasize—the spreading of cancer to other body parts.

Metric system—a method of measurement generally used to measure fluids.

Microbes—tiny organisms which can only be seen with a microscope.

Microorganisms—tiny organisms which can only be seen with a microscope, especially a bacteria.

Micturate—to pass the urine.

Minerals—substances that build body tissues and regulate body fluids.

Mitered corners—one type of corner used in the making of a hospital bed.

Modified Sippy diet—a diet consisting of half milk and half cream in small quantities every hour. Used in patients with ulcers.

Motor nerve—one containing motor fibers and conveying motor impulses.

Mucus—a viscid fluid secreted by mucous membranes and glands.

Muscular tissue—cells which have special ability to shorten and to lengthen.

Myocardial infarction—formation of an infarct in the heart muscle due to interruption of the blood supply to the area.

NPO—initials for nothing by mouth.

Neonate—name given to the newborn baby.

Neopathy—a new disease or a new complication in a disease.

Neoplasm—means new growth; another term for tumor.

Nephritis—inflammation of the kidney.

Nerve—axons and dendrites that are held together by connective tissues.

Nervous tissue—carries messages and regulates body functions.

Neuron—cell of the nervous system.

Nonexpendable—equipment that must be reused.

Nucleus—directs the activities of the cell.

Nutrient—foods which supply heat and energy, build and repair body tissue, and regulate body functions.

Nutrition—the process by which the body uses food for growth and repair and to maintain health.

Obese—overweight.

Obstruction—the blocking of a passageway.

Occult blood—blood in such minute quantity that it can only be recognized by microscope or chemical means.

Operative—pertaining to an operation.

Optic nerve—second cranial nerve. Special sense of sight.

Oral—concerning the mouth.

Oral hygiene—care of the mouth and teeth.

Orifice—body opening such as nose or mouth.

Orthopedic—concerning orthopedics; prevention or correction of deformities.

Orthopneic—positioning of a patient by adjusting the overbed table in such a way that the patient, supported by pillows, is able to lean on it.

Ossicles—any small bones, as one of the three bones in the ear.

Otitis media—inflamed condition of the media part of the ear.

Ovaries—the two glands in the female, producing the reproductive cell, the ovum, and two known hormones.

Oviducts—the two tubes extending laterally from the superior angles of the uterus which serve to convey the ovum from the ovary to the uterus.

Ovulation—the lunar monthly ripening and rupture of the mature graafian follicle and the discharge of the ovum from the cortex of the ovary, normally occurring 13 times a year.

Ovum—the female reproductive or germ cell.

Oxygen—a nonmetallic element occurring free in the atmosphere as a colorless, odorless, and tasteless gas.

Oxygenation—saturation with oxygen.

PBI—abbreviation for protein-bound iodine.

Pallor—less color than normal.

Pap smear—a simple test used to detect cancer of the cervix.

Paralysis—temporary suspension or permanent loss of function in a living part, especially loss of sensation or voluntary motion.

Paraplegia—paralysis of lower portion of the body and of both legs.

Parasite—an organism that lives within, upon, or at expense of another organism known as the host.

Parasympathetic—nerve fibers which carry impulses to control the usual functions of moderate heartbeat, digestion, elimination, respiration, and glandular activity.

Pathogens—microorganisms or substances capable of producing a disease.

Pathology—another name for disease.

Patience—the state, quality, ability, or fact of being patient.

Pelvic—pertaining to the hip area.

Penis—the male organ of copulation.

Pericardium—the membranes which surround the heart.

Peri light—another name for perineal lamp which is used to relieve pain of the perineum following birth.

Perineum—the region between the vulva and anus in a female or between scrotum and anus in a male.

Peristalsis—a progressive, wavelike movement which occurs involuntarily in hollow tubes of the body, especially the alimentary canal.

Pharnyx—the term for throat.

Physiology—the science of the function of the human body.

Pia mater—the innermost membrane that surrounds the brain and spinal cord.

Pinna—the auricle or projection part of the external ear.

Placenta—name given to the afterbirth.

Planes—imaginary lines that help to describe the relationship of one body part to another.

Plantar flexion—toes pointed down.

Plasma—fluid portion of the blood in which corpuscles are suspended.

Pleura—the membranes which surround the lungs.

Pneumonectomy—resection of lung tissue.

Pons—forms the brain stem.

Posterior—body parts behind the line (dorsal).

Postmortem—care given after death has occurred.

Postoperative—after a surgical operation.

Postpartum—after parturition; after birth.

Prenatal—before birth.

Preoperative—preceding an operation.

Pressure sores—another term for bedsores: decubiti.

Proctoscopy—instrumental inspection of the rectum.

Progesterone—a steroid hormone: female.

Prognosis—the probable outcome of a disease.

Pronation—palms of hands are down.

Prostatectomy—excision of part or all of the prostate gland.

Prostate gland—a male gland, partly glandular, partly muscular; surrounding the proximal portion of the male urethra and the neck of the bladder, consisting of a median lobe and two lateral lobes.

Prosthesis—the replacement of an absent part by an artificial substitute. An artificial organ or part.

Protein—the basic material of every body cell. An essential nutrient.

Protozoa—simple form of one-cell microbe.

Proximal—a term used to show the relationship of the part to its point of attachment to the body.

Pseudoanemia—a condition marked by paleness without true anemia.

Pubic—concerning the pubes.

Pulmonary artery—the large artery originating from the superior surface of the right ventricle.

Pupil—the opening of the iris.

Pyloric sphincter—the muscle at the exit point of the pylorus.

Pylorus—the narrow, tapered end of the stomach opening into the duodenum.

Quadriplegia—paralysis affecting all four limbs.

Radial artery—the artery near the radius. Used commonly to determine blood pressure.

Radial deviation—the wrists are turned toward thumb side.

Rales—fluid collected in the air passages causing bubbling type of respirations.

Range of motion exercises—types of joint motions.

Rate—valuation based on comparison with a standard.

Readiness—a ready quality or state.

Recovery room—location where surgical patients are taken after surgery. They return to their room when their condition stabilizes.

Rectal—pertaining to the rectum.

Rectocele—protrusion of posterior vaginal wall with anterior wall of rectum through the vagina.

Rectum—lower part of large intestine about 5″ (12 cm) long between sigmoid flexure and the anal canal.

Reflex—activities performed without conscious thought.

Renal calculi—stone in the kidney.

Renal colic—spasm in area near kidney accompanied by pain.

Retention—the inability to excrete urine that has been produced.

Retina—innermost or third tunic of the eyes which receives image formed by the lens and is the immediate instrument of vision.

Retrograde pyelogram—the moving backward of a roentgen picture of the ureter and renal pelvis.

Reverse isolation technique—requires that the environment, the patient and all objects coming in contact with the patient must be sterile or at least as free from microorganisms as possible.

Rhythm—a measured time or movement.

Rotation—joints are rolled away from center or toward center of body.

Rubra—unusual redness or flushing of the skin.

Saliva—the first digestive secretion emitted from the salivary glands into the mouth.

Saprophyte—organisms which live on dead matter or tissues.

Sclera—white of the eye.

Semicircular canals—the superior, posterior, and inferior passages forming the back part of the ear.

Sensory nerve—those nerves which control the senses.

Sensory receptor—enables one to be aware of surroundings.

Serum—the clear portion of any animal or plant fluid that remains after the solid elements have been separated out.

Sexually-transmitted disease (STD)—diseases which are transmitted sexually.

Siderails—a sliding metal bar (bars) that may be pulled up on each side of the bed which prevents the patient from falling out of bed.

Sign—any objective evidence of an abnormal nature in the body or its organs.

Simple fracture—the remaining of bones within the skin.

Simple goiter—thyroid gland hyperplasia unaccompanied by constitutional symptoms.

Sitz bath—a means of providing moist heat to the genital or anal area.

Skeletal muscle—muscles that stretch over joints.

Sperm—the male germ or reproductive cell.

Sphygmomanometer—instrument for determining arteriol pressure; blood pressure gauge.

Spirilla—spiral-shaped bacteria.

Spore—a dormant form of microbes which become active when conditions are favorable.

Sputum—matter brought up from the lungs: phlegm.

Sterility—inability to produce offspring.

Sterilize—to make articles safe for reuse.

Stethoscope—instrument used in auscultation to convey to the ear the sounds produced in the body.

Stimulant—any agent temporarily increasing functional activity.

Stool—another name for feces.

Strangulated hernia—one so tightly constricted that

gangrene results if operation does not relieve. Not reducible by ordinary means.

Stretcher—equipment used to transport a patient.

Stryker frame—a special kind of bed which is used when a patient can't be turned within the bed.

Subcutaneous—tissue that lies directly under the dermis.

Suppination—palms of hands are up.

Suppository—a device used to help the bowels eliminate feces.

Suppression—the inability to secrete urine by the kidneys.

Surgical bed—the bed used for surgery.

Sympathetic—in times of stress these nerve fibers are stimulated.

Sympathy—relationship between two organs or parts through which one unaffected part is affected or becomes disordered from disease in the other part without actual transmission of morbific cause.

Symptom—any perceptible change in the body or its functions which indicates disease or the kind or phases of disease.

Synapse—space between the axon of one cell and the dendrites of others.

Syphilis—an infectious, chronic, veneral disease characterized by lesions which may involve any organ or tissue. It usually exhibits cutaneous manifestations, relapses are frequent, and it may exist asymptomatic for years.

Systolic—pertaining to the systole. The point of maximum sound in blood pressure.

Tachycardia—an unusually fast heartbeat.

Tact—a delicate perception of the right thing to say or do without offending.

Tactile sense—perceptible to the touch.

Terminal cleaning—thorough cleaning of a room when a patient leaves the hospital.

Testes—the male gonads.

Testosterone—a steroid produced by the interstititial cells of Leydig; the male hormone.

Tetany—a nervous affection, characterized by intermittent toxic spasms, which are usually paroxysmal and involve the extremities.

Therapeutic—pertaining to results obtained from treatment. A healing agent.

Thoracic cavity—the space lying above the diaphragm and enclosed within the walls of the thorax.

Thrombocyte—platelet which is produced in the bone and is important in blood clotting.

Thrombophlebitis—the development of venous thrombi in the presence of inflammatory changes in the vessel wall.

Thrombus—a solid mass formed in the living heart or vessels from constituents of the blood.

Thyroxin—proprietary name for the active principle of the thyroid gland.

Toxin—microbes which produce poisons that travel to the central nervous system and cause damage.

Trachea—another term for windpipe.

Trauma—an injury to the body.

Tubercle—a small nodule, especially a circumscribed solid elevation of the skin or mucous membrane.

Tuberculosis—a lung disease caused by a microorganism, easily transmitted to others by sneezing and coughing.

Turning sheet—sheet used to turn a patient.

Tympanic membrane—membrane serving as the lateral wall of the tympanic cavity and separating it from the external acoustic meatus.

Ulcer—open sore caused by blood stoppage and broken skin.

Ulcerative colitis—ulceration of inner lining of colon with dilatation.

Ulnar deviation—wrists are turned toward the little finger side.

Ultraviolet—invisible heat rays beyond the spectrum at its violet end.

Umbilical cord—the attachment connecting the fetus with the placenta, artificially severed at birth of the child.

Umbilicus—depressed scar marking the site of entry of the umbilical cord in the fetus.

Urea—the diamide of carbonic acid found in blood, lymph, and urine.

Ureter—one of two tubes carrying urine from the kidneys to the bladder.

Urethra—a canal for the discharge of urine from the bladder to the outside.

Urgency—the need to urinate.

Uric acid—a crystalline acid occurring as an end-product of purine metabolism. It is formed from purine bases derived from nucleoproteins.

Urinal—a vessel for the urine (male).

Urinalysis—a laboratory test of urine.

Urinary bladder—receptacle for urine before it is voided.

Urine—the fluid secreted from the blood by the kidneys.

Uterus—the organ of gestation.

Vagina—a musculomembranous tube which forms the passageway between the uterus and the external orifice.

Vaginitis—inflammation of the vagina.

Vasoconstriction—when blood vessels constrict or become smaller when cold.

Vasodilation—blood vessels become larger when heat is applied.

Vein—a vessel which carries unaerated blood to the heart—except for the pulmonary vein which carries oxygenated blood directly from the lungs to the heart.

Veneral disease (VD)—one acquired ordinarily as a result of sexual intercourse with an individual who is affected.

Ventral—pertaining to the front side of the body.

Ventricle—a small cavity or chamber as in the brain or heart.

Venule—a small vein.

Vernix caseosa—a sebaceous deposit covering the fetus due to secretion of skin glands.

Vertigo—a sensation of rotation or movement of or about the person.

Virus—the specific living morbid principle by which an infectious disease is transmitted.

Visceral muscle—muscles that operate without our conscious control.

Vital signs—the patient's temperature, pulse, respiratory rate, and blood pressure readings.

Vitamins—substances that regulate body processes.

Void—the release of urine from the bladder.

Volume—the space occupied by a substance as measured by cubic units.

Voluntary—pertaining to or under control of the will.

Voluntary muscle—the ability to make our muscles contract and perform necessary movements.

Vomitus—act of ejecting matter from the stomach through the mouth.

Vulva—the external female genitalia.

Ward—rooms with more than two beds.

Wheelchair—a mobile chair for invalids, mounted on wheels.

Withhold—to keep a patient from being served food.

Acknowledgments

The authors would like to express their appreciation to the following hospitals for certain photos:

Memorial Hospital, Long Beach, CA for Figures 1-2, 1-3, 1-4, 1-5, 1-6, 1-7, 1-8, 4-1, 4-3, 4-12, 6-6, 7-3, 7-4, 8-1A and B, 9-1, 9-2, 9-4, 12-1, 12-4, 12-6, 13-1, 14-12, 15-1, 16-6, 24-6, 24-7A and B, 30-3, 31-4, 31-5, 31-6, 32-12, 32-15, 34-8, 34-12, 34-13, 34-14, 38-3, 38-4, 38-5, 38-6, 38-7, 38-8, 38-9, 38-10, 38-11, 38-12, 38-13, 38-14, and 38-15.

St. Mary's Hospital, Long Beach, CA for Figures 2-2, 3-4, 3-5, 8-1C, 12-5, 24-4, 27-1, 27-4, 28-13, 28-15, and 38-17.

Charter Suburbon Hospital, Paramount, CA for Figures 2-4, 2-5, 2-6, 3-2, 4-6, 5-1, 8-2, 11-12, 12-7, 13-2, 13-3A and B, 14-4, 14-5, 14-6, 14-13A and B, 14-14, 15-6A through E, 15-9, 18-3, 18-20, 20-4, 25-2, 27-8, 32-21A through C, 32-22, 32-23, 32-24, 32-25A and B, 32-26, 32-27, 32-28, 32-29, 32-30, 32-31, 32-32, 32-33, 32-34, 34-10, 36-4, 36-9, 39-1, 39-2A through E, 39-3A and B, and 39-4A through H.

Paramount General Hospital, Paramount CA for Figures 3-1, 3-3, 4-2, 4-4, 7-2, 7-5, 7-6, 7-7, 8-4, 10-9, 11-4A through C, 11-5, 12-3, 16-1, 16-3, 16-7, 16-8, 17-1, 17-2A through C, 17-3, 17-4, 18-1, 18-8, 18-10, 18-11, 18-12, 18-14, 19-1, 21-6, 22-5, 23-8, 25-3, 30-7, 30-11, 30-12, 33-7, 36-7, and 38-10.

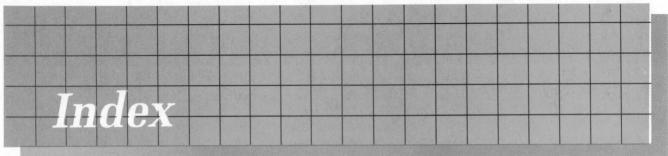

Index

492